AF556786

MOLECULAR ASPECTS OF CHEMOTHERAPY

MOLECULAR ASPECTS OF CHEMOTHERAPY

Proceedings of the Second International Symposium on Molecular Aspects of Chemotherapy

Gdańsk, Poland, July 5-8, 1988

Edited by

Edward Borowski

Technical University of Gdańsk, Gdańsk, Poland

and

David Shugar

Academy of Sciences, Warsaw, Poland

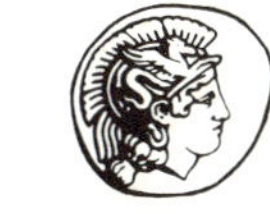

PERGAMON PRESS

Member of Maxwell Macmillan Pergamon Publishing Corporation

New York · Oxford · Beijing · Frankfurt

São Paulo · Sydney · Tokyo · Toronto

Pergamon Press Offices:

U.S.A.	Pergamon Press, Inc., Maxwell House, Fairview Park, Elmsford, New York 10523, U.S.A.
U.K.	Pergamon Press plc, Headington Hill Hall, Oxford OX3 0BW, England
PEOPLE'S REPUBLIC OF CHINA	Pergamon Press, Room 4037, Qianmen Hotel, Beijing, People's Republic of China
FEDERAL REPUBLIC OF GERMANY	Pergamon Press GmbH, Hammerweg 6, D-6242 Kronberg, Federal Republic of Germany
BRAZIL	Pergamon Editora Ltda, Rua Eça de Queiros, 346, CEP 04011, Paraiso, São Paulo, Brazil
AUSTRALIA	Pergamon Press Australia Pty Ltd., P.O. Box 544, Potts Point, NSW 2011, Australia
JAPAN	Pergamon Press, 8th Floor, Matsuoka Central Building, 1-7-1 Nishishinjuku, Shinjuku-ku, Tokyo 160, Japan
CANADA	Pergamon Press Canada Ltd., Suite 271, 253 College Street, Toronto, Ontario M5T 1R5, Canada

---

First edition 1990

Library of Congress Cataloging in Publication Data

International Symposium on Molecular Aspects of Chemotherapy (2nd : 1988 : Gdańsk, Poland)
Molecular aspects of chemotherapy : proceedings of the Second International Symposium on Molecular Aspects of Chemotherapy, Gdańsk, Poland, July 5-8, 1988 / edited by Edward Borowski and David Shugar.
p. cm.
Published as a supplement to the journal, Pharmacology & therapeutics.
ISBN 0-08-036848-4 :
1. Molecular pharmacology--Congresses. 2. Chemotherapy--Congresses. I. Borowski, Edward II. Shugar, D. (David). III. Pharmacology & therapeutics. IV. Title.
[DNLM: 1. Drug Therapy--congresses. WB 330 I632m 1988]
RM301.65.I58 1988
615.5'8--dc19
DNLM/DLC
for Library of Congress 89-2929
CIP

Printed in the United States of America

CONTENTS

LIST OF CONTRIBUTORS

Federico Arcamone
Menarini Richerche Sud
Pomezia, Italy

E. Michael August
Department of Pharmacology
Yale University School of Medicine
New Haven, CT

N. Bauman
Medical Research Division
Lederle Laboratories
American Cyanamid Company
Pearl River, NY

Evelyn Birks
Department of Pharmacology
Yale University School of Medicine
New Haven, CT

Neal Brown
Department of Pharmacology
University of Massachusetts Medical School
Worcester, MA

Angelika Chandra
Laboratory of Molecular Biology
Center of Biological Chemistry (ZBC)
University Medical School
Federal Republic of Germany

Prakash Chandra
Laboratory of Molecular Biology
Center of Biological Chemistry (ZBC)
University of Medical School
Federal Republic of Germany

Martin Charron
Centre de Recherche en Cancérologie
de L'Université Laval
Hotel-Dieu
Québec, Canada

George Deliconstantinos
Department of Experimental Physiology
University of Athens Medical School
Athens, Greece

Ilhan Demirhan
Laboratory of Molecular Biology
Center of Biological Chemistry (ZBC)
University Medical School
Federal Republic of Germany

Federico Focher
Department of Pharmacology
and Biochemistry
University of Zürich-Irchel
Zürich, Switzerland

Yvette Gaumont
Department of Biochemistry
Tufts University
Boston, MA

Thomas Gerber
Laboratory of Molecular Biology
Center of Biological Chemistry (ZBC)
University Medical School
Federal Republic of Germany

Graham W. Gooday
Department of Genetics and Microbiology
Marischal College
University of Aberdeen
Aberdeen, Scotland

Ronald Hancock
Centre de Recherche en Cancérologie
de L'Université Laval
Hotel-Dieu
Québec, Canada

Ulrich Hübscher
Department of Pharmacology and
Biochemistry
University of Zürich-Irchel
Zürich, Switzerland

Naseema Khan
Department of Pharmacology
University of Massachusetts Medical School
Worcester, MA

Thomas I. Kalman
State University of New York at Buffalo
Department of Medicinal Chemistry and
Biochemical Pharmacology
Buffalo, NY

David Kerridge
Department of Biochemistry
Cambridge University
Cambridge, United Kingdom

William D. Kingsbury
Department of Medicinal Chemistry
Smith Kline & French Laboratories
Swedeland, PA

Roy L. Kisliuk
Department of Biochemistry
Tufts University
Boston, MA

G.F. Kolar
Institute of Toxicology and Chemotherapy
German Cancer Research Center
Heidelberg, Federal Republic of Germany

Jerzy Konopa
Department of Pharmaceutical Technology and Biochemistry
Technical University of Gdansk
Gdansk, Poland

Herman Lambert
Centre de Recherche en Cancérologie de L'Université Laval
Hotel-Dieu
Québec, Canada

Margot Lemieux
Centre de Recherche en Cancérologie de L'Université Laval
Hotel-Dieu
Québec, Canada

Tai-Shun Lin
Department of Pharmacology
Yale University School of Medicine
New Haven, CT

Maria Elena Marongiu
Department of Pharmacology
Yale University School of Medicine
New Haven, CT

M.S. Marriott
Glaxo Group Research Ltd.
Greenford Road
Greeenford, United Kingdom

B. Rama Murthy
Department of Biochemistry
University of South Alabama
Mobile, AL

Madhavan G. Nair
Department of Biochemistry
University of South Alabama
Mobile, AL

R. Nilakantan
Medical Research Division
Lederle Laboratories
American Cyanamid Company
Pearl River, NY

Roumen Pankov
Institute of Molecular Biology
Academy of Sciences
1113 Sofia
Bulgaria

Normand Pepin
Centre de Recherche en Cancérologie de L'Université Laval
Hotel-Dieu
Québec, Canada

James R. Piper
Drug Synthesis Section
Southern Research Institute
Birmingham, AL

William H. Prusoff
Department of Pharmacology
Yale University School of Medicine
New Haven, CT

He-Ying Qian
Department of Pharmacology
Yale University School of Medicine
New Haven, CT

Franz A. Schmid
Laboratory for Molecular Therapeutics
Memorial Sloan-Kettering Cancer Center
New York, NY

Francis M. Sirotnak
Laboratory for Molecular Therapeutics
Memorial Sloan-Kettering Cancer Center
New York, NY

Anton Stütz
Sandoz Forschungsinstitut
Vienna, Austria

Robert Talanian
Department of Pharmacology
University of Massachusetts Medical School
Worcester, MA

Janet Thorndike
Department of Biochemistry
Tufts University
Boston, MA

Lutz F. Tietze
Institute of Organic Chemistry
University of Göttingen
Göttingen, Federal Republic of Germany

Thomas G. Wood
Department of Pharmacology
Yale University School of Medicine
New Haven, CT

George Wright
Department of Pharmacology
University of Massachusetts Medical School
Worcester, MA

R. Venkataraghavan
Medical Research Division
Lederle Laboratories
American Cyanamid Company
Pearl River, NY

PREFACE

The remarkable developments of the past few years in molecular biology and genetics have opened new vistas in the search and design of chemotherapeutic agents for treatment of bacterial, neoplastic, viral, and parasitic diseases. While serendipity and random screening continue to fulfill an important role in the search for new drugs, increasing attention is now being devoted to investigations on the mechanism of action of such drugs at the molecular level and utilization of the information so derived to improvements in existing drugs and the rational design of new ones.

This special edition contains most of the lectures delivered at the 2nd International Symposium on Molecular Aspects of Chemotherapy held in Poland in the historic and picturesque city of Gdańsk on the Baltic coast, July 5–8, 1988. It was organized by the Committee on Drug Research, Polish Academy of Sciences, and the Department of Pharmaceutical Technology and Biochemistry, Technical University of Gdańsk, under the auspices of the International Society of Chemotherapy.

The meeting brought together scientists from a variety of disciplines, ranging from quantum chemistry, CAD, and crystallography through chemistry, physical chemistry, biochemistry, and biophysics to enzymology, microbiology and virology.

The overall objective was to evaluate current progress and perspectives in mechanisms of inhibition of cellular function and metabolism at the molecular level. Time was also allotted to discussions on progress in molecular approaches to immune defense modulating agents, control of gene expression, and products of interest in a "nontoxic approach." While the meeting was devoted largely to problems of control in eukaryotic systems, novel concepts relating to control in prokaryotes were also included.

Specific topics covered in the various sessions included structural basis of biological properties of active agents; molecular mechanisms of drug-target interactions; new targets and drug prototypes, as well as rational drug design; and site-directed targeting. Lectures were presented in four sections: antiviral chemotherapy, antitumor chemotherapy, antifungal chemotherapy, and general. These were supplemented by presentations of 80 posters.

While of comparatively recent origin, the two Gdańsk symposia have aroused considerable interest, far beyond that originally envisioned by the organizers. The 1st International Symposium, held in 1984, was facilitated by the fact that it was organized as a postsymposium of the XVIth IUPAC (International Union of Pure and Applied Chemistry) Symposium on Chemistry of Natural Products in Poznan, Poland, following which some of the participants traveled to Gdańsk to join up with others who came specifically for the Gdańsk meeting. The *Proceedings* of the first symposium were published in the journal *Drugs under Experimental and Clinical Research*, Vol. 12, Nos. 6–7, 1986.

The enthusiasm of the participants of the foregoing meeting was such as to stimulate the organizers to arrange the 2nd International Symposium. In turn, the warm response to the present meeting resulted in the decision to organize such symposia in alternate years. Hence the 3rd International Symposium on Molecular Aspects of Chemotherapy will be held in Gdańsk in late September 1990, the precise date to be announced in the near future. It is further planned to expand the scope of the program to include such topics as chemotherapy of parasitic diseases in general, molecular aspects of design of antibacterial agents, drug biotechnology, molecular pharmacology, and some clinical aspects of chemotherapy.

Organization of the third symposium will be facilitated by formation of an International Advisory Committee, the membership of which will be given in the first circular. A list of invited speakers is now being prepared. However, the organizing committee warmly welcomes proposals from prospective participants for presentation of lectures. These proposals should be accompanied by a general outline of the topic to be covered and addressed to one of the undersigned.

Finally, we would like to express our appreciation to the International Society of Chemotherapy, under whose auspices these symposia are held; to the Committee on Drug Research, Polish Academy of Sciences and the Technical University of Gdańsk for organizational support, and to sponsors of the second symposium, as follows: Hoffman-La Roche (Switzerland), Beecham Research International (United Kingdom), Astra Alab AB (Sweden); and Institute of Pharmaceutical Industry, Tarchomin Pharmaceutical Works "Polfa," Starogard Pharmaceutical Works "Polfa," and Kutno Pharmaceutical Works "Polfa" (Poland).

Edward Borowski
Department of Pharmaceutical Technology and Biochemistry
Technical University of Gdańsk
11/12 Majakowskiego St.
80-952 Gdańsk, Poland

David Shugar
Institute of Biochemistry and Biophysics
Polish Academy of Sciences
36 Rakowiecka St.
02-532 Warsaw, Poland

CHAPTER 1

METHODS IN COMPUTER-ASSISTED DRUG DESIGN AND DISCOVERY

R. Nilakantan, N. Bauman, and R. Venkataraghavan

Medical Research Division, Lederle Laboratories, American Cyanamid Company, Pearl River, New York, United States

Abstract—The computer can be used by the medicinal chemist in establishing structure–activity correlations as the first step in the rational design of drugs. The method chosen depends upon the amount and nature of information available about the mechanism of action of the drug and its site of action. We discuss (1) statistical topological methods appropriate to large sets of compounds, (2) examples of detailed molecular modeling on small sets of compounds, and (3) automated methods for generation of novel structural candidates for synthesis.

1. INTRODUCTION

In the traditional pharmaceutical research setting, drugs are discovered by a process of random screening of compounds for various biological activities. Once a chemical entity has been identified as active, the medicinal chemist uses that structure as a framework and examines different structural variations. In exploring variations, the chemist uses a combination of intuition and deductive reasoning and constantly draws upon his or her knowledge of structure–activity correlations. However, there is often a very large amount of structural and biological information associated with a series of compounds, and it becomes difficult for the chemist to make all the correlations mentally. Nowadays, computers are used as an aid to the medicinal chemist in various stages of the drug discovery process. In this brief review, we shall describe some selected aspects of computer-assisted drug design.

2. TOPOLOGICAL METHODS

In most cases, we neither have detailed structural data on the target site of the drug nor do we know the mechanism of action. What we do have, however, is screening data (i.e., results of biological testing) on a large number of different molecules with known structures. In such cases, we use statistical methods to perceive structure–activity correlations. These methods are applied using two-dimensional representations (in the sense of a structure diagram drawn on paper) of the molecules. No three-dimensional data are used. The tacit assumption here is that the three-dimensional structure is to a large extent implicit in the structure diagrams of molecules. Such methods are called topological or graph-based methods, since they represent molecules as graphs. The use of computerized databases has an important role to play in the success of these methods. The advantages of these techniques are that they can be applied to large sets of molecules and are very fast. The important cautionary note is that these models are statistical and therefore "soft"; that is, they are essentially interpolative and have low predictive ability.

At Lederle, we have developed several topological structure–activity models as well as methods to discover novel variants of known structures (Carhart et al., 1985; Nilakantan et al., 1987). Two of the methods we use are called similarity probe and trend vector analysis.

The key to the topological methods is the resolution of each molecule into structurally defined "descriptors," that is, substructures that can be perceived from molecular structure.

2.1. SIMILARITY PROBE

Given a certain compound, the similarity probe technique tries to locate compounds in the database that are structurally similar to it. This can be done in an objective manner by resolving the probe molecule into its descriptors and then comparing these descriptors with the molecular descriptors of each compound in the database. We compute a similarity value for each, from the count of descriptors that the molecules have in common, using the formula

$$S = \frac{2C}{T}$$

where S is the calculated similarity value, C is the number of descriptors in common, and T is the total number of descriptors in the two molecules. The similarity value as defined lies between 0 and 1; it is 0 when two compounds share no descriptors in common and 1 when they are identical. This method, as implemented on our VAX 8600 computer, processes about 25,000 compounds per minute.

The approach we have given is independent of the type of descriptor. Indeed, one can choose any type of descriptor one wishes. It is important, however, to realize that the choice of descriptor will eventually decide the calculated degree of similarity between a pair of compounds. In our laboratory, we use two kinds of descriptors: atom pairs and topological torsions (Carhart et al., 1985; Nilakantan et al., 1987).

The atom pair is defined as a substructure composed of two nonhydrogen atoms and an interatomic separation measured in bonds along the shortest path connecting the two atoms. The description of each atom includes the element type, the number of heavy atom connections, and the number of pi electrons. The atom pair, it will be seen, can capture long-range structural correlations in molecules, since it includes all pairs of atoms in the molecule.

The topological torsion is defined as a linear sequence of four bonded nonhydrogen atoms, each described as in the atom pair. It is immediately seen that the topological torsion is a "local" descriptor in the sense that it is not altered by modifications in a distant part of the molecule. The atom pair and topological torsion descriptors magnify complementary aspects of molecular similarity.

2.2. TREND VECTOR ANALYSIS

The similarity probe method is useful when we have a known drug and are looking for novel structural variants of it. However, the method does not make use of any biological test data.

To make quantitative predictions of biological activity, we use a "training set," that is, a set of compounds whose structures and biological activities are known. Each compound is resolved into its descriptors; to each descriptor in the total training set we assign a coefficient proportional to the mean activity of all the compounds possessing this descriptor, less the mean activity of the whole training set. The set of coefficients, viewed as a vector, is called a trend vector, and may be thought of as a vector in very-high-dimensional space, pointing in the direction of the more active structures. The coefficients are *not* fitted by least squares analysis; they are a crude representation of the structure–activity trend, but less susceptible to spurious chance correlations than are fitted coefficients.

Before we proceed to make any predictions with this model, it is necessary to validate it by showing that it reflects a genuine dependence of activity on structure. To do this, we reassign the biological activities randomly among the set of compounds and recompute a (spurious) trend vector. This process is repeated several times. If the length of the real trend vector is significantly greater than the mean length of the spurious vectors, then the trend vector is considered to be meaningful. To use the trend vector to predict the biological activities of untested compounds, we sum, for each compound, the coefficients of the trend vector corresponding to the descriptors present in the compound, giving a predicted activity for that compound. The predicted activity can then be used to prioritize further screening of compounds.

Experimental evidence for the validity of this concept comes from studies such as the following:

We studied a set of about 4000 compounds tested for antihypertensive activity. The set was randomly divided into two sets of about 2000 compounds each. A trend vector was calculated using one of these two sets as the training set and applied to predict the antihypertensive activities of the other set. We used topological torsion descriptors for this example, but this could have been done with atom pairs as well.

Correctness of classification into active and inactive is not a suitable measure of the effectiveness of prediction; in pharmacological screening, the incidence of active compounds is often very low, below 1%, so that a worthless method that classified *all* compounds as inactive might achieve 99% correct prediction. What we want to know is how rapidly we would discover the active compounds if we test in accordance with our predictions as opposed to testing at random.

The trend vector was therefore used to reorder the compounds based on their predicted activity. If the trend vector were effective, we could test the compounds with high predicted activity and hope to find many more active compounds than if we had tested the same number at random. The effectiveness of the trend vector can be assessed by measuring the enhancement in hit-rate over random for various numbers of compounds tested. Figure 1-1 is a graph of the enhancement factor versus the percentage of compounds screened. The sharp peak in the graph indicates that at low levels of screening, the trend vector is very effective in enhancing the hit rate and enhanced effectiveness persists long enough to allow a reasonable harvest of actives.

3. SMALL-MOLECULE MODELING USING ACTIVE ANALOGS

Quite often we have detailed three-dimensional structural information on a small set of known drugs with the same therapeutic effect, but do not have structural information on the binding site. In such cases, one looks for common three-dimensional features among the drugs. It is assumed that these drugs are active because they are capable of engaging

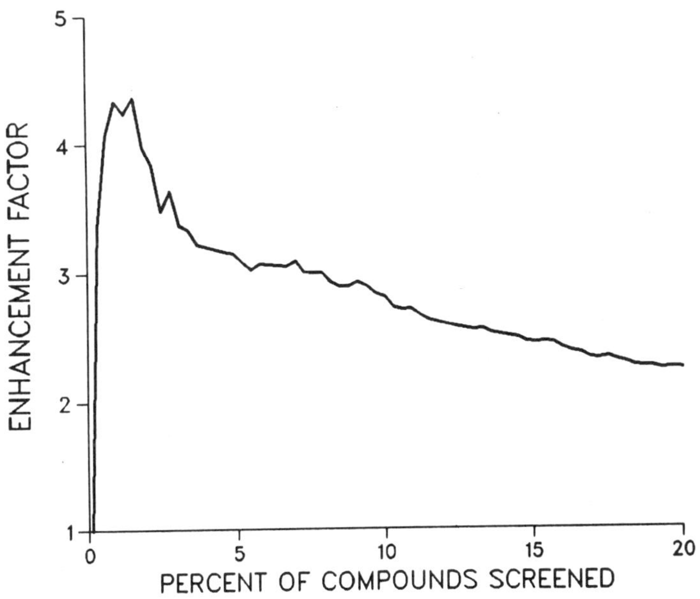

FIG. 1-1. Plot of the enhancement factor obtained as a function of percentages of the total number of compounds screened. The topological torsion descriptor was used in this calculation.

certain fixed groups in the receptor site; accordingly, it should be possible to align the drug molecules in some manner bringing their active functional groups into superposition. This can be done by systematic exploration of various conformations (Marshall et al., 1979) or by distance geometry techniques (Crippen, 1981; Sheridan et al., 1986). The determination of the active functional groups is not a mechanical task and has to be done based on a knowledge of the mechanism of action.

We give an example of the use of this approach to the design of reactivators of nerve-gas–inhibited acetyl cholinesterase. Nerve gases (chemical warfare agents) are organophosphorus compounds which react with acetyl cholinesterase by blocking a serine residue that is essential for enzyme activity. This prevents timely hydrolysis of acetylcholine, resulting in uncontrolled nerve stimulation and ultimately causing death. The best known therapeutic strategy for nerve-gas poisoning has been the use of reactivators of nerve-gas–inhibited acetyl cholinesterase.

A search of the literature showed that most of the potent reactivators of acetyl cholinesterase are pyridinium oximes (Hobbiger & Vojvodic, 1966; Erdmann & Engelhard, 1964). We examined the structures of the most potent of these oximes and tried to extract common structural features which could then be used as a framework to design more effective reactivators. Two classes of compounds were found, shown in Fig. 1-2. Both are bis-pyridinium oximes and differ essentially in the placement of the oxime group with respect to the pyridinium nitrogen; in one case it is *ortho* and in the other case it is *para*.

Since the oxime is the essential functional group, it is reasonable to assume that in the active bound states, the oximes of the two drugs would occupy the same site ("overlap") on the phosphorylated enzyme. The nonoxime ring presumably has a role in receptor recognition. Hence we assume that the two nonoxime rings would also overlap in the active conformation. If we could deduce the active conformations of the two drugs, their spatial

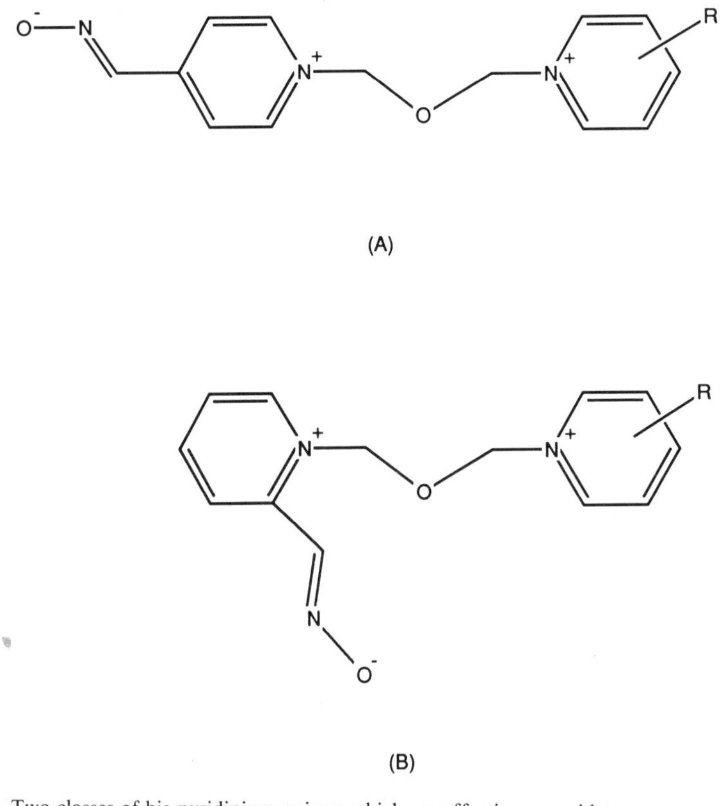

(A)

(B)

FIG. 1-2. Two classes of bis-pyridinium oximes which are effective as antidotes to nerve gas: (A) oxime group *para*- to the pyridinium nitrogen and (B) oxime group *ortho*- to the pyridinium nitrogen.

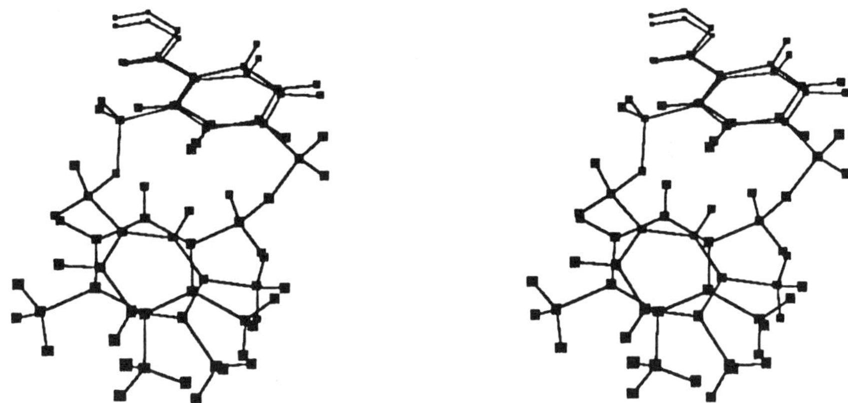

FIG. 1-3. Overlapped conformations of *ortho*- and *para*-bis-pyridinium oxime skeletons. Note that the two oxime groups are perfectly overlapped while the two nonoxime rings are approximately overlapped.

overlap could suggest ideas for the design of new drugs which contain features from both molecules. Now, the question reduces to one of finding conformations of the two drugs such that the oxime group and the nonoxime ring of one molecule overlap with the corresponding parts of the other.

We built three-dimensional models for the *ortho*- and *para*-bis-pyridinium oximes using the CHEM-X* molecular modeling program. These models were refined by a few cycles of simple molecular mechanics. To find conformations of the two drugs where the oxime groups and the nonoxime rings overlap, we used a modification of the distance geometry method (Crippen, 1981). The distance geometry method allows us to generate conformations of molecules subject to a set of distance constraints, specified as a set of lower and upper distance limits for pairs of atoms. In our slightly modified version of this method, called the "ensemble" approach (Sheridan et al., 1986), we consider the molecules to be overlapped as a single combined molecule in which the lower and upper distance limits of atoms to be brought into coincidence have been set to 0 (within a small tolerance). Other implicit and explicit constraints are also expressed as upper and lower distance bounds. The method selects sets of interatomic distances randomly within the specified bounds and goes on to generate conformations satisfying those distance constraints. Typically, the solution is not unique, so we generate several sets of conformations and look for conformational classes.

In the present example, it turned out that there was a unique overlapping conformation for the two molecules (Fig. 1-3), suggesting that this is the active conformation of these molecules. Our next step was to seek ways of producing a rigidified analog which would preserve the orientation of the active groups in the molecule. Examination of the overlapped molecules led us to design two semirigid analogs, shown in Fig. 1-4. In each case there is a third ring between the two pyridinium rings, which imposes conformational constraints on the molecule. Thus it is likely that these molecules show increased activity.

4. MACROMOLECULAR MODELING

Very often, drug targets are enzymes or other proteins. There are several instances when we know the mechanism of action of a drug, the nature of the target protein, and its amino acid sequence. However, we do not have three-dimensional X-ray crystal structure data on the protein. Prediction of the three-dimensional structure of a protein starting from the

*CHEM-X, created by E. K. Davies, Chemical Crystallography Laboratories, Oxford University, developed and distributed by Chemical Design Ltd., Oxford, United Kingdom.

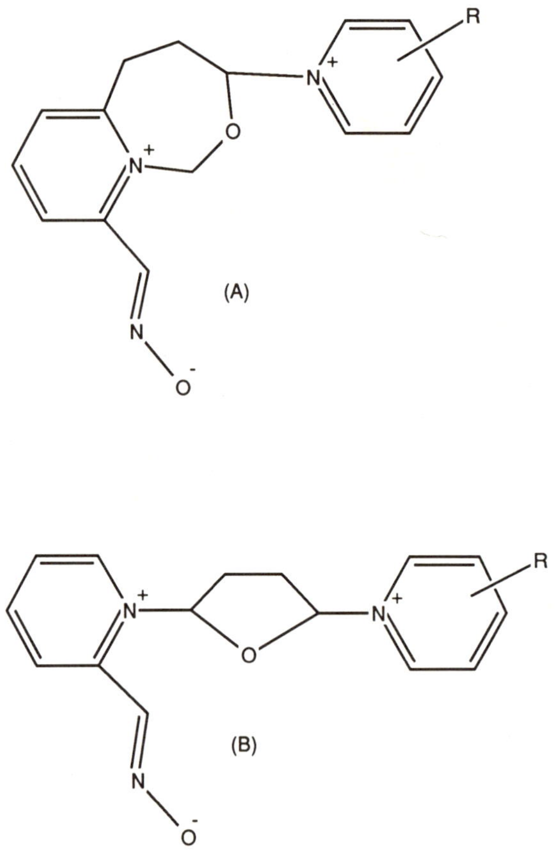

FIG. 1-4. Two types of semirigid analogs designed as antidotes to nerve gas with (A) a seven-membered rigidifying ring and (B) a five-membered rigidifying ring.

amino acid sequence is usually not possible because of the large number of ways of folding a polypeptide chain. Sometimes, however, we have access to three-dimensional data on a related protein, that is, a protein with a significant sequence homology. When two proteins are related closely in sequence, they are also generally closely related in structure. Hence, it may be possible to arrive at the structure of a protein when the structure of a closely related protein is known. In our example, we discuss a model building study of human renin (Dixon et al., 1985), an aspartic protease.

Renin is an important enzyme in the renin–angiotensin system which regulates blood pressure. Renin cleaves the alpha-globulin angiotensinogen to produce the decapeptide angiotensin I. Angiotensin-converting enzyme removes the C-terminal dipeptide yielding the potent vasoconstrictor angiotensin II. Thus, the inhibition of renin or angiotensin-converting enzyme would be expected to have an antihypertensive effect. Indeed, the well-known drug captopril is an inhibitor of angiotensin-converting enzyme. Inhibitors of renin would also be expected to have a similar effect. There is hence a large effort by many pharmaceutical companies to produce an effective renin inhibitor.

Several groups have generated approximate structures for human renin (Carlson et al., 1982; Blundell et al., 1983) using the amino acid sequence of mouse renin (Panthier et al., 1982; Misono et al., 1982). Our model was built using the human renin sequence (Imai et al., 1983) and the crystal structure of penicillopepsin (James & Sielecki, 1983), an acid protease from *Penicillium janthinellum*. The technique, known as protein extension (Feldmann et al., 1985), involves the following steps: (1) alignment of the two sequences, (2) alteration of the side chains and insertion and deletion of backbone segments wherever required, and (3) relaxation by some form of energy optimization. The alignment and alteration of side chains were performed using software supplied by R. J. Feldmann. The insertion of backbone segments involves looping out the extra piece and linking the ends in a stereochemically satisfactory manner. Similarly, deletion involves bringing together two loose ends and sealing them in a stereochemically acceptable manner.

The energy optimization was performed using the molecular mechanics program AMBER (Assisted Model Building with Energy Refinement) (Singh et al., 1986). The resulting structure had no obvious defects. The renin structure has a long active-site cleft, which contains two aspartate residues which are involved in peptide bond hydrolysis. A heptapeptide segment of the natural substrate of renin was docked into the active site to examine the ligand–receptor interactions. The initial crude docking was followed by energy optimization. The N-terminal segment of the substrate was in an extended conformation. Around the middle of the substrate there was a bend, and then the C-terminal segment continued in an extended conformation. There was good hydrophobic/hydrophilic matching between the enzyme and the substrate segment. These aspects of interaction between the heptapeptide and the enzyme are in general agreement with X-ray data on binding of substrates to aspartic proteases (Bott et al., 1982; James et al., 1982).

We have used this model to examine various candidate renin inhibitors. We assess the fit of these molecules based on stereochemistry as well as hydrophobic/hydrophilic compatibility. This model serves as a basis for our effort at rational design of inhibitors of human renin.

5. MODELING DRUG-RECEPTOR INTERACTIONS

Sometimes we have a good idea of the structure of the receptor and of the drug, but do not have X-ray data on their interaction. In these cases, it is often possible to use indirect evidence and computer methods to arrive at a likely model for the interaction. We give as an example a study (Balaji et al., 1985) of the interaction with DNA of two anticancer drugs: mitoxantrone (Murdock et al., 1979) and bisantrene (Murdock et al., 1982). Figure 1-5 shows the chemical structures of these two drugs.

Electron micrographs reveal an elongation of DNA upon binding of these drugs. This is consistent with the hypothesis that these drugs are intercalating agents (Lerman, 1961; Freifelder, 1971). It was seen in electron micrographs that mitoxantrone (but not bisantrene) had the property of creating lacelike networks in circular DNA. These networks were thought to arise because the side chains of mitoxantrone cross-linked adjacent DNA molecules. We undertook a detailed energy analysis of the interaction of DNA with these two drugs so that we could explain the above observations and also have a framework for future drug design efforts.

It can be seen that the drug–DNA complex has several degrees of freedom, and it is not

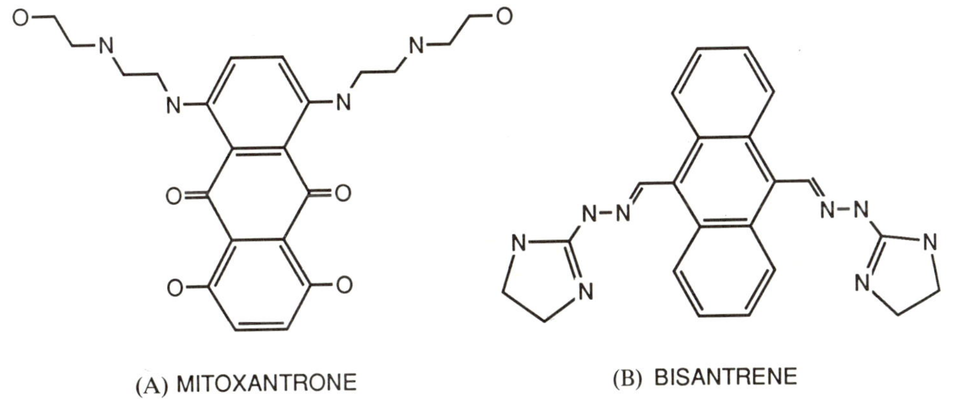

(A) MITOXANTRONE

(B) BISANTRENE

FIG. 1-5. Chemical structure of two anticancer agents: (A) mitoxantrone and (B) bisantrene.

possible to explore all the possible conformations and modes of interaction of drug and DNA. However, it is possible to make several reasonable simplifying assumptions which make the modeling practical. We used a base-paired DNA tetramer for our studies. The intercalation site was between the central base pairs, which had a separation of 0.676 nm as observed in crystal structures of drug–DNA intercalation complexes (Neidle, 1979; Neidle & Berman, 1982). Various DNA conformations were generated by varying the deoxyribose sugar geometry and the backbone geometry. The drug molecules were built using fragments derived from the Cambridge Crystal File (Allen et al., 1979).

Conformational potential energy calculations were carried out using coulombic electrostatic, London dispersion, van der Waals repulsive, induced dipole, torsional, hydrogen bonding, and bond length and bond angle distortion terms (Olson & Flory, 1972; McGuire et al., 1972; Levitt, 1983). We first considered the energy of interaction of the tricyclic ring systems of each drug with DNA, ignoring the side chains on the drugs. We calculated the energy of interaction as a function of depth of penetration of the ring system into the DNA molecule. At this stage, it was found that penetration from the major groove side and from the minor groove side were about equally favorable. Once approximate intercalation geometries were obtained, we added the side chains and completed the minimization. Once the side chains were added, mitoxantrone and bisantrene showed differences in their preferred binding modes. The energy calculations showed that mitoxantrone intercalates from the minor groove side and its side chains remain free for hydrogen bonding to adjacent DNA molecules. This could explain the observation of lacelike networks as described earlier. Bisantrene, on the other hand, seems to prefer entry from the major groove side. Furthermore, it has no available hydrogen bonding groups which could cross-link with adjacent DNA molecules.

6. NEW DIRECTIONS IN DRUG DESIGN

We have discussed topological methods for calculating structural similarity and for establishing structure–activity correlations. We have also discussed how we could use these methods to select candidate compounds from a large database. Now, we ask ourselves whether we could come up with totally novel compounds that would rank high in a trend vector model or would show high similarity to a known drug.

We have implemented a graphical design system which allows a chemist to draw a structure and modify it, under guidance of a trend vector; that is, with each change in structure there is immediate feedback telling the designer whether the change was favorable or unfavorable. In principle, one would like to design a molecule rich in "active" descriptors and poor in "inactive" ones. It is very difficult to do this directly, as there are many interdependencies among the descriptors.

We have therefore used an alternative approach, which takes full advantage of the speed of the computer in performing simple repetitious tasks. In essence, myriad structures are assembled at random and then screened with the trend vector and similarity probes described earlier.

We have implemented a random compound generator which selects fragments from a MACCS* database and assembles them. Selection probabilities are assigned to the various fragments in the database in accordance with the desired frequency of their occurrence. These weights and various other adjustable parameters have been fine-tuned so that we can generate compounds which closely resemble compounds from our own corporate database, and yet 99% are new. Some of these generated compounds may be chemically nonsensical, but this is not important. Periodically we generate a set of 10,000 random compounds and evaluate them against a panel of trend vectors. We also calculate their similarity values to a set of chosen drugs. Most of the unreasonable structures are rejected in the selection process. The highest ranking 0.1% of the compounds are printed as a bulle-

*MACCS is the trade name for a chemical database management system supplied by Molecular Design Ltd., San Leandro, California.

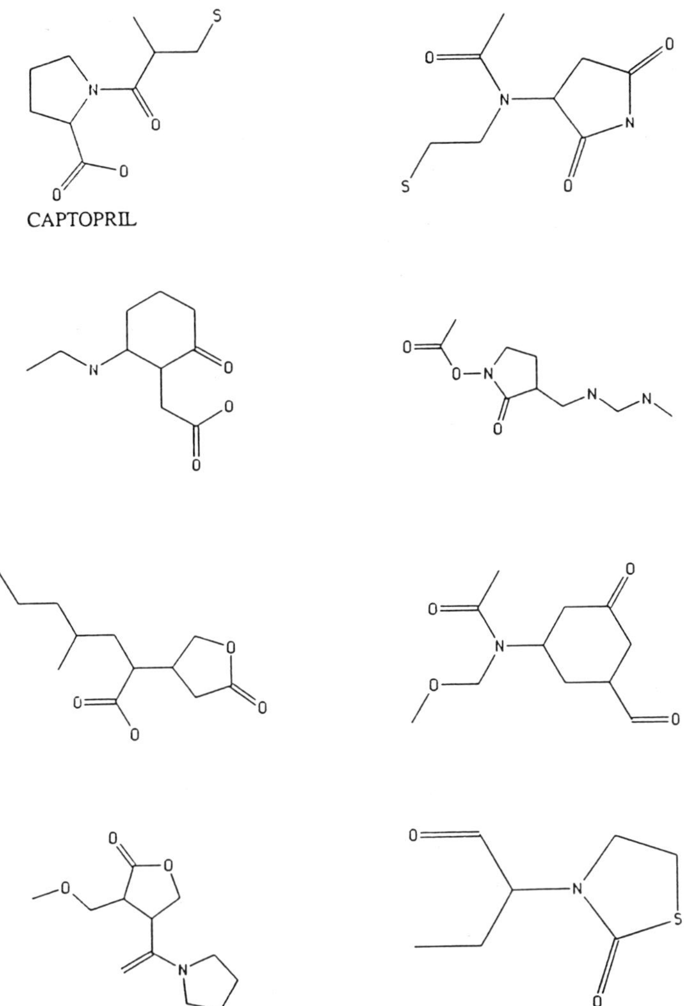

FIG. 1-6. A sample page from the random compound bulletin showing captopril and randomly generated structures similar to it. The similarity probe was done using atom pair descriptors, but could as well have been done with topological torsions.

tin. Figure 1-6 shows a sample page from the bulletin with a set of randomly generated compounds selected for their similarity to captopril, a well-known antihypertensive drug. Although not close analogs, these structures may be suggestive.

Thus this method produces novel structures associated with potential biological activities. Of course, their realization as compounds must await the initiative of the synthetic chemist.

Acknowledgments—We wish to acknowledge the contribution of former colleagues Dr. R. Carhart, Dr. D. H. Smith, Dr. J. S. Dixon, and Dr. V. N. Balaji. This work was supported in part by the U.S. Army Medical Research and Development Command, Contract No. DAMD17-84-C-4111.

REFERENCES

Allen, F. H., Bellard, S., Brice, M. D., Cartwright, B. A., Doubleday, A., Higgs, H., Hummelink, T., Hummelink-Peters, B. G., Kennard, O., Motherwell, W. D. S., Rodgers, J. R., and Watson, D. G. (1979). The Cambridge crystallographic data center: Computer-based search, retrieval, analysis, and display of information. *Acta Crystallogr.* **B35**: 2331–2339.

Balaji, V. N., Dixon, S. J., Smith, D. H., Venkataraghavan, R., and Murdock, K. C. (1985) Design of anticancer drugs using modeling techniques. *Ann. N.Y. Academy Sci.* **439**:140–161.

Blundell, T., Sibanda, B. L., and Pearl, L. (1983) Three dimensional structure, specificity, and catalytic mechanism of renin. *Nature* **304**: 273–275.

Bott, R., Subramaniam, E., and Davies, D. R. (1982) Three-dimensional structure of the complex of the *Rhizopus chinensis* carboxyl proteinase and pepstatin at 2.5 Å resolution. *Biochemistry* **21**: 6956–6962.

Carhart, R. E., Smith, D. H., and Venkataraghavan, R. (1985) Atom pairs as molecular features in structure-activity studies: Definition and applications. *J. Chem. Inf. Comput. Sci.* **25**: 64–73.

Carlson, W., Feldmann, R. J., and Haber, E. (1982) Three-dimensional structure of renin and implications for the binding of renin inhibitors. *Circulation* **66**: II–287.

Crippen, G. M. (1981) in *Distance geometry and conformational calculations*. New York: Research Studies Press.

Dixon, J. S., Sheridan, R., Venkataraghavan, R., and Kuntz, I. D. (1985) Methodology for protein design. *190th ACS National Meeting*, Abstract number 49, Chicago, Illinois.

Erdmann, W. D., and Engelhard, H. (1964) Pharmacologic–toxicologic investigations of a new esterase reactivator; the dichloride of bis(4-hydroxyiminomethylpyridiniomethyl) ether. *Arzneim. Forsch.* **14**: 5–11.

Feldmann, R. J., Bing, D. H., Potter, M., Mainhart, C., Furie, B., Furie, B. C., and Caporale, L. H. (1985) On the construction of computer models of proteins by the extension of crystallographic structures. *Ann. N.Y. Acad. Sci.* **439**: 12–43.

Freifelder, D. (1971) Electron microscopic study of the ethidium bromide–DNA complex. *J. Mol. Biol.* **60**: 401–402.

Hobbiger, F., and Vojvodic, V. (1966) The reactivating and antidotal actions of N,N′-trimethylenebis(pyridinium 4-aldoxime) (TMB-4) and N,N′-oxydimethylenebis(pyridinium 4-aldoxime) (Toxogonin) with particular reference to their effect on phosphorylated acetylcholinesterase in the brain. *Biochem. Pharmacol.* **15**: 1677–1690.

Imai, T., Miyazaki, H., Hirose, S., Hori, H., Hayashi, T., Kageyama, R., Ohkubo, H., Nakanishi, S., and Murakami, K. (1983) Amino acid sequence of mouse submaxillary gland renin. *Proc. Natl. Acad. Sci. USA* **80**: 7405–7409.

James, M. N. G., and Sielecki, A. R. (1983) Structure and refinement of Penicillopepsin at 1.8 Å resolution. *J. Mol. Biol.* **163**: 299–361.

James, M. N. G., Sielecki, A., Salituro, F., Rich, D. H., and Hofmann, T. (1982) Conformational flexibility in the active sites of aspartyl proteinases revealed by a pepstatin fragment binding to penicillopepsin. *Proc. Natl. Acad. Sci. USA* **79**: 6137–6141.

Lerman, L. S. (1961) Structural considerations in the interaction of deoxyribonucleic acid and acridines. *J. Mol. Biol.* **3**: 18–30.

Levitt, M. (1983) Computer simulations of DNA double helix dynamics. *Cold Spring Harbor Symposia on Quantitative Biology* **XLVII**: 251–262.

Marshall, G. M., Barry, C. D., Bosshard, H. E., Dammkoehler, A., and Dunn, D. A. (1979) The conformational parameter in drug design: The active analog approach. *Computer-assisted drug design*, E. C. Olson and R. E. Christoffersen, eds., ACS Symp. Series 112, American Chemical Society, Washington, DC, pp. 205–226.

McGuire, R. F., Momany, F. A., and Scheraga, H. A. (1972) Energy parameters in polypeptides. V. An empirical hydrogen bond potential function based on molecular orbital calculations. *J. Phys. Chem.* **76**: 375–393.

Misono, K. S., Chang, J., and Inagami, T. (1982) Amino acid sequence of mouse submaxillary gland renin. *Proc. Natl. Acad. Sci. USA* **79**: 4858–4862.

Murdock, K. C., Child, R. G., Fabio, P. F., Angier, R. B., Wallace, R. E., Durr, F. E., and Citarella, R. V. (1979) Antitumor agents. 1. 1,4-Bis[(aminoalkyl)amino]-9,10-anthracenediones. *J. Med. Chem.* **22**: 1024–1032.

Murdock, K. C., Child, R. G., Lin, Y.-I., Warren, J. D., Fabio, P. F., Lee, V. J., Izzo, P. T., Lang, S. A., Angier, R. B., Citarella, R. V., Wallace, R. E., and Durr, F. E. (1982) Antitumor agents. 2. Bisguanyl hydrazones of anthracene-9,10-dicarboxaldehydes. *J. Med. Chem.* **25**: 505–518.

Neidle, S. (1979) The molecular basis for the action of some DNA-binding drugs. *Progr. Med. Chem.* **16**: 151–221.

Neidle, S., and Berman, H. M. (1982) In *Molecular structure and biological activity*, J. F. Griffin and W. L. Duax, eds., pp. 287–302. New York: Elsevier.

Nilakantan, R., Bauman, N., Dixon, J. S., and Venkataraghavan, R. (1987) Topological torsion: A new molecular descriptor for SAR applications. Comparison with other descriptors. *J. Chem. Inf. Comput. Sci.* **27**: 82–85.

Olson, W. K., and Flory, P. J. (1972) Spatial configuration of polynucleotide chains. II. Conformational energies and the average dimensions of polyribonucleotides. *Biopolymers* **11**: 25–56.

Panthier, J. J., Foote, S., Chambraud, B., Strosberg, A. D., Corvol, P., and Rougeon, F. (1982) Complete amino acid sequence and maturation of the mouse submaxillary gland renin precursor. *Nature* **298**: 90–92.

Sheridan, R. P., Nilakantan, R., Dixon, S., and Venkataraghavan, R. (1986) The ensemble approach to distance geometry: Application to the nicotinic pharmacophore. *J. Med. Chem.* **29**: 899–906.

Singh, U. C., Weiner, P. K., Caldwell, J. W., and Kollman, P. A. (1986) AMBER (UCSF Version 3.0), Dept. Pharmaceutical Chemistry, University of California, San Francisco.

CHAPTER 2

OVERVIEW OF MOLECULAR ASPECTS OF ANTIVIRAL DRUG ACTION AND DESIGN

William H. Prusoff, Tai-Shun Lin, E. Michael August, Thomas G. Wood,
Maria Elena Marongiu, Evelyn Birks, and He-Ying Qian
Department of Pharmacology, Yale University School of Medicine, New Haven, Connecticut, United States

Abstract—The molecular basis for the antiviral activity of the seven compounds approved for clinical use in the United States is reviewed. However, none is without some problems, and hence there is a need for improved agents as well as a need for drugs or vaccines for viral infections for which we do not at present have effective therapy. Two approaches to the design of a drug are presented. One, the *empirical approach*, involves repeated structure modification of a lead compound to optimize activity. The second, or *rational approach*, requires a sophisticated knowledge of the target structure and the biochemical pathways involved to arrive at a candidate compound. The advantages and difficulties associated with these approaches are discussed.

It has been estimated that only about 1% of compounds that have antiviral activity in cell culture are also active in animal systems. Of those that have good antiviral activity and acceptable toxicity in animals, only a few become antiviral drugs for use in humans. The objective of antiviral drug development is the synthesis of a potent compound with high bioavailability and little or no toxicity, and one that will maintain an effective concentration at the target site for the time required to exert its antiviral activity. As of today, only seven antiviral compounds have been approved for clinical use in humans by the Food and Drug Administration in the United States (Figure 2-1). The molecular basis for their antiviral activity has been recently reviewed (DeClercq & Walker, 1988; Cheng & Prusoff, 1986; Prusoff & Lin, 1988), and the present discussion of the molecular basis for antiviral activity will be restricted to these seven drugs.

1. ANTIVIRAL COMPOUNDS APPROVED FOR CLINICAL USE IN HUMANS

1.1. Amantadine

Amantadine is used for therapy and prophylaxis of respiratory infections caused by the influenza A virus. The compound is well absorbed upon oral administration and has a mean half-life of about 15 hours, with about 86% appearing unchanged in the urine within 4 days. There is no evidence that metabolic alteration is required for amantadine to exert its antiviral activity.

The molecular basis for its antiviral activity is not clear, although several hypotheses have been proposed (references cited in Prusoff et al., 1985; Prusoff & Lin, 1988). More recently, Hay and colleagues (1985, 1986) reported that, depending on the strain of influenza virus, amantadine inhibits either the initiation of infection or of virus assembly. They identified the membrane-associated portion of the M_2 protein to be the critical target. Amantadine is believed to interfere specifically with either the function of this viral membrane protein or its interaction with haemagglutinin. However, the specific mechanism whereby amantadine affects the M_2 protein or its function is yet to be elucidated.

An earlier hypothesis concerns the ability of amantadine, as a primary amine, to increase the pH of endosomes. Such an increase would prevent the acid-catalyzed conformational protein rearrangements required of the viral capsid for fusion with the endosomal membrane for uncoating of the virus. However, much higher concentrations of amantadine are required to affect the pH than to affect the M_2 protein (Hay et al., 1986).

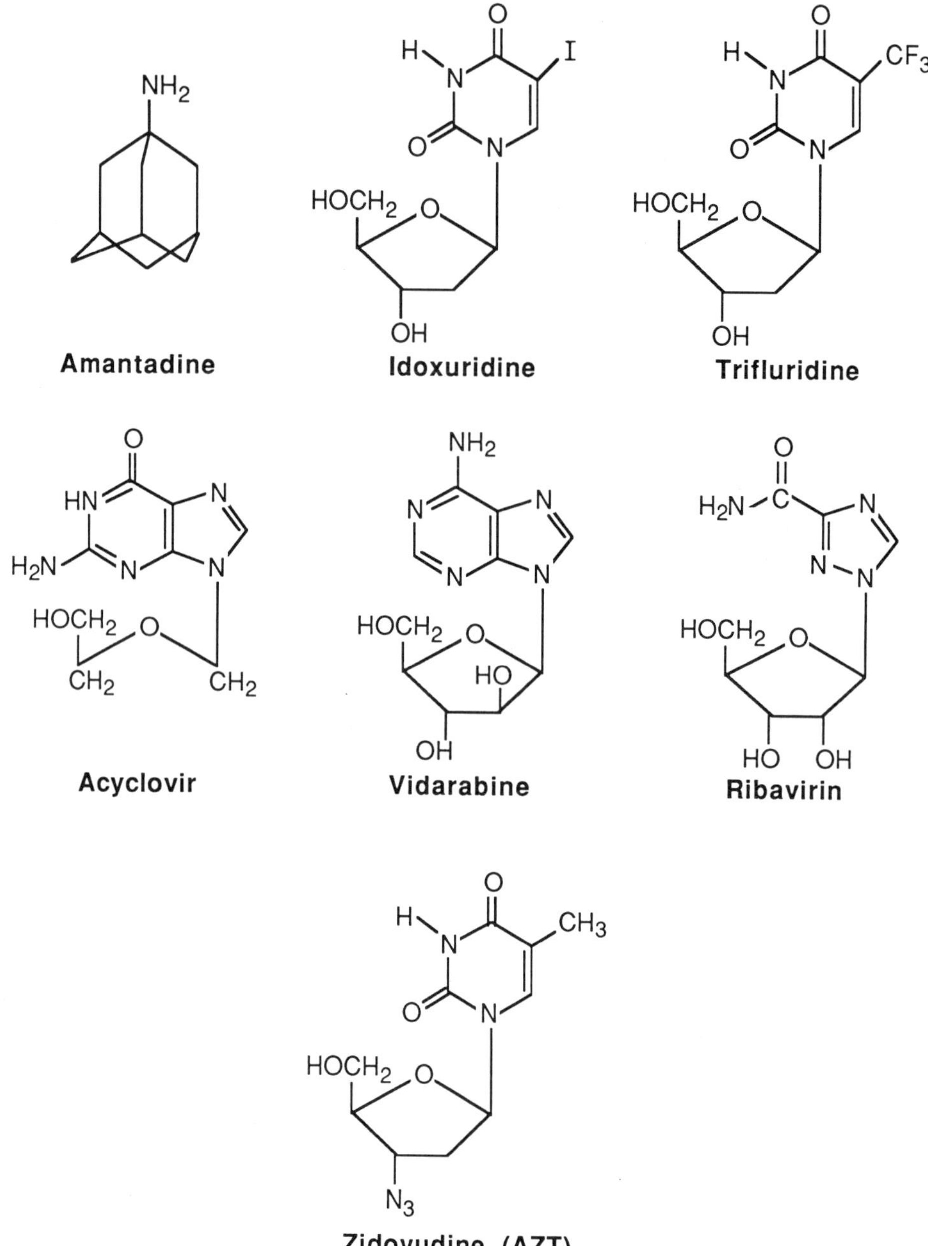

FIG. 2-1. Antiviral agents approved for clinical use.

1.2 IDOXURIDINE

Idoxuridine (5-iodo-2′-deoxyuridine, IdUrd) is an analog of thymidine, and its use in the United States is restricted to topical therapy of herpes keratitis. IdUrd is phosphorylated to the corresponding monophosphate (IdUMP) by cellular, as well as viral-encoded, thymidine kinase. IdUMP can interact with thymidylate synthetase, the consequence being dehalogenation with formation of dUMP and subsequent methylation to form dTMP. For this reason IdUrd labeled with radioactive iodine, but not tritium- or carbon-labeled IdUrd, is a good marker for incorporation studies of IdUrd into DNA. IdUMP is further phosphorylated by cellular enzymes to the corresponding di- and triphosphate analogs (IdUDP, IdUTP). IdUTP is a good substrate for both cellular- and viral-encoded DNA polymerases and hence is incorporated into cellular as well as viral DNA. The incorporation into cellular DNA of uninfected cells may result in cytotoxicity, and hence its use clinically is restricted to topical administration (Calabresi et al., 1961; Boston Interhospital Virus Study Group, 1975).

A direct correlation exists between the extent of viral inhibition and incorporation of IdUrd into the DNA of herpes simplex virus (Fischer et al., 1980). Incorporation of IdUrd into HSV-1 DNA produced no apparent effect on the physical integrity of the substituted DNA; however, a similar substitution with the 5′-amino analog of IdUrd (AIdUrd) produced both single- and double-strand breaks in the viral DNA (Fischer et al., 1980). Pronounced effects on viral gene expression were produced as a consequence of incorporation of IdUrd into the DNA of herpes simplex virus. The formation of polyadenylated RNA was markedly decreased and that of nonpolyadenylated RNA was profoundly increased when HSV-1 was grown in the presence of IdUrd (Otto et al., 1984) or of AIdUrd (Zucker et al., 1988). The consequence of these RNA effects is expressed during protein synthesis, specifically a variable reduction of late β- and γ- but not early α-proteins, and in addition progeny virions had altered protein patterns (Otto et al., 1982).

1.3. Trifluridine

5-Trifluoromethyl-2′-deoxyuridine (CF_3dUrd), like IdUrd, is in clinical use only for topical therapy of herpes keratitis. It is phosphorylated by cellular- as well as a viral-encoded thymidine kinase to the monophosphate (CF_3dUMP). As the monophosphate it interacts with thymidylate synthetase, thereby inhibiting the formation of dTMP via the *de novo* pathway, and in addition it is further phosphorylated to the di- and triphosphate (CF_3dUTP). The triphosphate analog competes with dTTP for incorporation into viral DNA, the consequence being loss of viral infectivity (Heidelberger & King, 1979; Carmine et al., 1982).

1.4. Vidarabine

Vidarabine (9-β-D-arabinofuranosyladenine; adenine arabinoside, araA) is of value for therapy of herpes keratitis, herpes encephalitis, varicella zoster, and neonatal herpes. It is converted by cellular enzymes to the mono-, di-, and triphosphate analogs. There are multiple sites of inhibition, but the specific site responsible for viral inhibition is yet to be established. As the triphosphate, ara ATP causes inhibition of several enzymes: ribonucleoside-diphosphate reductase, RNA-dependent RNA polymerase, viral and cellular DNA polymerases, and terminal deoxynucleotidyl transferase. In addition, araA is incorporated into both viral and cellular DNA. Incorporation of a single molecule of araA slows DNA elongation, thereby behaving as a pseudoterminator of DNA polymerase α and β; however, a similar effect with herpes virus DNA polymerase requires incorporation of two or more molecules of araA into the viral nucleic acid (Reid et al., 1988). AraA in the unphosphorylated form inhibits S-adenosylhomocysteine hydrolase, the consequence being an accumulation of S-adenosylhomocysteine, which in turn inhibits essential S-adenosylmethionine-dependent methylation reactions (North & Cohen, 1979; Drach, 1983).

1.5. Acyclovir

9-(2-Hydroxyethoxymethyl) guanine (acyclovir, ACV) is in clinical use for therapy of herpes keratitis, herpes encephalitis, varicella zoster, neonatal herpes, and genital herpes and as a prophylactic repressor of herpes virus reactivation in patients receiving immunosuppressive drugs. ACV is activated in the herpes virus infected cell by a viral-encoded thymidine kinase, which accounts for its low toxicity in uninfected tissues. Those viruses that do not induce a viral-encoded thymidine kinase are resistant to ACV. After conversion to the monophosphate (ACV-MP), cellular enzymes continue the phosphorylation to the di- and triphosphate analogs. Not only is ACV-TP a competitive inhibitor of the utilization of dGTP for synthesis of DNA, but also ACV is incorporated into the growing viral DNA, resulting in a 3′-termination of the DNA chain elongation (Elion, 1982; Furman et al., 1979). A consequence of viral growth in the presence of ACV is a marked reduction in the synthesis of HSV-1 γ-proteins, but not of α- or β-proteins (Furman & McGuirt, 1983).

1.6. Ribavirin

Ribavirin (1-β-D-ribofuranosyl-1,2,4-triazole-3-carboxamide, virazole) inhibits a wide variety of DNA and RNA viruses, but it is approved in the United States only for therapy of severe respiratory infections in infants and children caused by the respiratory syncytial virus (RSV). Several reviews have appeared recently (Robins, 1986; Gilbert & Knight, 1986).

Ribavirin is phosphorylated to the mono-, di-, and triphosphate (Rib-TP) in both the RSV-infected and -uninfected cells (Smee & Mathews, 1986). The monophosphate of ribavirin (Rib-MP) is a potent inhibitor of the enzyme inosinate dehydrogenase, which is responsible for the conversion of inosinate (IMP) to xanthylate (XMP), the immediate precursor of guanylate (GMP). This results in depletion of both GTP and dGTP pools. In addition, the triphosphate of ribavirin inhibits the mRNA guanyltransferase enzyme with resultant blocking of the initial step in the capping of virus-specific mRNA, that is, the transfer of GMP from GTP to the 5′-terminus of viral mRNA. In addition, the enzyme N^7-methyl transferase, which is responsible for transfer of the methyl moiety from S-adenosylmethionine to the N^7 of the terminally added GMP, is also blocked (Robins, 1986). Inhibition of the capping or methylation reactions should result in a detrimental effect on translation of viral mRNA. In addition, a direct effect of ribavirin triphosphate on influenza virus RNA polymerase and on vesicular stomatitis virus transcription by ribavirin diphosphate has been reported (Eriksson et al., 1977; Wray et al., 1985a,b; Toltzis et al., 1988).

1.7. Azidothymidine

3′-Azido-3′-deoxythymidine (azidothymidine, AZT, retrovir) is an analog of thymidine which is in clinical use for therapy of acquired immune deficiency syndrome (AIDS). AZT is metabolized to the 5′-mono-, di-, and triphosphate analogs to the same extent in HIV-1 infected and uninfected cells (Furman et al., 1986). Furman and colleagues (1986) found the K_m and V_{max} for the phosphorylation of dThd and AZT by thymidine kinase to be similar. Although the K_m of AZT-MP for thymidylate kinase was twice that for dTMP, the V_{max} was only 0.3% of that for dTMP. The consequence is an increase in the pool of dTMP and a markedly reduced intracellular pool of dTTP (Furman et al., 1986). Thus the rate limiting step in the metabolism of AZT is the phosphorylation of AZT-MP by thymidylate kinase to the diphosphate of AZT (AZT-DP). The triphosphate of AZT is a potent inhibitor of the HIV-encoded reverse transcriptase (Furman et al., 1986), and if incorporated into DNA would function, as does acyclovir, as a terminator of DNA chain elongation.

Although these seven compounds are in clinical use as approved drugs for therapy of viral infections, none are without some problems. Thus, not only do we need improved drugs to circumvent these problems, but also we need drugs to attack viral infections for which we do not at present have clinically useful drugs or vaccines. There are a number of very effective antiviral agents in cell culture and animal models which could be clinically useful, if we could devise procedures for their preferential uptake into the infected cell or restrict their action to only the infected cell. This is not a trivial task.

2. EMPIRICAL APPROACH TO DRUG DESIGN

The design of a drug can be approached by one of two strategies: rational or empirical. The *empirical* approach has been very successful in providing most of the drugs we have today and will be relied upon for years to come. The empirical approach is also called the *practical* approach and involves repeated structure modification of a lead compound, and evaluation of activity, to produce a continual improvement until optimization is achieved. The lead compound may have been obtained from random screening or biochemical knowledge, and the structural modifications made are dependent upon the chemist's experience and intuition as well as serendipity. The probability of producing an active compound can be improved by combining structure–activity relationships with computer graphic model building.

An example of the empirical approach is structural modification of Idoxuridine (5-iodo-2′-deoxyuridine), which was the first nucleoside to demonstrate clinically useful antiviral activity (Prusoff, 1988). Thus, replacement of the iodine atom in the 5-position of the pyrimidine moiety with the $-CF_3$ group produced 5-trifluoromethyl-2′-deoxyuridine (Trifluridine) (Fig. 2.1).

Another example of the empirical approach is the design and synthesis by DeClercq and colleagues (1986) of a novel series of phosphonylmethoxyalkyl derivatives of purines and pyrimidines. Figure 2-2 shows one such compound, (S)-9-(3-hydroxy-2-phosphonylmethoxypropyl) adenine, [(*S*)-HPMPA], a combination of two antiviral agents which separately have different mechanisms of action. Phosphonoformate is an inhibitor of HSV-1 DNA polymerase, and the acyclic adenosine is an inhibitor of S-adenosylhomocysteine hydrolase, the consequence being inhibition of essential methylation of viral mRNA. (S)-HPMPA is phosphorylated to the mono- and diphosphates and inhibits HSV-1 DNA synthesis; the precise mechanism is under study (Votruba et al., 1987).

A number of antiviral compounds have been developed which fortuitously take advantage of a viral-encoded thymidine kinase for preferential activation by phosphorylation in the infected cell (Fig. 2-3). Thymidine kinase encoded by the herpes virus genome is critical for the activation of a number of antiviral agents with diverse structures and which are not substrates for cellular thymidine kinase. The virus-induced enzyme differs from the comparable host cell thymidine kinase in molecular weight, substrate specificity, electrophoretic mobility, isoelectric point, and immunological properties (Kit, 1979).

The thymidine kinase encoded by HSV-1 catalyzes the phosphorylation of not only thymidine, but also deoxycytidine (Jamieson et al., 1974) as well as a host of nucleoside analogs, some of which are seen in Figure 2-3. The enzyme will also catalyze the phosphorylation of thymidine-5′-phosphates (Chen & Prusoff, 1978) as well as some other nucleoside-5′-phosphates such as (E)-5-(2-bromovinyl)-2′-deoxyuridine-5′-monophosphate, BrVdUMP (Fyfe, 1982), and even 5′-phosphonoamidates (Chen & Prusoff, 1978). Kinetic studies of HSV-1–encoded TK-TMP kinase support the conclusion that phosphorylation of dThd and dTMP share the same active site, or two sites exist but they overlap (Chen et al., 1979). However, the TK encoded by HSV-2 phosphorylates dTMP very poorly and that of BrVdUMP insignificantly (Fyfe, 1982). In view of these activities, it would be well worth examining the substrate properties of this enzyme. Modifications that have produced alternate substrates for the viral thymidine kinase which have antiviral activity include (1) replacement of a pyrimidine by a purine as in acyclovir or ganciclovir (DHPG); (2)

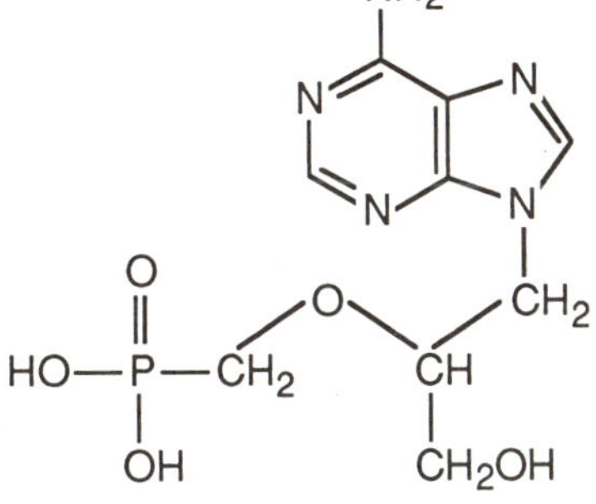

FIG. 2-2. Structure of (S)-9-(3-hydroxy-2-phosphonylmethoxypropyl) adenine, (S)-HPMPA.

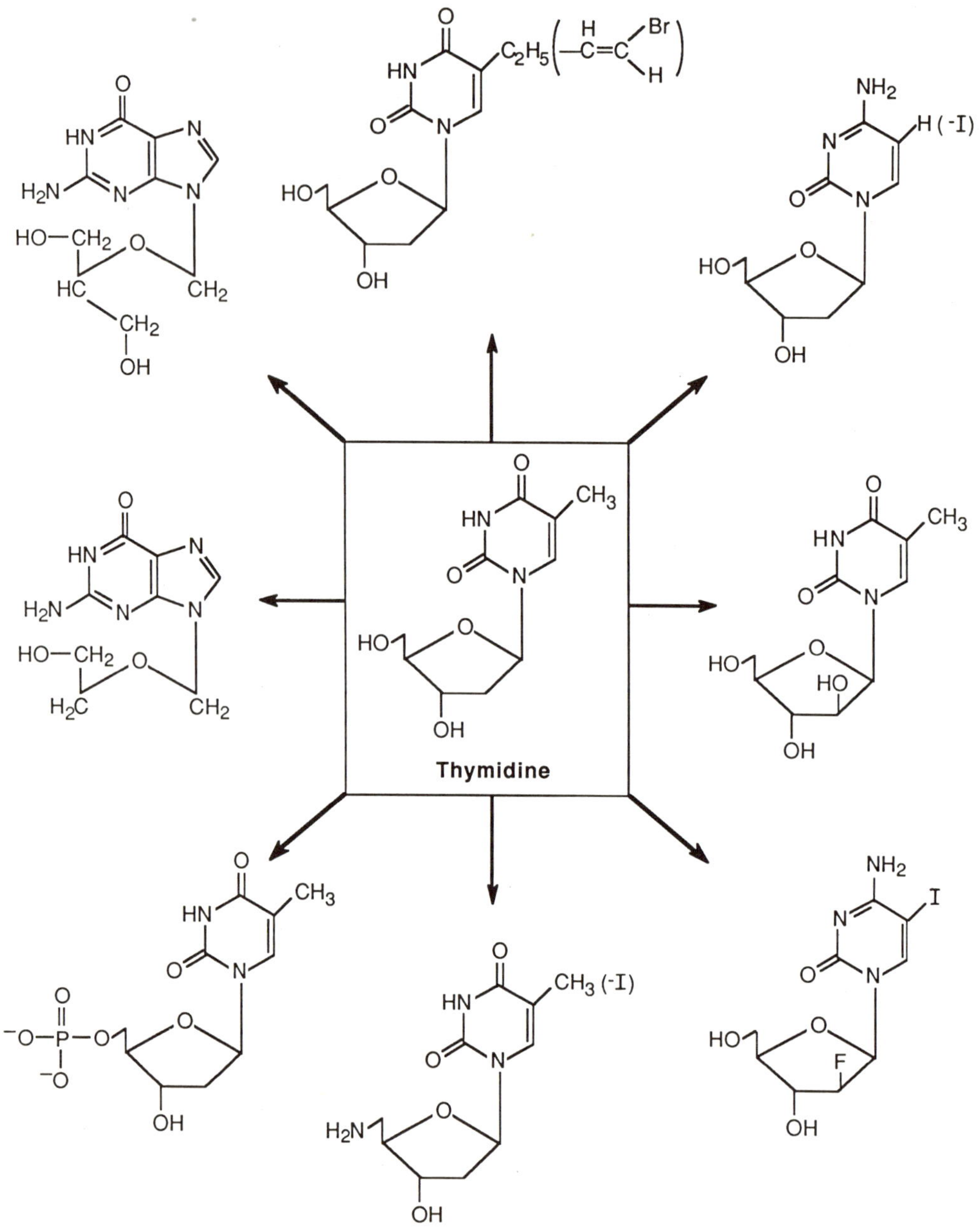

FIG. 2-3. Substrates for herpes simplex virus type 1 thymidine kinase.

replacement of the methyl moiety of dThd by ethyl, propyl, or a 2-bromovinyl moiety; (3) replacement of the deoxyribose by an arabinose as in thymine arabinoside (ara T) or 1-(2-deoxy-2-fluoro-β-D-arabinofuranosyl)-5-iodocytosine (FIAC); (4) replacement of deoxyribose by an acyclic moiety as in acyclovir or DHPG; or (5) replacement of the 5′—OH by an amino group as in 5-iodo-5′-amino-2′,5′-dideoxyuridine (AIdUrd) or 5′-amino-5′-deoxythymidine (AdThd).

A simple structural modification may not produce the desired end product because any modification of structure will produce changes in size, shape, electronic distribution, partition coefficient, solubility, pKa, chemical reactivity, metabolism, and hydrogen bonding capabilities. The hope is that the change being made will result in improved potency, selectivity, duration of action, bioavailability, and reduced toxicity (Baldwin, 1987).

3. RATIONAL APPROACH TO DRUG DESIGN

The second approach to drug design is the *rational* approach, which is intellectually more satisfying, but much more difficult. Nevertheless, we believe we are making rapid progress in this direction, and it will, in the near future, be the productive way to go. The rational approach requires a sophisticated knowledge of the target structure—be it an active site of an enzyme, a receptor, or a macromolecule such as DNA, RNA, or regulatory protein—as well as a knowledge of the biochemical pathways involved.

However can we acquire the knowledge required for the rational approach? The target to be attacked must first be identified, and then the next step is to determine the structural, spatial, and electronic requirements for a compound to interact uniquely with the target receptor. The targets that merit consideration are those that are unique to the virus under consideration.

Whereas the viral thymidine kinase catalyzes reactions that normally occur in the uninfected cell (dThd → dTMP), there are also several viral-encoded enzymes that are essential for viral replication and catalyze reactions that are unique to the virus-infected cell. These enzymes are excellent targets for the design of an antiviral drug. The RNA transcriptase of the influenza virus, the RNA replicase of the enteroviruses and rhinoviruses, and the reverse transcriptase of the retroviruses (HIV-1) are examples of enzymes with unique activity. The problem is to design a compound that uniquely inhibits the enzyme.

Another category of viral-encoded enzymes exists which are essential for viral replication but catalyze reactions for which there is a counterpart in the uninfected cell. The herpes virus–encoded DNA polymerase is a DNA polymerase preferentially inhibited by phosphonoformate (Oberg, 1983a). In addition, there are a number of viral-encoded proteases which are under active study for design of a compound that will specifically, or at least preferentially, inhibit its function and thereby prevent viral replication (Korant, 1981; Korant et al., 1984). Analyses of the HIV-1 protease are in progress with the object to develop a specific inhibitor of this viral-encoded enzyme (Debouck et al., 1987; Mous et al., 1988). These enzymes also constitute ideal targets for antiviral drug development (Cheng et al., 1985; Oberg, 1983b).

Today we have the potential to determine not only the three-dimensional atomic structure of target sites such as enzymes, or receptors, or viruses, or macromolecules, but also how antiviral agents or drugs interact with these targets by use of X-ray crystallography and NMR. The complete three-dimensional structure of human rhinovirus-14 has been determined by use of the Cyber 205 supercomputer into which X-ray pictures of the crystallized virus were loaded, and the site of attachment of an antiviral agent known to prevent uncoating was elucidated (Smith, T. J., et al., 1986, Rossmann et al., 1987).

X-ray crystallography provides unambiguous information about shapes and interactions of molecules in the solid state, and high-resolution NMR provides information about structures in solution, such as the nature of the drug when it is bound to a macromolecule. A problem with X-ray crystallography, however, is the requirement that the target be in the crystalline state. The crystals once obtained can now be bombarded with X-rays, which cast diffraction shadows. These shadows are converted into numbers and funneled into a computer that determines the structure of the molecule. Another computer then displays the information on a screen, and the image can be twisted, inverted, and enlarged. The chemist can interchange parts of a molecule, atoms, or other fragments to find the combination that best gives the desired result. Thus, knowledge of how the atoms are arranged, when combined with molecular modeling and interactive computer graphics, can afford the design of specific drugs. The use of computer models also enables calculation of the strength of interaction between a drug and its receptor as well as the rates of biological reactions (Burgen et al., 1986; Williams & Malick, 1987).

The design of specific enzyme inhibitors on a rational basis was reviewed by Stark and Bartlett (1983). They discussed multisubstrate analogs, transition-state analogs, affinity labels, and suicide inhibitors, as well as approaches to designing such inhibitors through use of computer modeling and energy minimization programs. Ideally one would like to know the X-ray crystal structure of the enzyme. Using these data, computer graphics techniques allow the visualization of the three-dimensional arrangement of ligand binding sites as well as how the enzyme and ligand interact sterically and electronically.

If a protein is in the crystalline state, it is possible to combine subzero temperature studies of enzyme–substrate interaction (cryoenzymology) (Fink, 1977) with X-ray diffraction to provide structural information with high resolution. A major problem has been to obtain large amounts of protein and prepare single crystals of protein large enough that the three-dimensional structure could be elucidated by X-ray diffraction. Littke and John (1984) recently reported the successful formation of single crystals of β-galactosidase and lysozyme under conditions of microgravity that were 27 and 1000 times larger, respectively, than those obtained under normal gravitation. Large amounts of protein are required for crystallization and can today be obtained by genetic engineering, for example, by use of bacteria in which the appropriate gene has been inserted. If successful, the protein will be subjected to X-ray analysis, the objective being the development of new drugs. Even though a drug is designed based on the X-ray structure of the macromolecule, this does not ensure its clinical utility. There are problems of absorption, distribution, metabolism, excretion, and unpredictable toxicities. But this is true of any new compound.

Another approach for rational design of antiviral drugs is based on our understanding of gene structure and function. Some success has already been achieved in the synthesis of "antisense" oligodeoxyribonucleotides, whose base pairs are complementary to critical regions of the viral genome or mRNA, and following specific hybridization block their expression (Green et al., 1986; Weintraub et al., 1985; Loose-Mitchell, 1988; Knorre & Vlassov, 1985; Knorre et al., 1985; Blake et al., 1985; Cazenave et al., 1986; Helene et al., 1985; Toulme et al., 1986; Stein & Cohen, 1988).

Zamecnik and Stephenson (1978) found that a single-stranded 13-base oligodeoxyribonucleotide, complementary to a region of the terminally redundant sequences of Rous sarcoma virus, inhibited viral production in cell culture. More recently, Zamecnik and colleagues (1986) reported that the replication and expression of the AIDS virus HIV-1 was inhibited by an antisense synthetic oligonucleotide, and To and colleagues (1986) found the replication of avian retroviruses in cell cultures could be inhibited by an antisense RNA.

Izant and Weintraub (1984) and Kim and Wold (1985) reported that antisense RNA can inhibit the expression of herpes virus—and of cellular thymidine kinase, respectively. Studies by Izant and Weintraub (1984) showed that an artificial antisense RNA gene could be used to regulate the expression of a selected herpes virus gene. They injected a mixture of plasmids containing the sense and antisense HSV-TK genes into mouse LTK^- cells. Expression of the antisense viral TK gene significantly decreased the activity of herpes thymidine kinase, compared to that from cells which received only the sense viral TK gene. This inhibitory effect of the antisense viral TK gene was specific to the herpes TK expression, since it had no effect on the expression of chicken TK gene, when a similar experiment was performed.

However, there are several problems in the use of antisense oligonucleotides:

1. High concentrations required
2. Rapid degradation by nucleases in plasma and cells
3. Transport into cells

This challenge has been met by several groups.

P. O. P. Ts'o et al. (1983) decreased sensitivity to enzyme degradation by converting the phosphodiester linkage between nucleosides to either phosphotriesters or to alklyl phosphonates. Also the methyl phosphonates, being less polar, are transported more readily into cells (Aris et al., 1986; Miller et al., 1981; Smith, C. C., et al., 1986). They found that an oligodeoxyribonucleoside methyl phosphonate that is complementary to a section of HSV-1 mRNA, and has a chain length of 8-nucleotidyl units, produced a two-log reduction in virus yield.

Several other approaches have been described to circumvent or at least decrease the problems of degradation of synthetic oligonucleotides, as well as how to increase the stability of the interaction with the target mRNA or gene. Thuong and colleagues (1987) conjugated acridine derivatives via a pentamethylene tether to either the 3′ or 5′ end of the oligonucleotide. Thus, they retained the binding specificity toward the complementary sequence, while the intercalating acridine provided additional binding energy to stabilize the hybrid complex. In addition, the acridine decreased susceptibility to exonuclease degradation and also facilitated cellular uptake. Furthermore, because of the increased binding stability, the size of the oligonucleotide can be shortened (Asseline et al., 1984a,b; Helene et al., 1985).

These workers also prepared a hepta-oligodeoxyribonucleotide–acridine conjugate which was complementary to a part of the 3′-terminal sequence common to the eight viral RNAs of the influenza-type A virus. This influenza A–antisense oligodeoxynucleotide inhibited the viral cytopathic effect in cell culture, and specificity was established, since influenza B was not affected (Zerial et al., 1987). *Exo*nuclease degradation was blocked by the terminal acridine (Asseline et al., 1984a,b), and protection from *endo*nuclease can be achieved by modification of the phosphodiester linkage (Miller et al., 1979) or of the sugar configuration (Morvan et al., 1986).

Helene and coworkers also found that the α-oligonucleotides are more resistant to both exo- and endonuclease degradation than are the normal β-oligonucleotides. The α-polymer binds strongly to the complementary β-polymer (Thuong et al., 1987) and also has a half-life markedly longer than the β-oligomers in *Xenopus* oocytes (Cazenave et al., 1987).

Imbach and associates have published a series of papers concerned with the synthesis and characterization of α-anomeric oligodeoxyribonucleotides (Helene & Thuong, 1988; Sun et al., 1987; Gagnor et al., 1987; Morvan et al., 1988; Helene et al., 1988; Praseuth et al., 1987). Studies of translation in a cell-free system indicated that the α-oligonucleotides failed to inhibit translation (Gagnor et al., 1987).

Transport of oligodeoxyribonucleotides into cells is a problem, and this has partially been improved by decreasing enzymic degradation and decreasing the polarity of these polyanions as described earlier. Another approach is that described by Lemaitre and colleagues (1987). They synthesized a 15-mer oligodeoxyribonucleotide which was complementary to the initiation region of the vesicular stomatitis virus-N-protein-mRNA. Cytidine was covalently linked to the 3′-terminus, and the 2′,3′-bond of the attached cytidine was oxidatively cleaved and reacted with the epsilon amino moiety of polylysine, forming an N-morpholine ring linking the oligomer to polylysine. Whereas most oligomers previously evaluated for antiviral activity required concentrations of 50–100 μM, Lemaitre and colleagues (1987) demonstrated potent antiviral activity against the vesicular stomatitis virus at a concentration of 0.1 μM.

Thus, it appears that solutions to the problems of stability, transport, and activity are well on the way. However, the ultimate concern is what other problems need to be solved for use *in vivo*?

Another very exciting approach, with great potential, is that described by Moser and Dervan (1987), Youngquist and Dervan (1987), and Iverson and Dervan (1987); reviewed by Baum (1988); and adopted by Miller and Ts'o (1987). The technique is termed "affinity cleaving" and involves the synthesis of a 12–15-mer oligodeoxyribonucleotide that is complementary to a specific sequence of double-stranded DNA and is conjugated with a DNA-cleaving moiety. The objective is to destroy a specific gene. The complex reacts at a specific site in the DNA forming a triple helix.

The synthetic oligo-conjugate contains two domains: One binds to a specific sequence of DNA, and the other cleaves the DNA. The cleaving function is ethylenediaminetetraacetic acid (EDTA) with chelated ferrous ion (Fe II). Under appropriate redox conditions, Fe^{++} generates highly reactive hydroxyl radicals from oxygen. The hydroxyl radical ($\cdot$OH), being short-lived, oxidizes only those deoxyribose groups that are close to where it is bound in the DNA. The consequence is cleavage on both strands of DNA. The objective of this approach is a rational chemotherapeutic approach for inactivation of specific genes. Can this approach be used to attack the latency problem with herpes, varicella, or the AIDS viruses? Can other cleaving functions be attached which are not dependent on redox potential?

Miller and Ts'o (1987) cited unpublished data of L. Aurelian, and also of M. Colvin, which reports that an oligodeoxyribonucleotide–EDTA–Fe^{++} complex, targeted against the splice junction of HSV–mRNA 4 and 5, when applied in the form of a cream to the infected ear of a mouse, decreased the viral yield. The yield of virus in both skin region and ganglia region of the ear was reduced. When labeled with tritium and injected into the tail vein of a mouse, it appeared in all organs and tissues except the brain.

Another approach to prevent recurrences is to deliver the antiviral drug by retrograde axonal transport to the cell body of the ganglion. Horseradish peroxidase, a low-molecular-weight (40,000 daltons) protein, has been shown to be transported to the trigeminal ganglion of mice when applied topically to the eye or nose of mice (Fox & White, 1980; Kristensson, 1978). So far, it has only been shown that Idoxuridine, when complexed to horseradish peroxidase, can be so transported to the ganglia (Haschke et al., 1980). Can a complementary oligonucleotide be so transported?

Another intriguing approach is based on the reports by Croen and colleagues (1987) and Gordon and colleagues (1988) who found a large amount of an "antisense" transcript, encoded by a region of herpes virus DNA, in human trigeminal ganglia, which was recovered at autopsy of subjects with *no* clinical evidence of active herpetic infection. If this "antisense" RNA, or its encoded protein, is involved in maintaining the latent state, then it constitutes a good target to prevent reactivation of the virus. This transcript is an immediate early protein known as the infected-cell protein number zero (ICP-0). Herpes simplex virus type 1 latency-associated transcripts have been also found in latently infected sensory ganglia in animals (Spivack & Fraser, 1988, and references cited by Gordon et al., 1988).

The precise mechanism for inhibition of viral replication by oligonucleotides, however, may be more complex than inhibition of transcription or translation. Matsukura and colleagues (1987) at the National Institutes of Health found phosphorothioate analogs of oligodeoxynucleotides were potent inhibitors of the AIDS virus at a concentration of 0.5 μM, comparable to that of dideoxycytidine. They found significant inhibition of purified HIV reverse transcriptase. Therefore, these compounds may have multiple sites of inhibition, which may vary with the specific composition and length. Similarly, Chang and Stoltzfus (1987) present data to support antisense RNA inhibition of virus replication to have a site of inhibition in addition to translation, such as blocking viral RNA packaging or transport from nucleus to cytoplasm.

4. CONCLUSION

We have discussed some molecular aspects for the antiviral action of seven clinically approved drugs as well as several strategies for antiviral drug design. There are many other strategies or combination of strategies that encompass both rational and empirical approaches. Some of the strategies mentioned may appear to be wild, but we should have faith, because the future may indeed bring some of these strategies into reality. This may require combining the talents of an organic chemist, a biochemist, a biophysical chemist, a crystallographer, a computer scientist, a theoretician, and perhaps an astronaut. Such a combination of talents should overcome the problems inherent in these futuristic hopes. Finally, as of today, serendipity has not been eliminated in any of the empirical or so-called rational approaches, but as Sir Arnold Burgen (1986) stated at the conclusion of a paper on rational drug design: "BUT ONE DAY!!!"

Acknowledgment—The research emanating from our laboratories was supported by U.S. Public Health Service, grants CA-05262 and AI 26055, from the National Cancer Institute.

REFERENCES

Aris, C. H., Blake, K. R., Miller, P. S., Reddy, M. P., and Ts'o, P. O. P. (1986) Inhibition of vesicular stomatitis virus protein synthesis and infection by sequence-specific oligodeoxyribonucleoside methylphosphonates. *Biochemistry* **25**: 6268–6275.

Asseline, U., Delarue, M., Lancelot, G., Toulme, F., Thuong, N. T., Montenay-Garestier, T., and Helene, C. (1984a) Nucleic acid-binding molecules with high affinity and base sequence specificity: Intercalating agents covalently linked to oligodeoxynucleotides. *Proc. Natl. Acad. Sci. USA* **81**: 3297–3301.

Asseline, U., Toulme, F., Thuong, M. J., Delarue, M., Montenay-Garestier, J., and Helene, C. (1984b) Oligodeoxynucleotides covalently linked to intercalating dyes as base sequence-specific ligands. Influence of dye attachment site. *EMBO J.* **3**: 795–800.

Baldwin, J. J. (1987) Drug design. In *Drug discovery and development*, M. Williams and J. B. Malick, eds., pp. 33–71. Clifton, NJ: Human Press.

Baum, R. M. (1988) Mechanism of sequence-specific DNA recognition elucidated. Synthetic oligonucleotides, peptides and antibiotic analogs can recognize specific DNA sequences up to 15 base pairs in length. *Chem. Engineer. News*, Jan. 4, pp. 20–26.

Blake, K. R., Murakami, A., Spitz, S. A., Glave, S. A., Reddy, M. P., T'so, P. O. P., and Miller, P. S. (1985) Hybridization arrest of globin synthesis in rabbit reticulocyte lysates and cells by oligodeoxyribonucleoside methyl phosphonates. *Biochemistry* **24**: 6139–6145.

Boston Interhospital Virus Study Group and the NIAID-Sponsored Cooperative Antiviral Clinical Study. (1975) Failure of high-dose 5-iodo-2′-deoxyuridine in the therapy of herpes simplex virus encephalitis, evidence of unacceptable toxicity. *New Engl. J. Med.* **292**: 599–603.

Burgen, A. S. V. (1986) The road to rational design. In *Innovative approaches in drug design*, A. F. Harms, ed., pp. 1–7. Amsterdam: Elsevier.

Burgen, A. S. V., Roberts, G. C. K., and Tute, M. S. (eds.) (1986) *Molecular graphics and drug design.* New York: Elsevier.

Calabresi, P., Cardoso, S. S., Finch, S. C., Kligerman, M. M., von Essen, C. F., Chu, M. Y., and Welch, A. D. (1961) Initial clinical studies with 5-iodo-2′-deoxyuridine. *Cancer Res.* **21**: 550–559.

Carmine, A. A., Brogden, R. N., Heel, R. C., Speight, J. M., and Avery, G. S. (1982) Trifluridine, a review of its antiviral activity and therapeutic use in the topical treatment of viral eye infections. *Drugs* **23**: 329–353.

Cazenave, C., Chevrien, M., Thuong, N. T., and Helene, C. (1987) Rate of degradation of (α)- and (β)-oligodeoxynucleotides in *Xenopus* oocytes. Implications for anti-messenger strategies. *Nucleic Acid Res.* **15**: 10507–10521.

Cazenave, C., Loreau, N., Toulme, J. J., and Helene, C. (1986) Anti-messenger oligodeoxynucleotides: Specific inhibition of rabbit β-globin synthesis in wheat germ extracts and *Xenopus* oocytes. *Biochimie* **68**: 1063–1069.

Chang, L.-J., and Stoltzfus, C. M. (1987) Inhibition of Rous sarcoma virus replication by antisense RNA. *J. Virology* **61**: 921–924.

Chen, M. S., and Prusoff, W. H. (1978) Association of thymidylate kinase activity with pyrimidine deoxyribonucleoside kinase induced by herpes simplex virus. *J. Biol. Chem.* **253**: 1325–1327.

Chen, M. S., Walker, J., and Prusoff, W. H. (1979) Kinetic studies of herpes simplex virus type 1-encoded thymidine and thymidylate kinase, a multifunctional enzyme. *J. Biol. Chem.* **254**: 10747–10753.

Cheng, Y.-C., and Prusoff, W. H. (1986) Antiviral chemotherapy. In *Handbook of chemotherapeutic agents*, M. Verderame, ed., Vol. II, pp. 207–338. Boca Raton, FL: CRC Press.

Cheng, Y.-C., Grill, S. P., Nutter, L. M., Bastow, K. F., Frank, K. E., and Chiou, J.-F. (1985) Deoxynucleotide metabolism of herpes virus and the implication in chemotherapy. In *Herpes virus and virus therapy: Pharmacological and clinical approaches*, R. Kono and A. Nakajima, eds., pp. 41–43. Amsterdam: Elsevier.

Croen, K. D., Ostrove, J. M., Dragovic, L. J., Smialek, J. E., and Straus, S. E. (1987) Latent herpes simplex virus in human trigeminal ganglia. Detection of an immediate early gene "anti-sense" transcript by *in situ* hybridization. *New Engl. J. Med.* **317**: 1427–1432.

Debouck, C., Gorniak, G., Strickler, J. E., Meek, T. D., Metcalford, B. W., and Rosenberg, M. (1987) Human immunodeficiency virus protease expressed in *Escherichia coli* exhibits autoprocessing and specific maturation of the gag precursor. *Proc. Natl. Acad. Sci. USA* **84**: 8903–8906.

DeClercq, E., and Walker, R. T. (eds.). (1988) *Antiviral drug development.* New York: Plenum Press.

DeClercq, E., Holy, A., Rosenberg, I., Sakuma, T., Balzarini, J., and Maudgal, P. C. (1986) A novel selective broad-spectrum anti-DNA virus agent. *Nature* **323**: 464–467.

Drach, J. C. (1983) Purine nucleoside analogs as antiviral agents. In *Targets for the design of antiviral agents*, R. T. Walker and E. DeClercq, eds., pp. 231–257. London: Plenum Press.

Elion, G. B. (1982) Mechanism of action and selectivity of acyclovir. *Amer. J. Med.* **73**(1a): 7–13.

Eriksson, B., Helgstrand, E., Johannson, N. G., Larsson, A., Misiorny, A., Noren, J. O., Phillipson, L., Stenberg, K., Stening, G., Stridh, S., and Oberg, B. (1977) Inhibition of influenza virus ribonucleic acid polymerase by ribavirin triphosphate. *Antimicrob. Agents Chemother.* **11**: 946–951.

Fink, A. L. (1977) Cryoenzymology: The study of enzyme mechanisms of subzero-temperatures. *Acc. Chem. Res.* **10**: 233–239.

Fischer, P. H., Chen, M. P., and Prusoff, W. H. (1980) The incorporatin of 5-iodo-5′-amino-2′,5′-dideoxyuridine and 5-iodo-2′-deoxyuridine into herpes simplex virus DNA—relationship between antiviral activity and effects on DNA structure. *Biochim. Biophys. Acta.* **606**: 236–245.

Fox, J. S., and White, D. O. (1980) Delivery of antiviral chemotherapeutic agents to neurons by retrograde axonal transport. *Medical Hypothesis* **6**: 773–779.

Furman, P. A., Fyfe, J. A., St. Clair, M. H., Weinhold, K., Rideout, J. L., Freeman, G. A., Nusinoff-Lehrman, S., Bolognesi, D. P., Broder, S., Mitsuya, H., and Barry, D. W. (1986) Phosphorylation of 3′-azido-3′-deoxythymidine and selective interaction of the 5′-triphosphate with human immunodeficiency virus reverse transcriptase. *Proc. Natl. Acad. Sci. USA* **83**: 8333–8337.

Furman, P. A., and McGuirt, P. V. (1983) Effect of acyclovir on viral protein synthesis in cells infected with herpes simplex virus type 1. *Antimicrob. Agents Chemother.* **23**: 332–334.

Furman, P. A., St. Clair, M. H., Fyfe, J. A., Rideout, P. M., Keller, P. M., and Elion, G. B. (1979) Inhibition of herpes simplex virus-induced DNA polymerase activity and viral replication by 9-(2-hydroxyethoxymethyl)guanine and its triphosphate. *J. Virol.* **32**: 72–77.

Fyfe, J. A. (1982) Differential phosphorylation of (E)-5-(2-bromovinyl)-2′-deoxyuridine monophosphate by thymidylate kinases from herpes simplex viruses types 1 and 2 and varicella zoster virus. *Molec. Pharm.* **21**: 432–437.

Gagnor, C., Bertrand, J. R., Thener, S., Lemaitre, M., Morvan, F., Rayner, B., Malvy, C., Lebleu, B., Imbach, J. L., and Paoletti, C. (1987) α-DNA VI: Comparative study of α- and β-anomeric oligodeoxyribonucleotides in hybridization to mRNA and in cell-free translation inhibition. *Nucleic Acid Res.* **15**: 10419–10436.

Gilbert, B. E., and Knight, V. (1986) Biochemistry and clinical applications of ribavirin. *Antimicrob. Agents Chemother.* **30**: 201–205.

Gordon, Y. J., Johnson, B., Romanowski, E., and Araullo-Cruz, T. (1988) RNA complementary to herpes simplex virus type 1 ICP-0 gene demonstrated in neurons of human trigeminal ganglia. *J. Virology* **62**: 1832–1835.

Green, P. J., Pines, O., and Inouye, M. (1986) The role of antisense RNA in gene regulation. *Ann. Rev. Biochem.* **55**: 569–597.

Haschke, R. H., Ordronneau, J. M., and Bunt, A. H. (1980) Preparation and retrograde axonal transport of an antiviral drug/horseradish peroxidase conjugate. *J. Neurochem.* **35**: 1431–1435.

Hay, A. J., Zambon, M. C., Wolstenholme, A. J., Skehel, J. J., and Smith, M. H. (1986) Molecular basis of resistance of influenza A viruses to amantadine. *J. Antimicrobiol. Chemother.* **18** (Suppl. B): 19–29.

Hay, A. J., Wolstenholme, A. J., Skehel, J. J., and Smith, M. H. (1985) The molecular basis of the specific anti-influenza action of amantadine. *EMBO J.* **4**: 3021–3024.

Heidelberger, C., and King, D. H. (1979) Trifluorothymidine. *Pharmacol. Ther.* **6**: 427–442.

Helene, C., Praseuth, D., Doan, T. L., Chassignol, M., Decout, J.-L., Habhoub, N., L'homme, J., and Thuong, N. T. (1988a) Sequence-targeted photosensitized reactions in nucleic acids by oligo-α-deoxynucleotides and oligo-β-deoxynucleotides covalently linked to proflavin. *Biochemistry* **27**: 3031–3038.

Helene, C., and Thuong, N. T. (1988b) Oligo-[α]-deoxynucleotides covalently linked to intercalating agents, DNA and RNA binding properties. *Biochemical Pharmacology* **37**: 1797–1798.

Helene, C., Montenay-Garestier, T., Saison, T., Takasugi, M., Toulme, J. J., Asseline, U., Lancelot, G., Maurizot, J. C., Toulme, F., and Thuong, N. T. (1985) Oligodeoxynucleotides covalently linked to intercalating agents: A new class of gene regulatory substances. *Biochimie* **67**: 777–783.

Iverson, B. L., and Dervan, P. B. (1987) Nonenzymatic sequence-specific cleavage of single-stranded DNA to nucleotide resolution. DNA methyl thioether probes. *J. Amer. Chem. Soc.* **109**: 1241–1243.

Izant, J. G., and Weintraub, H. (1984) Constitutive and conditional suppression of exogenous and endogenous genes by antisense RNA. *Science* **229**: 345–352.

Jamieson, A. T., Gentry, G. A., and Subak-Sharpe, J. H. (1974) Induction of both thymidine and deoxycytidine kinase activity by herpes viruses. *J. Gen. Virol.* **24**: 465–480.

Kim, S. K., and Wold, B. J. (1985) Stable reduction of thymidine kinase activity in cell expressing high levels of anti-sense RNA. *Cell* **42**: 129–133.

Kit, S. (1979) Viral-associated and -induced enzymes. *Pharmacol. Ther.* **4**: 501–585.

Korant, B. D. (1981) Inhibition of viral protein cleavage. In *Design of inhibitors of viral functions*, K. Gauri, ed., pp. 37–47. New York: Academic Press.

Korant, B. D., Lonberg-Holm, K., and LaColla, P. (1984) Picornaviruses and togaviruses: Targets for design of antivirals. In *Targets for the design of antiviral agents*, E. DeClercq and R. T. Walker, eds., pp. 61–98. New York: Plenum Press.

Knorre, D. G., and Vlassov, V. V. (1985) Complementary-addressed (sequence specific) modification of nucleic acid. *Prog. Nucleic Acid Res. Molec. Biol.* **32**: 291–320.

Knorre, D. G., Vlassov, V. V., and Zarytova, V. F. (1985) Reactive oligonucleotide derivatives and sequence-specific modification of nucleic acids. *Biochmie* **67**: 785–789.

Kristensson, K. (1978) Retrograde transport of macromolecules in axons. *Ann. Rev. Pharmac. Toxicol.* **18**: 97–110.

Lemaitre, M., Bayard, B., and Lebleu, B. (1987) Specific antiviral activity of a poly (L-lysine)-conjugated oligodeoxyribonucleotide sequence complementary to vesicular stomatitis virus N protein mRNA site. *Proc. Natl. Acad. Sci. USA* **84**: 648–652.

Littke, W., and John, C. (1984) Protein single crystal growth under microgravity. *Science* **225**: 203–204.

Loose-Mitchell, D. S. (1988) Antisense nucleic acids as a potential class of pharmaceutical agents. *TIPS* 9:45–47.

Matsukura, M., Shinozuka, K., Zon, G., Mitsuya, H., Reitz, J., Cohen, S., and Broder, S. (1987) Phosphorothioate analogs of oligodeoxynucleotides: Inhibitors of replication and cytopathic effects of human immunodeficiency virus. *Proc. Natl. Acad. Sci. USA* **84**: 7706–7710.

Miller, P. S., and Ts'o, P. O. P. (1987) A new approach to chemotherapy based on molecular biology and nucleic acid chemistry: Matagen (masking tape for gene expression). *Anti-Cancer Drug Design* **2**: 117–128.

Miller, P. S., McParland, K. B., Jayaraman, K., and Ts'o, P. O. P. (1981) Biochemical and biological effects of nonionic nucleic acid methylphosphonates. *Biochemistry* **20**: 1874–1880.

Miller, P. S., Yano, J., Yano, E., Carroll, C., Jayaraman, K., and Ts'o, P. O. P. (1979) Nonionic nucleic acid analogs. Synthesis and characterization of dideoxyribonucleoside methylphosphonates. *Biochemistry* **18**: 5134–5143.

Morvan, F., Rayner, B., Leonetti, J.-P., and Imbach, J.-L. (1988) α-DNA VII. Solid phase synthesis of α-anomeric oligodeoxyribonucleotides. *Nucleic Acids Research* **16**: 833–847.

Morvan, F., Rayner, B., Imbach, J.-L., Chang, D.-D., and Lown, J. W. (1986) α-DNA I. Synthesis, characterization by high-yield H-NMR, and base-pairing properties of the unnatural hexadeoxyribonucleotide α-[d(CpCpTpTpCpC)] with its complement β-[d(GpGpApApGpG)]. *Nucleic Acid Res.* **14**: 5019–5035.

Moser, H. E., and Dervan, P. B. (1987) Sequence-specific cleavage of double helical DNA by triple helix formation. *Science* **238**: 645–650.

Mous, J., Heimer, P., and Le Grice, F. J. (1988) Processing protease and reverse transcriptase from human immunodeficiency virus type 1 polyprotein in *Escherichia coli. J. Virology* **62**: 1433–1436.

North, T. W., and Cohen, S. (1979) Aranucleosides and aranucleotides in viral chemotherapy. *Pharmcol. Ther.* **4**: 81–108.

Oberg, B. (1983a) Antiviral effects of phosphonoformate (PFA, foscarnet sodium). *Pharmacol. Ther.* **19**: 387–415.

Oberg, B. (1983b) Inhibition of virus specific enzymes. In *Problems of antiviral therapy*, C. Stuart-Harris and J. Oxford, eds., pp. 35–69. London: Academic Press.

Otto, M. J., Goz, B., and Prusoff, W. H. (1984) Antiviral activity of iodinated pyrimidine deoxyribonucleosides. In *Antiviral drugs and interferon: The molecular basis of their activity*, Y. C. Becker, ed., pp. 11–38. Hingham, MA: Martinus Nijhof.

Otto, M. J., Lee, J. J., and Prusoff, W. H. (1982) Effects of nucleoside analogues on the expression of herpes simplex type 1 induced proteins. *Antiviral Res.* **2**: 267–281.

Praseuth, D., Chassignol, M., Takasugi, M., LeDoan, T., Thuong, N., and Helene, C. (1987) Double helices with parallel strands are formed by nuclease-resistant oligo-α-deoxynucleotides and oligo-α-deoxynucleotides covalently linked to an intercalating agent with complementary oligo-β-deoxynucleotides. *J. Mol. Biol.* **196**: 939–942.

Prusoff, W. H. (1988) Idoxuridine or how it all began. In *Clinical use of antiviral drugs*, pp. 15–24. Boston: Martinus Nijhoff.

Prusoff, W. H., and Lin, T.-S. (1988) Experimental aspects of antiviral pharmacology. In *Antiviral drug development*, E. DeClercq and R. T. Walker, eds., pp. 173–202. New York: Plenum Press.

Prusoff, W. H., Zucker, M., Mancini, W. R., Otto, M. J., Lin, T.-S., and Lee, J. J. (1985) Basic biochemical and pharmacological aspects of antiviral agents. *Antiviral Res. Suppl.* **1**: 1–10.

Reid, R., Mar, E.-C., Huang, E.-S., and Topal, M. D. (1988) Insertion and extension of acyclic, dideoxy, and ara nucleotides by herpesviridae, human α and human β polymerases. *J. Biol. Chem.* **263**: 3898–3904.

Robins, R. K. (1986) Synthetic antiviral agents. *Chem. Engineer. News*, Jan. 27, pp. 28–40.

Rossman, M. G., Arnold, E., Griffith, J. P., Kamer, G., Luo, M., Smith, J., Vriend, G., Rueckert, R. R., Sherry, B., McKinlay, M. A., Diana, G., and Otto, M. (1987) Common cold viruses. *TIBS* **12**: 313–318.

Smee, D. F., and Mathews, T. R. (1986) Metabolism of ribavirin in respiratory syncytial virus—infected and uninfected cells. *Antimicrob. Agents Chemother.* **30**: 117–121.

Smith, C. C., Aurelian, L., Reddy, M. P., Miller, P. S., and Ts'o, P. O. P. (1986) Antiviral effect of an oligo(nucleoside methyl-phosphonate) complementary to the splice junction of herpes simplex virus type 1 immediate early pre-mRNAs 4 and 5. *Proc. Natl. Acad. Sci. USA* **83**: 2787–2791.

Smith, T. J., Kremer, M., Luo, M., Vriend, G., Arnold, E., Kamer, G., Rossman, M. G., McKinlay, M. A., Diana, G. D., and Otto, J. (1986) The site of attachment in human rhinovirus 14 for antiviral agents that inhibit uncoating. *Science* **233**: 1286–1293.

Spivack, J. G., and Fraser, N. W. (1988) Expression of herpes simplex virus type 1 latency-associated transcripts in the trigeminal ganglia of mice during acute infection and reactivation of latent infection. *J. Virology* **62**: 1479–1485.

Stark, G. R., and Bartlett, P. A. (1983) Design and use of potent, specific enzyme inhibitors. *Pharmac. Ther.* **23**: 45–78.

Stein, C. A., and Cohen, J. S. (1988) Oligodeoxynucleotides as inhibitors of gene expression: A review. *Cancer Res.* **48**: 2659–2668.

Sun, H.-S., Asseline, U., Rouzaud, D., Montenay-Garestier, T., Thuong, N. T., and Helene, C. (1987) Oligo-[α]-deoxynucleotides covalently linked to an intercalating agent. Double helices with parallel strands are formed with complementary oligo-[β]-deoxynucleotides. *Nucleic Acids Research* **15**: 6149–6158.

Thuong, N. T., Asseline, U., Roig, V., Takasugi, M., and Helene, C. (1987) Oligo(α-deoxynucleotide)s covalently linked to intercalating agents: Differential binding to ribo- and deoxyribopolynucleotides and stability towards nuclease digestion. *Proc. Natl. Acad. Sci. USA* **84**: 5129–5133.

To, R. Y. L., Booth, S. C., and Neiman, P. E. (1986) Inhibition of retroviral replication by anti-sense RNA. *Molec. Cell Biol.* **6**: 4758–4762.

Toltzis, P., O'Connell, K., and Patterson, J. L. (1988) Effect of phosphorylated ribavirin on vesicular stomatitis virus transcription. *Antimicrob. Agents Chemother.* **32**: 492–497.

Toulme, J. J., Krish, H. M., Loreau, N., Thuong, N. T., and Helene, C. (1986) Specific inhibition of mRNA translation by complementary oligonucleotides covalently linked to intercalating agents. *Proc. Natl. Acad. Sci. USA* **83**: 1227–1231.

Ts'o, P. O. P., Miller, P. S., and Greene, J. J. (1983) Nucleic acid analogs with targeted delivery on chemotherapeutic agents. In *Development of target-oriented anticancer drugs*, Y.-C. Cheng, B. Goz, and K. A. Minkoff, eds., pp. 189–206. New York: Raven Press.

Votruba, I., Bernaerts, R., Sakuma, T., DeClercq, E., Merta, A., Rosenberg, I., and Holy, A. (1987) Intracellular phosphorylation of broad-spectrum anti-DNA virus agent (S)-9-(3-hydroxy-2-phosphonylmethoxypropyl)adenine and inhibition of viral DNA synthesis. *Molec. Pharmacol.* **32**: 524–529.

Weintraub, H., Izant, J. G., and Harland, R. M. (1985) Anti-sense RNA as a molecular tool for genetic analysis. *Trends Genet.* **1**: 22–25.

Williams, M., and Malick, J. B. (1987) *Drug discovery and development*. Clifton, NJ: Humana Press.

Wray, S., Gilbert, B. F., and Knight, V. (1985a) Effect of ribavirin triphosphate on primed generation and elongation during virus transcription *in vitro*. *Antiviral Res.* **5**: 39–48.

Wray, S., Gilbert, B. F., Noall, M. W., and Knight, V. (1985b) Mode of action of ribavirin: Effect of nucleotide pool alterations on influenza virus ribonucleoprotein synthesis. *Antiviral Res.* **5**: 29–37.

Youngquist, R., and Dervan, P. B. (1987) A synthetic peptide binds 16 base pairs of T,T double helical DNA. *J. Amer. Chem. Soc.* **109**: 7564–7566.

Zamecnik, P. C., Goodchild, J., Taguchi, Y., and Sarin, P. S. (1986) Inhibition of replication and expression of human T-cell lymphotropic virus type III in cultured cells by exogeneous synthetic oligonucleotides complementary to viral RNA. *Proc. Natl. Acad. Sci. USA* **83**: 4143–4146.

Zamecnik, P. C., and Stephenson, M. L. (1978) Inhibition of Rous sarcoma virus replication and cell transformation by a specific oligodeoxynucleotide. *Proc. Natl. Acad. Sci. USA* **75**: 280–284.

Zerial, A., Thuong, N. T., and Helene, C. (1987) Selective inhibition of the cytopathic effect of type A influenza virus by oligodeoxynucleotides covalently linked to an intercalating agent. *Nucleic Acid Res.* **15**: 9909–9919.

Zucker, M. L., Dube, S., and Prusoff, W. H. (1988) The effect of 5′-amino-5′-deoxythymidine on the pattern of polyadenylation of herpes simplex virus type 1 ribonucleic acid. *Virus Res.* **9**: 221–232.

CHAPTER 3

MOLECULAR MECHANISMS FOR THE CONTROL OF HUMAN IMMUNODEFICIENCY VIRUS INFECTION

PRAKASH CHANDRA, ANGELIKA CHANDRA, ILHAN DEMIRHAN, AND THOMAS GERBER
Laboratory of Molecular Biology, Center of Biological Chemistry (ZBC), University Medical School, Federal Republic of Germany

Abstract—Compared to other T-cell lymphotropic human retroviruses, human T-cell leukemia/lymphoma virus type 1 (HTLV-I) and type 2 (HTLV-II), the acquired immunodeficiency syndrome (AIDS)-associated virus, human immunodeficiency virus type 1 (HIV-1), is a nontransforming cytopathic virus without immortalizing activity. Hence, its replication is an important event in the manifestation of this disease, and the interruption of viral replication offers an important strategy for the control of AIDS. Unlike most retroviruses, HIV-1 and other AIDS-associated viruses possess a set of accessory genes which autoregulate the functional activity of structural genes and thereby control virus replication. The implication of these regulatory genes as potential targets and other strategies for designing inhibitors of virus replication are described.

1. INTRODUCTION

Acquired immune deficiency syndrome (AIDS) was first recognized in 1981 as an unexplained progressive immunodeficiency disorder associated with opportunistic infections (*Morbid Mortal Rep.*, 1981a) and Kaposi's sarcoma (*Morbid Mortal Rep.*, 1981b). Not knowing the nature of the etiological agent at that time, therapeutic approaches were devised to treat the opportunistic infections and/or Kaposi's sarcoma, reconstituting the immunological status by bone marrow transplantation or adaptive transfer of immune competent cells and by immunological enhancement using cytokines such as interleukin (IL-2) and interferons, or immunogenic adjuvants. Identification of a virus, associated with AIDS in 1983 (Barre-Sinoussi et al., 1983) and 1984 (Feorino et al., 1984; Popovic et al., 1984; Robert-Guroff et al., 1985), provided important strategies in the diagnosis and treatment of this disease. The virus, earlier called LAV (Barre-Sinoussi et al., 1983), HTLV-III (Popovic et al., 1984; Robert-Guroff et al., 1985) or ARV (Levy et al., 1984) is now designated as HIV-1 (human immunodeficiency virus type 1) and belongs to the subfamily lentiviriae of retroviruses.

Confirmation of the role of HIV and other associated retroviruses in the development of AIDS and related conditions opened exciting new avenues of research: (1) Experiments were designed to identify the cells which harbor, and are most likely affected by, the virus and to learn the fate of infected cells in the body. (2) Molecular biologists began analyzing gene sequences and looking for differences in the genomic organization of these viruses to other known retroviruses. Each new discovery gave a better understanding of the kinds of approaches required to block HIV-1 infection and limit the spread of the disease. The most important and fascinating aspects of these discoveries was the knowledge that this class of viruses has a unique genomic organization. Unlike animal retroviruses, these viruses possess a set of accessory genes which autoregulate their replication. We know that HIV-1 has six regulatory genes. Some of these genes have a negative regulatory function (i.e., inhibition of the virus replication) while others function as positive regulators of the virus replication. To understand their functional activity and to develop specific strategies to block virus replication, we shall briefly discuss the role of these genes in the replicative cycle of HIV-1.

2. GENOMIC ORGANIZATION

The AIDS virus, HIV-1, is an exogenous virus without any cell-derived sequences, as shown by the lack of hybridization of its genome to uninfected cell DNA (Hahn et al., 1984). Unlike other retroviruses which have a site-specific integration of their proviral

DNA, HIV-1 DNA has two functional components in the infected cell: One exists as a polyclonally integrated provirus, the other as unintegrated superhelical or linear viral DNA. The persistence of a large amount of unintegrated viral DNA is unusual, but it has been shown for other cytopathic retroviruses, such as spleen necrosis virus (Keshet & Temin, 1979), some strains of avian leukosis virus (Weller et al., 1980), and visna virus (Clements & Naryano, 1981). The genomic organizations of HIV-1 and HIV-2 are shown in Fig. 3-1.

In addition to the usual retroviral genes, **gag**, **pol**, and **env**, which encode proteins that constitute the virus structure, these viruses have a set of five (HIV-1) to six (HIV-2) regulatory genes. Very recently, the presence of another regulatory gene in HIV-1 has been reported (Haseltine, 1988). This gene, **vpu**, is located between the **tat** and **env** genes, and is absent in HIV-2. For comparison, the organization of human T-cell leukemia/lymphoma viruses types I and II (HTLV-1 and HTLV-II) is also shown in Fig. 3-1. Although these viruses have a different pathogenic effect in that they belong to the oncogenic class of retroviruses inducing leukemia and lymphoma in humans, they exhibit the same cellular specificity as the immunodeficiency viruses. All these viruses infect T4 cells and use the CD4 receptor as the target. Interestingly, HTLV-I and HTLV-II also possess some accessory genes which regulate virus replication. However, the genome of immunodeficiency viruses possesses more regulatory genes. The products of these genes are not present in the virus itself. The regulatory genes encode their proteins in the infected cell, and these contribute to the expression of structural genes at different levels of molecular processing. The functional role of structural genes **gag**, **pol**, and **env** is to encode proteins which form different regions of the virus. Each of these genes encodes a primary product, a polyprotein, which then is processed to structural or functional antigens. A summary of these products encoded by various structural genes is given in Table 3-1.

The proteins encoded by some accessory genes are now well characterized, and this has helped a great deal in understanding how these genes regulate virus replication. The products of regulatory genes are summarized in Table 3-2.

Now let us consider what kind of regulatory mechanisms are operated by these accessory genes. Each of these operational processes could serve as a potential target for designing specific inhibitors of virus replication. For this reason, the functional role of each of these genes will be considered separately.

One of the regulatory genes located at the 3′-end of the viral genome, called 3′-open

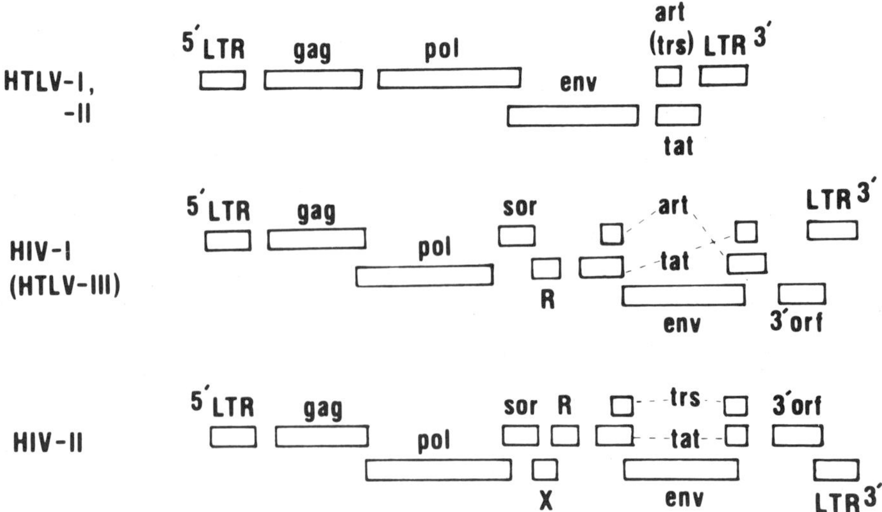

FIG. 3-1. Genomic organization of human T-cell lymphotropic viruses. A new nomenclature for the regulatory genes has been recently recommended (Gallo et al., 1988). The new designations are as follows: *art* = *rev*, *sor* = *vif*, *R* = *vpr*, *3′-orf* = *nef*, *X* = *vpx*, and *tat* = *tat*.

TABLE 3-1. *Products of the Structural Genes*

Gene	Primary product	Structural proteins	Region
gag	p 55	p17, p24, p 9/7	Core
pol	p 98	p66/p53 (RT)* p34 (integrase) prt (protease)	Capsid
env	p 160	gp 120 gp 41	Envelope

TABLE 3-2. *Products of the Regulatory Genes*

Gene	Product	Location	Function
sor (*vif*)	p 23	Cytoplasm Inn. Memb.	Postbinding infection
tat (*tat*)	p 14	Nucleus cytoplasm	Transactivation (transcription/posttranscription)
trs/art (*rev*)	p 18	Nucleus	Posttranscription processing
3′-*orf* (*nef*)	p 27	Cytoplasm	Negative regulation of virus replication
R (*vpr*)	p 10	?	?

Designations in parentheses have recently been proposed by Gallo et al. (1988).

reading frame (**3′-orf**) or **nef**, has a negative effect on HIV replication. Deletions in the 3′-**orf** gene lead to replication of the virus increased 5- to 10-fold. It encodes a polypeptide of 260 amino acids which is myristylated at the N-terminal, and also phoshorylated at a residue close to the N-terminal, like pp^{60} sarc. The question we may pose is: Why is the product of this gene myristylated and at the same time phosphorylated? Phosphorylation at position 15—a threonine—is also present in the EGF receptor. A second phosphorylation site involves serine which is not yet quite localized. The phosphorylation at residue 15 is enhanced by phorbol esters, suggesting that this is mediated by protein kinase C. And, finally, it has been shown that the 27k protein exhibits GTP binding and GTPase activities (Guy et al., 1987). Recent findings (Guy et al., 1987) suggest that the **3′-orf** gene exerts an indirect effect on virus replication by altering the level of expression of the viral receptor, T4 antigen. Thus, the loss of **3′-orf** activity may be critical to activation of HIV-1 replication *in vivo*. It would be interesting to examine whether the presence or absence of a stop codon in the **3′-orf** gene correlates with the stage of HIV-1 infection in humans.

The role of the **sor** gene has been examined by a series of proviral genomes of HIV-1 that either lacked the coding sequences for **sor** or contained point mutations in **sor**, constructed by Fisher and colleagues (1987) and Strebel and colleagues (1987). Normal amounts of **gag**-, **pol**-, and **env**-derived proteins were produced by the mutants, and assays in both lymphoid and nonlymphoid cells indicated that their transactivating capacity was intact and comparable with the wild type (Fisher et al., 1987). A mutant virus deficient in **sor** gene was shown to produce virion particles normally (Strebel et al., 1987); however, the particles were 1000-fold less infective than the wild type. These data suggest that **sor** influences generation of infectious virus at a novel, posttranscriptional stage and that its action is independent of the regulatory genes **tat** and **trs/art**.

The structure and function of the **R** gene is not yet known. Recent results from Wong-Staal and colleagues (1987) indicated that it encodes a protein of 80–100 amino acids and that this gene is highly conserved, not only among various HIV-1 isolates but also in the distantly related ungulate lentivirus, visna. The fact that some, but not all, HIV-1 infected patients have antibodies that recognize **R** gene product indicates that it may have an important function in the pathogenesis of HIV-1 infection.

The next accessory gene which is important for the expression of structural genes, particularly the **env** gene, is called **trs** or **art**. These names were coined by two research groups with different views regarding its mode of action. Wong-Staal and coworkers (Feinberg et al., 1986) named it **trs** to document its role as a transregulator of splicing, whereas Haseltine's group (Sodrosky et al., 1986) named it **art** for anti-repression transactivator. According to Haseltine and coworkers, the unspliced messenger RNA for HIV-1 structural proteins contains a regulatory sequence that would inhibit the synthesis of proteins if its effect is not countered by the **art** gene product. Because **trs/art** and **tat** genes overlap (in different reading frames) with each other, and with envelope gene, it has been difficult to completely dissect the functional role of their products (see also Fig. 3-1). Studies of **tat** or **art/trs** proviral deletion mutants have been difficult to interpret because of the possibility of more than one functional unit being altered simultaneously and because other viral genes may influence the results. However, site-directed mutagenesis of **trs/art** has shown that a chain termination mutation early in this gene results in an increase in transcription of viral mRNA, as measured by nuclear transcription experiments, but only one major species of viral mRNA (1.8 kilobases) was detected and little or no viral structural proteins were made. Thus **trs** gene product is essential for expression of viral structural proteins but, at the same time, may have a transregulatory negative effect on the transcription of regulatory genes (Reza-Sadai et al., 1988). On the other hand, a recent study by Rosen and colleagues (1988) shows that sequences located within the coding region of the envelope gene exert a negative effect on the expression of heterologous genes and that the negative effect of these sequences can be relieved by the **art/trs** gene product. Whatever may be the modus operandi for this gene, mutations in this gene lead to total inhibition of expression of **gag** and **env** genes. For this reason, manipulations in its regulatory function could serve as a potential target for developing antiviral compounds.

Perhaps the most important of all the regulatory genes is the **tat** gene, which is responsible for the expression of all other genes. The term **tat** was coined to designate the transactivator of transcription. The transactivating sequences have been localized to nucleotides 5406 and 5607 of the HIV-1 genome. This region contains the N-terminal segment of the **tat** reading frame, which potentially encodes a protein of 72 or 86 amino acids, depending upon the use of alternative RNA splicing pathways. The transactivator is the protein product of **tat** gene, which has been identified as a 15-kd polypeptide in HIV-1–infected cells requiring only 56 amino acids for activity. The domain essential for transactivation has some characteristic features which are suggestive of a potential nucleic acid-binding protein. First, the functional domain in **tat** protein has an abundance of basic over acidic residues, which could mediate binding to the negatively charged backbone of the DNA segment, designated as TAR sequence located within the HIV-1 LTR. Second, the functional domain also contains a cluster of seven cysteine residues which may comprise a metal-binding domain important to nucleic acid binding. The differential ability of HIV-1 (**tat**) and HIV-2 (**tat**) to transactivate some of the same LTRs (Emerman et al., 1987) supports the binding of **tat** protein to specific sequences in LTR.

The functional role of the **tat** gene has been studied intensively (Reza-Sadai et al., 1988; Rosen et al., 1988; Arya et al., 1985; Rice & Matthews, 1988; Emerman et al., 1987; Muesing et al., 1987), and the data can be summarized as follows: Analysis of both steady-state viral messenger RNA and nascently transcribed RNA clearly demonstrates that the **tat** gene product plays a major role in transcriptional activation (Reza-Sadai et al., 1988), since its abrogation resulted in a great reduction of both. Furthermore, **tat** also has a role in posttranscriptional activation (Feinberg et al., 1986; Sodrosky et al., 1986). Feinberg and colleagues (1986) reported that a mutant deleted in the splice acceptor site of **tat** expressed greatly reduced **tat** activity. Cells transfected with this genome expressed correspondingly lower levels of viral mRNA. Similarly, a mutant with a single amino acid change in **tat**, with reduced transactivation activity, was much more compromised in protein expression than in viral mRNA expression (Reza-Sadai et al., 1988). Therefore, **tat** may enhance both transcriptional and posttranscriptional events, depending upon the cellular localization of the **tat** protein (Okomoto & Wong-Staal, 1986). For example, Felber and colleagues (1985)

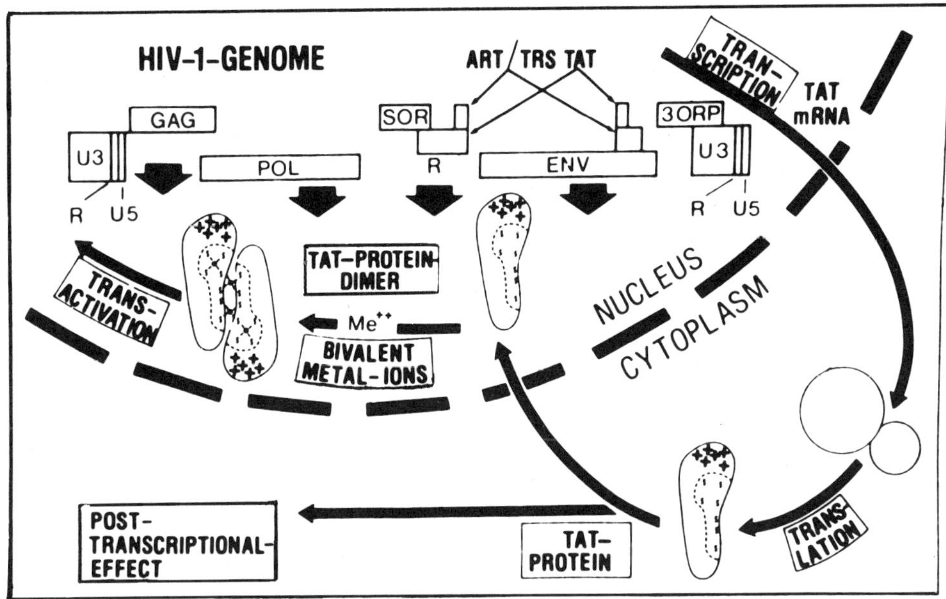

FIG. 3-2. Model for the bimodal function of the transactivator protein. The formation of *tat* protein dimer for metal binding is based on data reported by Frankel et al., personal communication.

showed that the transactivator protein of HTLV-I was restricted to the nucleus in transiently transfected, low-expressing cells, but spilled over to the cytoplasm in a stable high-expressing cell line. If the analogy holds for HIV-1, **tat** may first be found in the nucleus where it exerts its transcriptional effect and then in the cytoplasm where it may activate a step or steps leading to protein production. This bimodal function of the **tat** protein is shown in Fig. 3-2.

3. REPLICATIVE CYCLE

HIV-1 infection begins with a specific interaction between the virus envelope (glycoprotein, gp 120) and a receptor on the cell that is being infected, a cell-surface protein present on T4 cells, called CD4 antigen. The CD4 antigen is present in high concentrations on helper T cells and to a lesser extent on macrophages, endothelial cells, antibody-producing B cells, and nonneural brain cells (Perry & Gordon, 1987). Maddon and colleagues (1987) have shown that insertion of CD4 antigen into epithelial cells makes them susceptible to infection by HIV-1 (Maddon et al., 1987). After its entry into the cell, the virus is uncoated, and a series of metabolic events takes place. In the cytoplasm, reverse transcriptase transcribes the genomic RNA of the virus to form the proviral DNA transcript. This enzyme is novel to all retroviruses, and no similar reaction is known to occur in normal uninfected cells. Reverse transcriptase is a multifunctional enzyme, with at least four domains that mediate RNA-dependent DNA polymerase activity, RNase-H activity, DNA-dependent DNA polymerase activity, and a site for nucleic acid binding. All these domain-mediated functional activities offer attractive targets for inhibiting the synthesis of DNA in retroviruses. The final product of the reactions mediated by reverse transcriptase is a linear duplex DNA. This linear DNA is longer than the 35s subunit of genomic RNA and contains long terminal repeats [the composition of which can be written as 5′-U3-TR-U5-3′ present at both ends. The LTR of HIV-1 has a number of regulatory elements: enhancer element (−104 to −80), according to nucleotide positions of the clone BH 10 (Ratner et al., 1985)], the target region for the transactivator protein, the TAR sequence from position −17 to +80 (Rosen et al., 1985), and three Sp1 binding sites from −77 to −45, as demonstrated by DNA footprinting (Jones et al., 1986). Thus, LTR of HIV-1 is a mediator of the functional activity of regulatory gene products which control virus replication.

The role of the accessory genes in regulating virus replication has been described in the last section. The following scenario can be envisioned from all this knowledge. After infection, a basal level of viral transcription in an activated T4-positive cell first allows the synthesis of **tat** protein, which will initiate viral transcription and expression of the other regulatory proteins. However, no viral structural proteins would be expressed until a threshold level of **trs/art** product is accumulated. The expression of **trs** and **3′-orf** would in turn decrease the level of virus production. The negative feedback controls would also explain the long and variable latency for disease induction. Host and environmental factors may influence the negative control by inhibiting overexpression of negative regulatory genes, and this may lead to virus production, resulting in acceleration of the clinical course of the disease. There is recent evidence that concomitant infections with other viruses can enhance virus replication. Herpes simplex virus type 1 (HSV-1) and some of its immediate early genes have been shown to transactivate the promoter of HIV-1, and thereby stimulate HIV-1 production. Deletion mutants within HIV-1 LTR showed that the target for HSV stimulation is distinct from **tat** responsive sequences and maps near the Sp1 binding sites (Ostrove et al., 1987). A similar type of transactivation of the HIV-1 promoter was shown by early gene products of human cytomegalovirus (Davis et al., 1987). Siekevitz and colleagues (1987) have shown that the transactivator protein from HTLV-I, and several T-cell specific mitogens, can transactivate the promoter of HIV-1. Nabel and Baltimore (1987) have produced evidence that a nuclear factor χB (NFKB), a factor present only in activated T-cells, can stimulate virus production by transactivating the promoter of HIV LTR. In summary, all these results implicate the role of other viruses and mitogenes in HIV-1 replication via the transregulatory mechanism operated through the LTR region. These protein–nucleic acid interactions offer very attractive sites for chemical manipulation to influence virus replication.

The proviral DNA synthesized in the cytoplasm of the infected cell enters the nucleus, is circularized, and is then integrated into the host genome. The proviral DNA can also be present in the unintegrated form and can replicate in the cytoplasm. This situation is unique for AIDS-associated and a few other viruses, as discussed in the earlier section. The infection of target cells by HIV-1 and various steps in its replication are schematically shown in Fig. 3-3.

4. POTENTIAL TARGETS FOR THE ANTIVIRAL CHEMOTHERAPY OF ACQUIRED IMMUNODEFICIENCY SYNDROME

Therapeutic intervention can be envisaged at various stages in the replicative cycle of the virus. Some of these strategies are summarized as follows:

1. Blocking penetration of the target cell membrane by the virus
2. Blocking virus uncoating inside the cell membrane
3. Formation of DNA provirus
   a. Inhibitors of reverse transcriptase
   b. Inhibitors of the endonuclease coded by the **pol** gene
4. Transcriptional and posttranscriptional events
   a. Inhibition of transregulatory processes
      Blocking **trs/art** gene expression
      Blocking **tat** gene expression
      Modification of **trs** and **tat** gene products
   b. Protein processing by the **pol** gene coded protease
   c. Translation of the functional v-mRNA
   d. Assembly of proteins and RNA
5. Preventing nuclear factor χB (NFKB) synthesis: NFKB is found in antibody-producing B-cells. This protein has now been found in activated T4 cells, but not in resting cells.

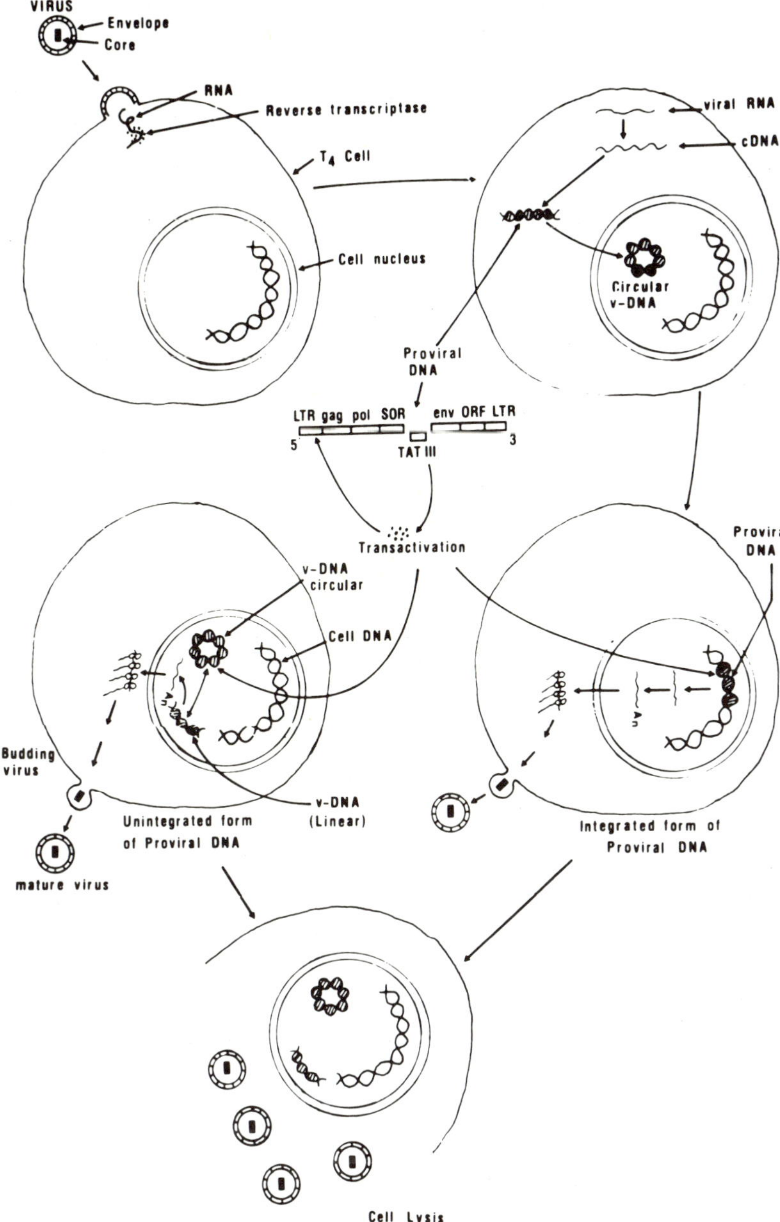

FIG. 3-3. Replicative cycle of human immunodeficiency virus type 1 (HIV-1).

The penetration or attachment of the virus to T4 cell membrane can be inhibited by monoclonal antibodies that block the receptor site specifically or by a soluble form of CD4 antigen which may bind the virus. A number of such studies have been recently reported (Fisher et al., 1988; Hussey et al., 1988; Deen et al., 1988; Traunecker et al., 1988; Clapham et al., 1988) which demonstrate that soluble T4 antigen inhibits HIV-1 infectivity. Since HIV entry to nonlymphoid cells might be mediated by receptors other than CD4, including the infection of monocytes via Fc receptors, it is important to know whether the soluble CD4 inhibition of HIV infection applies solely to CD4-mediated entry (Weiss, 1988). Another approach would be to use agents that destroy the integrity of the viral envelope by puncturing it and thus making it inactive or less infective. One such agent, AL-721, has been shown to interfere with HIV-1 infection and replication (Sarin et al., 1985). Chemical modification of the virus membrane proteins is another approach to affect penetration and infectivity of HIV-1. The envelope glycoprotein, gp 120, of HIV-1 is a highly glycosylated molecule with 24 candidate N-linked glycosylation sites according to the predicted amino acid sequence. The oligosaccharides of this protein are likely to be prominent structures on the virus surface and are therefore important in the attachment process. The N-linked glycoprotein processing inhibitors tunicamycin (precursor synthesis), castanospermine (glucidase I), 1-deoxynojirimycin (glucidase I), and bromoconduritol (glucidase II) were examined for anti-HIV-1 activity (Haseltine, 1988; Montefiori et al., 1988). The infectivity and cytopathicity of HIV-1 were attenuated when virus was synthesized in the presence of tunicamycin, castanospermine, and 1-deoxynojirimycin, but bromoconduritol had no effect. However, none of these inhibitors reduced virus production in acutely infected cells. These studies conclude that inhibitors of glycosylation are important in exploring the possibility of blocking infectivity of the virus. The nature of the disease has intensified the search for potential inhibitors of HIV-1 replication which can be used clinically. Two approaches have been, so far, rewarding, rewarding in the sense that future work along these lines may lead to the development of clinically usable drugs with lower toxicity. We will now focus our attention on the processes of reverse transcription and transactivation.

5. REVERSE TRANSCRIPTION

For some years now, we have been interested in designing a specific inhibitor of reverse transcriptase (Chandra, P., & Bardos, 1972; Chandra, P., et al., 1972a,b,c,d,e,f; Chandra, P., 1974; Chandra, P., et al., 1974; Chandra, P., et al., 1975; Chandra, P. et al., 1977a,b,c; Ebener, 1977; Chandra, P., 1979; Chandra, P., & Mildner, 1979a,b; Chandra, P. et al., 1979; Mildner and Chandra, 1979; Chandra, P., et al., 1984; Chandra, P., et al., 1985). Recent studies from our laboratory (Chandra, P., et al., 1986; Chandra, A., et al., 1986a,b; Chandra, P., et al., 1987) have shown that the reverse transcriptase purified from HIV-1–infected cells, or HIV-1 virions has some novel features which could be important in designing specific inhibitors of the enzyme. For this reason we will first describe the characterization of HIV-1 reverse transcriptase.

5.1. CHARACTERIZATION OF HIV-1 REVERSE TRANSCRIPTASE

The enzyme from HIV-1–infected H9 cells or HIV-1 virion suspensions was purified by successive chromatography on DEAE-cellulose (DEAE 23 and DEAE 52) and phosphocellulose columns. A single-peak of high reverse transcriptase activity was eluted from phosphocellulose column at salt concentrations of 0.175 M KCl. This peak of activity was unable to transcribe the template primers $(dC)_n \cdot (dG)_{12}$ and $(dA)_n \cdot (dT)_{12}$, indicating that no DNA-dependent DNA polymerase activities were present in this fraction. A quantitative analysis of the enzyme activity at various purification steps showed a 120- to 140-fold purification, starting from the crude fraction obtained after centrifugation at 170,000 × g (Chandra, P., et al., 1985). Assays were performed with the same batch of enzyme using the same concentration. Viral 70s RNA was tested in the presence of three other cold dNTPs with the indicated radioactive dNTP. DNA polymerase activity was measured by adding 20 μl of the enzyme fraction to a volume of 30 μl, which gave a final concentration of 50 mM tris-HCl buffer (pH 7.9), 50 mM KCl, divalent cations as indicated, 1 mM dithiothreitol, 20 μM each of the complementary dNTPs cold or ^{3}H-labeled and 1.25 μg template primer as indicated (Table 3-3).

The purified and concentrated enzyme was tested with various template primers in the presence of different concentrations of divalent cations. These assays are useful in deriving information as to whether cellular DNA polymerases are present and whether the enzyme has a type specificity; for example, mammalian viruses of the C-type have ionic requirements different from those of viruses belonging to the B-type. As follows, from Table 3-3, the purified enzyme transcribes $(rA)_n \cdot (dT)_{12}$, $(rAm)_n \cdot (dT)_{12}$, $(rC)_n \cdot (dG)_{12}$, and $(rCm)_n \cdot (dG)$ primer alone with either cation gives no activity.

TABLE 3-3. *Template Primer Requirements of the Purified Reverse Transcriptase from HIV-1*

Template primer	^{3}H-labeled substrate	Enzyme activity per hour (pmol/μg protein h)	
		Mg^{2+} (mM)	Mn^{2+} (mM)
$(rA)_n \cdot (dT)_{12}$	dTTP	15.45(0.5)	0.23(0.05)
$(rAm)_n \cdot (dT)_{12}$	dTTP	0.18(3.0)	94.77(0.05)
$(rC)_n \cdot (dG)_{18}$	dGTP	273.90(15.0)	0.74(0.075)
$(rCm)_n \cdot (dG)_{18}$	dGTP	38.17(3.0)	89.03(0.2)
70 S RNA (SSAV)	dGTP	1.79(10.0)	0
70 S RNA + $(dT)_{12}$	dGTP	4.78(10.0)	0
$(dT)_{12}$	dGTP	0.01(0.5)	0

Assays were performed with the same batch of enzyme using the same concentration. Viral RNA (70 S) was tested in the presence of three other cold dNTPs with the indicated radioactive dNTP. DNA polymerase activity was measured by adding 20 μl of the enzyme fraction to a volume of 30 μl, which gave a final concentration of 50 mM tris-HCl buffer (pH 8.0), 50 mM KCl, divalent cations (as indicated), 1 mM dithiothreitol, 20 μM each of the complementary dNTP, or ^{3}H-labeled substrate and 1.25 μg template primer (as indicated).

The pattern of template primer utilization by the enzyme distinguishes it from terminal deoxynucleotidyltransferase and host DNA polymerases. Another property unique to reverse transcriptase is its capacity to catalyze transcription of the viral RNA (70s RNA). This was confirmed for the HIV-1 enzyme using purified 70s RNA from SSAV.

Except for the transcription of 2′-O-methylated templates, $(rAm)_n \cdot (dT)_{12}$, and $(rCm)_n \cdot (dG)$, all other template primers require Mg^{++} for optimal activity. The fact that $(rC)_n \cdot (dG)_{12}$-dependent activity is severalfold higher than that catalyzed by $(rA)_n \cdot (dT)_{12}$ and is strictly magnesium dependent constitutes a novel feature of the HIV-1 enzyme, compared to known properties of other C-type virus reverse transcriptases. In this respect, the enzyme resembles more closely reverse transcriptases from B- and D-type viruses.

To study the cross-reactivity between antigens of HIV-1 and other related viruses, we have recently generated hybridoma clones (mouse/mouse) which secrete monoclonal antibodies to p24, p31, gp41, gp 120, and p51/66 reverse transcriptase. Here, we will describe the serological analysis of reverse transcriptases purified from HTLV-I, and HTLV-II, and HIV-1, using monoclonal antibodies to HIV-1 reverse transcriptase; the hybridoma clone carries the designation 4F8. The supernatant fluid obtained from this clone was screened by ELISA using disrupted HIV-1 virions as antigen. Wells were coated overnight with lysates of density-banded HTLV-I, HTLV-II, and HIV-1 containing different amounts of antigen. The remaining protein-binding sites were saturated with 1% BSA in PBS. Then 50 μl of the hybridoma supernatant was added to each well and incubated for 1 hour at 37°C. The immunoreactivity was measured by adding affinity-purified goat antimouse IgG/IgM conjugated with β-galactosidase, using p-nitrophenyl-μ-galactopyranoside as substrate. The activities were measured at 405 nm in an ELISA reader.

The results demonstrate that viral proteins from HTLV-I and HTLV-II do not bear any cross-reactive epitope to antibodies secreted by the clone 4F8 (Table 3-4). As a control in these experiments, BSA was used. On the other hand, a concentration-dependent cross-reactivity is exhibited by the viral antigens from HIV-1 against antibodies secreted by clone 4F8.

Following the procedure just described, wells of 96-well plastic trays were coated overnight with reverse transcriptases purified from HTLV-I, HTLV-II, and HIV-1. To document the specificity of clone 4F8 for reverse transcriptase, another hybridoma clone secreting monoclonal antibodies against the gp 120 antigen of HIV-1, designated 1A6, was included in this experiment. It follows from Table 3-5 that no cross-reaction between reverse transcriptases of HTLV-I and HTLV-II was observed toward antibodies to HIV-1 (clone 4F8). In the same experiment, the antibodies secreted by the clone 1A6 showed no cross-reactivity toward the reverse transcriptase from HIV-1.

The specificity of antibodies secreted by the clone 4F8 for HIV-1 reverse transcriptase was further documented by immunoblotting. The electrophoretic separation of lysates from

TABLE 3-4. *Serological Relationship Between Human T-lymphotropic Retroviruses Defined by Monoclonal Antibodies*

	$E_{405} \times 10^3$ at various virus (protein) concentrations (ng/well)							
Experiment	0(PBS/BSA)	15	30	60	125	250	500	1000
HTLV-I	57	63	63	55	57	55	67	53
HTLV-II	64	69	64	51	63	77	60	50
HTLV-III	50	60	61	54	75	96	198	288

Supernatant fluid obtained from clone 4F8 was screened by ELISA using disrupted HTLV-III as antigen. Wells of a 96-well plastic tray were coated overnight with HTLV-I, HTLV-II, and HTLV-III lysates containing different amounts of antigen. After saturation of the remaining protein-binding sites with 1% BSA, 50 μl of culture supernatant from 4F8 was added to each well. The cross-reactivity was measured by adding antimouse IgG + M conjugated with β-galactosidase, using p-nitrophenyl-β-D-galactopyranoside as substrate. The activities were measured in an ELISA reader at 405 nm.

TABLE 3-5. *Serological Relationship Between Reverse Transcriptases from Human T-lymphotropic Viruses Defined by Monoclonal Antibodies to HIV-1 Reverse Transcriptase*

	$E_{405} \times 10^3$ at various RT concentrations (protein) (ng/well)							
Experiment	0(PBS/BSA)	15	30	60	125	250	500	1000
HTLV-1 RT								
(4F8)	51	56	44	48	47	68	48	39
(1A6)	45	44	41	45	56	56	53	39
HTLV-II RT								
(4F8)	45	45	56	46	54	61	51	39
(1A6)	49	42	42	48	53	55	50	42
HTLV-III RT								
(4F8)	55	44	49	70	82	154	231	287
(1A6)	44	50	56	52	50	53	55	42

Following the procedure described in the text, wells were coated overnight with various amounts of reverse transcriptases purified from HTLV-I, HTLV-II, and HTLV-III. The clone 1A6, serving as negative control, secretes antibodies against glycoprotein gp120.

HTLV-I (lane 1), HTLV-II (lane 2), and HIV-1 (lane 3) are shown in Fig. 3-4(A); lane 4 shows the separation of affinity-purified M_r markers (phosphorylase b = 96 kd, BSA = 66 kd, ovalbumin = 43 kd, carbonic anhydrase = 30 kd, soybean trypsin inhibitor = 20.1 kd, and α-lactalbumin = 14.4 kd). Figure 3-4(B) depicits the immunoblots of HTLV-I (lane 1), HTLV-II (lane 2), and HIV-1 (lane 3), incubated with monoclonal antibodies secreted by clone 4F8 and developed with goat antimouse horseradish peroxidase conjugated antibodies using 4-chloro-1-naphthol as substrate. There is no cross-reacting band seen on HTLV-I and HTLV-II strips. The strip with HIV-1 shows two prominent bands in the region of M_r 51 kd and 66 kd. To separate the two reactivities, the clone 4F8 was subjected to repeat cycling; even after the fourth cycling the two reactivities remain. This indicates that both the reactive antigens, 51 kd and 66 kd, have a common epitope recognized by the same determinant.

To elucidate the biochemical nature of 4F8 antibodies' interaction to HIV-1 reverse transcriptase, we have measured the catalytic activity of reverse transcriptase in the presence of antibodies (Fig. 3-5).

Antibodies secreted by clone 4F8 are unable to neutralize the enzymatic activity. Measurement of residual activity by immunoprecipitation of the antigen–antibody complex, however, shows a concentration-dependent inhibition of enzyme activity. These data indicate that the antibodies secreted by clone 4F8 are not directed toward the active center of HIV-1 reverse transcriptase.

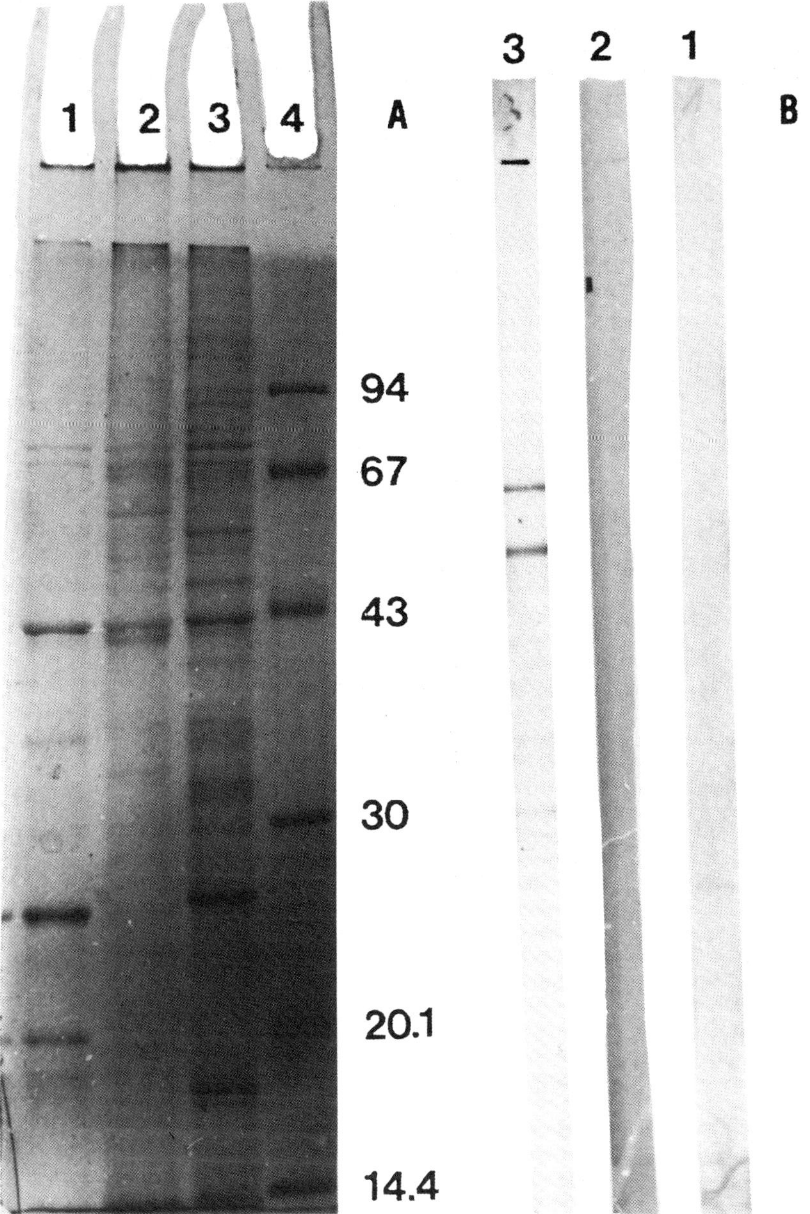

FIG. 3-4. (A) SDS polyacrylamid gel electrophoresis of virus lysates. A 100 μl virus suspension containing 50 mM tris-HCl (pH 6.8), 1% SDS, and 0.1% DTT was boiled for 5 minutes, then 20 μl bromphenolblue (0.1%) stained glycerol was added. An amount of 15 μl of this suspension was used per slab. Lanes 1, HTLV-1; 2, HTLV-II; 3, HIV-1; 4, M_r markers: 94 kd, phosphorylase b, 66 kd, bovine serum albumine, 43 kd, ovalbumine, 30 kd, carbonic anhydrase, 20.1 kd, soybean trypsin inhibitor, 14.4 kd, α-lactalbumin. (B) Immunoblot transfer analysis of antigenic cross-reactivities of HTLV-1, HTLV-II, and HIV-1 toward antibodies secreted by the clone 4F8. Lanes 1, HTLV-1; 2, HTLV-II; 3, HIV-1.

The biochemical and immunological data presented suggest that two forms of reverse transcriptase activities having a common epitope to the antibodies secreted by clone 4F8 are nonneutralizing, but specific for HIV-1 reverse transcriptase. Thus, the reverse transcriptase of HIV-1 is serologically different from those of HTLV-I and HTLV-II. Immunoblotting shows two forms of the enzyme of M_r, 51 kd and 66 kd. There are two possible mechanisms to explain this heterogeneity of HIV-1 reverse transcriptase: one possibility is that the product of the **pol** gene is a polyprotein, which is processed at different sites producing two forms of the molecule; the other explanation is that the parent enzyme of

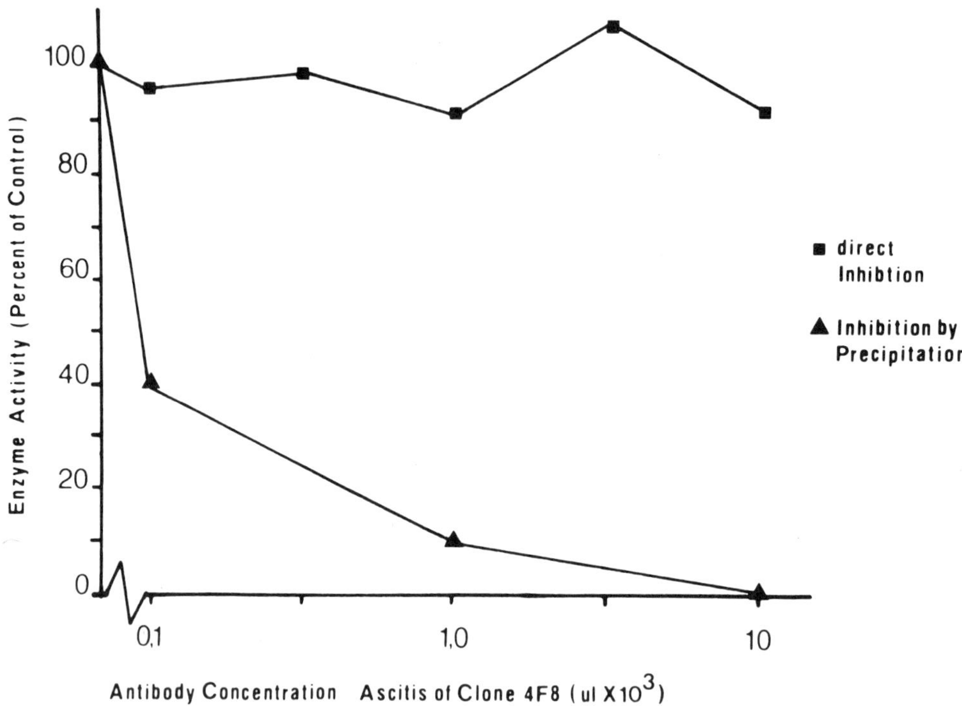

FIG. 3-5. Catalytic activity of HIV-1 reverse transcriptase in the presence of antibodies secreted by the hybridoma clone 4F8. Ascites prepared from clone 4F8 was used as the source of antibodies. Neutralizing activity was measured by preincubating 20 μl of enzyme with 20 μl of the properly diluted ascites fluid overnight. Of this 10 μl was used to assay the enzyme activity. To measure the residual activity, 10 μl of the enzyme was incubated with 10 μl of properly diluted ascites overnight at 4°C. To this 100 μl of magnetic conjugate of goat antimouse IgG (Biomag M 4400, Sebak, Aidenbach, FRG) was added, and the tubes were placed on a magnetic separation device (Sebak). After 1 hr, 30 μl aliquots were pipetted from the supernatant and assayed for the residual enzyme activity. All estimations were done in triplicate. In the control experiments, 1:100 dilution of ascites from another clone which showed no cross-reactivity to reverse transcriptase was used.

66 kd is processed by a protease associated to the HIV-1 genome. Experimental evidence is in favor of the second possibility. We have recently shown that HIV-1 reverse transcriptase can be separated by isoelectric focusing into two peaks with isoelectric points of 5.75 and 6.25 (Fig. 3-6).

These differences are probably due to cleavage of roughly 100 amino acids from the carboxyl end by a specific protease. The characterization of two enzymes separated by isoelectric focusing should help answer these questions. The studies reported in this section conclude that HIV-1 has two catalytically active reverse transcriptases which can be biochemically separated on preparative isoelectric focusing columns. We believe that the presence of two catalytically active reverse transcriptases may account for the genomic heterogeneity of HIV-1, especially in the **env** region.

The two enzymic activities separated on preparative isoelectric focusing columns were tested serologically against the monoclonal antibodies secreted by the hybridoma clone 4F8. Both activities have the same affinity profiles against the monoclonal antibodies to reverse transcriptase (Fig. 3-7).

5.2. REVERSE TRANSCRIPTASE INHIBITORS

The strategic role of nucleic acids, or nucleic acid polymerases, as targets involves two distinct features. The investigational drug must have the capacity to recognize distinct bases or base-pair sequences, either by directed interaction between functional groupings on the base-pairs and the drug molecule, or indirectly via recognition of the conformational pe-

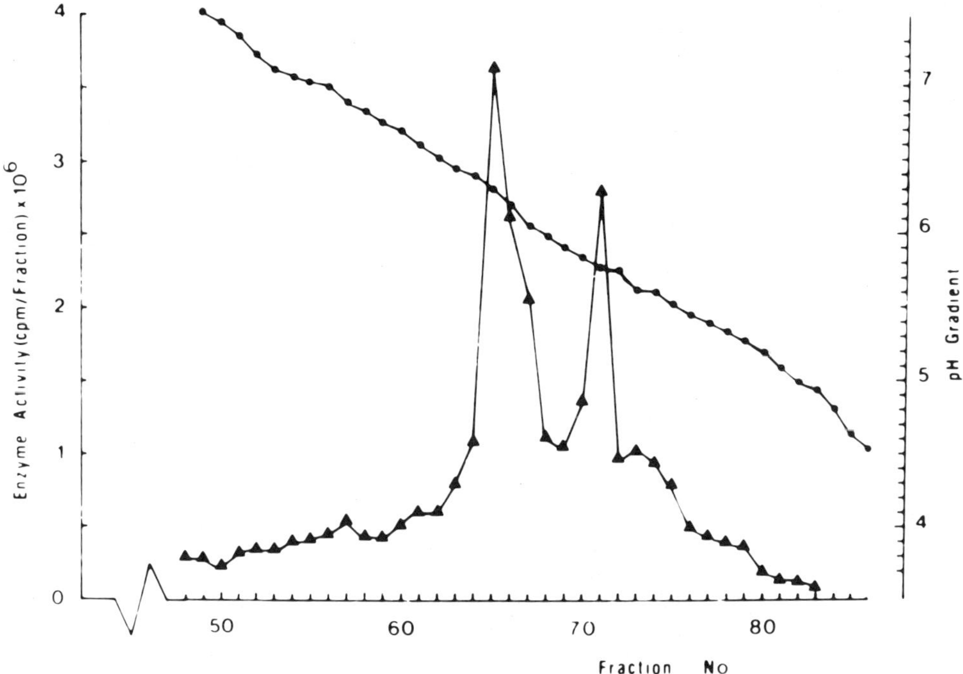

FIG. 3-6. Profile of DNA polymerase activities after electrofocusing of the HIV-1 enzyme eluted from a phosphocellulose column. The enzyme activity of the eluted fractions was measured in the presence of $(rC_n)\cdot(dG)_{12}$ using Mg^{++} (15 mM).

culiarity of the nucleic acid molecule. The other alternative is the specific affinity of the drug for one or the other nucleic acid polymerizing enzymes. From the strategic standpoint, this is a more specific approach, since a number of enzymes are involved in the polymerization of nucleic acids.

RNA-directed DNA synthesis is unique to the life cycle of retroviruses. No similar reaction is known to occur in normal uninfected cells. Reverse transcriptase is a multifunctional enzyme, with at least four domains that mediate RNA-dependent DNA polymerase activity, RNase H activity, DNA-dependent DNA polymerase activity, and a nucleic acid binding site. All these domain-mediated functional activities offer attractive targets for inhibiting the synthesis of DNA in retroviruses. The final product of the reactions mediated by reverse transcriptase is a linear duplex DNA. This linear DNA is longer than the 35s subunit of genomic RNA and contains long terminal repeats (the composition of which can be written as 5′-U3-TR-U5-3′) present at both ends. The process of reverse transcription offers a unique target for drug design, and the number of compounds reported to inhibit this process has exceeded expectations. However, the critical analysis of the **en bloc** progress leaves a big gap. The *in vitro* assay systems used for reverse transcriptase determination reveal a variety of substrates, template primers, and interacting compounds which can modulate the catalytic rate of DNA synthesis (Chandra et al., 1979). Some examples of this type of modulation are the detergent effect on the activity of rifamycins, influence of divalent cations (Mg^{++} or Mn^{++}) on the rate of DNA synthesis with different substrates and the role of chelating agents or cation binders in buffer, and the interaction of thiols with some potential inhibitors or their direct influence on measured DNA synthesis. Thus slight variations in assay conditions may lead to wrong interpretations with respect to the specificity of a particular inhibitor in the viral DNA polymerase system.

The second problem is the interpretation of the enzymatic data with respect to the antiviral activity of these inhibitors (Chandra, P., et al., 1977a). This is particularly the case with those compounds that exert their inhibitory action by complexing with one or more synthetic templates. Such an effect cannot be very specific for the viral enzyme. Drugs

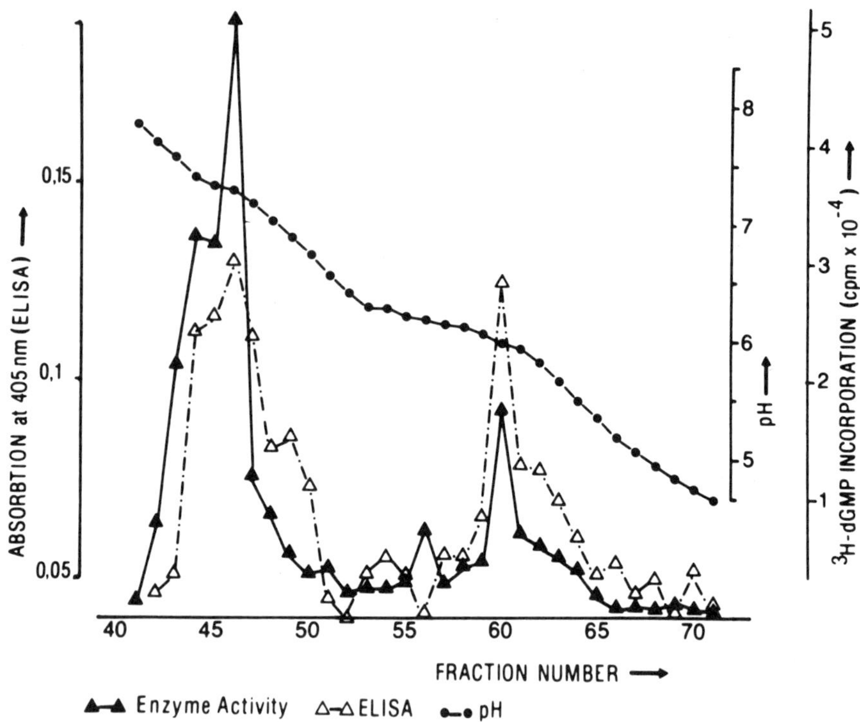

FIG. 3-7. Serological profiles of reverse transcriptase activities from HIV-1 against monoclonal antibodies secreted by clone 4F8.

exhibiting cytotoxic effects to the extent of causing a delayed death or those which intervene in the replicative cycle of the host cell may give erroneous information about the specific antiviral activity of the compound. Thus antiviral studies *in vitro* should be carried out under conditions and at inhibitor concentrations which have little or no effect on the replicative cycle of the cell.

The strategy for designing the inhibitors is largely dependent on the type of process to be investigated. Depending upon the mode of action, there are several possibilities for the design of such compounds: (1) enzyme-binding compounds, (2) substrate analogs, (3) template-primer analogs, (4) template-binding compounds, and (5) divalent cation-binding agents. Most of the compounds reported in the literature (for review, see Chandra et al., 1979) inhibit by binding to the template. The compounds which act by binding to the template are not specific to reverse transcriptase inhibition; cellular DNA polymerases are also inhibited. For this reason, they exhibit cytotoxicity. Molecular manipulations of parent compounds have proved to be very useful in several instances in the development of inhibitors of viral DNA synthesis which exhibit a low cytotoxicity and, at the same time, a higher antiviral potential. This is evidenced from our earlier studies on distamycin derivatives (Chandra, P., 1972a,b), tilorone congeners (Chandra, P., et al., 1972d; Chandra, P., 1974; Chandra, P., et al., 1974), diamidine phenylindol derivatives (Chandra, P., and Mildner, 1979a,b; Mildner and Chandra, 1979), and daunomycin derivatives (Chandra, P., et al., 1972b,c,e). These studies have been reviewed extensively (Chandra, P., et al., 1972f; Chandra, P., et al., 1979) and will not be discussed here.

The second approach, which has proved to be more useful and relatively specific in developing such inhibitors, is to design compounds that bind to the viral enzyme. Our efforts to develop compounds that inhibit the viral DNA polymerase reaction by directly interacting with the enzyme led to the discovery of a polycytidylic acid analog, containing 5-mercapto-substituted cytosine bases, a partially thiolated polycytidylic acid. This compound, MPC, was found to inhibit retroviral DNA polymerase in a very specific manner (Chandra, P., and Bardos, 1972; Chandra, P., et al., 1972f; Chandra, P., et al., 1975;

Chandra, P., et al., 1977a,b,c; Chandra, P., 1979; Chandra, P., et al., 1979). We have therefore analyzed the effect of partially thiolated polycytidylic and polyuridylic acid probes on the catalytic activities of reverse transcriptase and DNA polymerase β, purified from HIV-1–infected H9 cells (Chandra, P., et al., 1985).

As seen from Table 3-6, aphidicolin, a specific inhibitor of eukaryotic DNA polymerase α, has no effect on the catalytic activity of DNA polymerase β and the reverse transcriptase. By contrast, the catalytic activity of HIV-1 reverse transcriptase is strongly inhibited by modified poly(U) and poly(C), containing 5-mercapto-substituted pyrimidines; at as small a concentration as 1 μg, HIV-1 reverse transcriptase loses almost 90% of its catalytic activity in the presence of 5-mercapto-polyuridylic acid (SH = 4%) or in the presence of MPC (SH = 15% and 30%).

Mitsuya and colleagues (1984) have reported the protection of T-cells *in vitro* against infectivity and cytophatic effect of HIV-1 by suramin (synonyms are Germanin, Bayer 205, Naganol, and Antrypol), an antitrypanosomal drug. The development of suramin dates back to the initial discovery of Paul Ehrlich in 1904 (Ehrlich & Shiga, 1904), who discovered that the sulfonate derivative of aminonaphthalene, trypan red, has a high therapeutic activity against trypanosomal infections. The effect of suramin on the catalytic activities of DNA polymerase α and HIV-1 reverse transcriptase is shown in Table 3-7.

DNA polymerase α was a highly purified preparation from human placenta (Chandra et al., 1985). As follows from the results, suramin inhibits both enzymatic activities very strongly, with no preference for reverse transcriptase. As evident from its structure, suramin has a high binding capacity to proteins due to sulfonic acid residues present in the molecule. Thus, it does not offer any rationale for specificity toward any particular pro-

TABLE 3-6. *Effect of Thiolated Polynucleotides on DNA-Polymerase β and Reverse Transcriptase Activities from HIV-1–Infected H9 Cells*

Inhibitor	Concentration* (μg)	Enzyme activity (percent of control) $(dA)_n \cdot (dT)_{12}$	$(rC)_n \cdot (dG)_{18}$
None	—	100 (14.028)†	100 (20.130)†
Aphidocolin	10	92.4	123
Poly-U(4-thio)	10	91.5	113
Poly-U(5-thio)			
(SH = 4%)	0.1	80.0	38.5
	1.0	64.0	12.61
Poly-C(5-thio)			
(SH = 15%)	0.1	97.0	46.89
	1.0	90.0	16.07
(SH = 30%)	0.1	90.0	38.49
	1.0	72.0	11.06

*Denotes μg/reaction mixture (50 μl).
†Denotes pmol dNMP incorporation/μg protein/hr.

TABLE 3-7. *Inhibition of DNA-Polymerase α and Reverse Transcriptase Activities from HIV-1 by Suramin*

System	^{3}H-dNMP incorporation (percent of control) $(dA\text{-}dT)_n \cdot (dA\text{-}dT)_n$	$(rC)_n \cdot (dG)_n$
Complete	100 (9.414)*	100 (67.719)*
Germanin*		
0.1 μg†	33	27.8
1.0 μg	10.6	0.82
10.0 μg	0	0.23

*Denotes pmol dNMP incorporation/μg protein/hr.
†Amount added to the reaction mixture (50 μl).

tein. It is known to have a high binding affinity to serum albumin, which is perhaps responsible for irreversible damage to the kidney. In clinical trials suramin showed a transient reduction in virus expression and severe toxic side effects, including anemia, proteinuria, haptic failure, and agranulocytosis (Broder et al., 1985; Levine et al., 1986). After treatment with suramin was discontinued, virus expression returned to pretreatment levels. Due to its toxic side effects, and its inability to suppress virus expression, clinical trials with this compound have been suspended.

Another class of compounds which inhibit reverse transcriptase, and are being clinically used, are the chain terminators. The important members of this group, 3′-azido-3′-deoxythymidine (AzT) and 2′,3′-dideoxy derivatives of cytidine and adenosine (ddC and ddA), have been shown to be clinically effective but endowed with too many side effects (Richman et al., 1987a,b; Fischl et al., 1987; Yarchoan and Broder, 1987).

An important issue in the development of nucleoside analogs as inhibitors of HIV-1 replication has recently been underlined by the studies of Richman and colleagues (1987b). They have shown that the primary human monocyte-derived macrophages lack nucleoside kinase activities for thymidine, deoxycytidine, and uridine; adenosine kinase activity was present but only at 50% of the level found in CEM cells. Since macrophages serve as a reservoir for immunodeficiency viruses, the inability of nucleoside analogs to inhibit virus multiplication in macrophages offers severe disadvantages in their clinical application (Richman et al., 1987b). In a recent study, Perno and colleagues (1988) elegantly demonstrated that the inhibitory effect of nucleoside analogs is dependent on the differentiation stage of macrophages. Thus, the loss of kinase activities in terminally differentiated macrophages may limit the application of nucleoside analogs in the antiviral treatment of AIDS.

6. INHIBITORS OF TRANSACTIVATION

The mechanism of transactivation and its importance in regulating gene expression have been described. The **tat** protein has a stretch of highly basic amino acids (2 lysines and 6 arginines within 9 residues) that could participate in nucleic acid binding, for example, to the TAR region of HIV-1 LTR. It also contains a cluster of cystein residues (7 cysteines within 16 residues), and a sequence comparison from several HIV-1 isolates shows that the cysteines are perfectly conserved. Mutation of any of these cysteine residues leads to total inactivation of the **tat** function. Potential metal-binding proteins have a characteristic feature in having cysteine-rich regions at the binding site (Berg, 1986). Since **tat** is essential for HIV-1 replication, it provides an attractive target for drug design. D-penicillamine (DPA), an amino acid analog of cysteine, is known to interact with cysteine-rich proteins (Chandra, P., & Koch, 1975; Wacker et al., 1966; Wacker et al., 1971). This interaction occurs by the formation of interdisulfide bonds between D-penicillamine and cystine or cysteine, and such D-penicillamine–protein complexes are highly stable, as suggested by the fact that cystine or cysteine added after D-penicillamine cannot remove the drug from proteins (Planas-Bohne, 1981). The chelation of metals by D-penicillamine is the basis of its application in the treatment of Wilson's disease (Walshe, 1956). The interaction of D-penicillamine with cysteine-rich proteins, and its chelating potential, motivated us to examine its effect on the replication of HIV-1 (Chandra, P., & Sarin, 1986).

The effects of D- and L-penicillamine (LPA) on the replication of HIV-1 in H9 cells was determined as a function of drug concentration by measuring the expression of viral proteins p17 and p24 in an immunofluorescence assay procedure using monoclonal antibodies. Figure 3-8 shows a concentration-dependent inhibition of p17 expression by both the compounds L-penicillamine (filled circles) and D-penicillamine (open circles). At lower concentrations L-penicillamine is more effective than D-penicillamine. However, to obtain total inhibition, a drug concentration of 40 μg/ml was needed for both the isomers.

The cytotoxicity of D-penicillamine is very low (Chandra, P., & Sarin, 1986); concentrations up to 200 μg/ml do not inhibit the growth of uninfected H9 cells. At 500 μg/ml, D-penicillamine shows a 32% inhibition of cell growth. In a limited clinical trial on asymp-

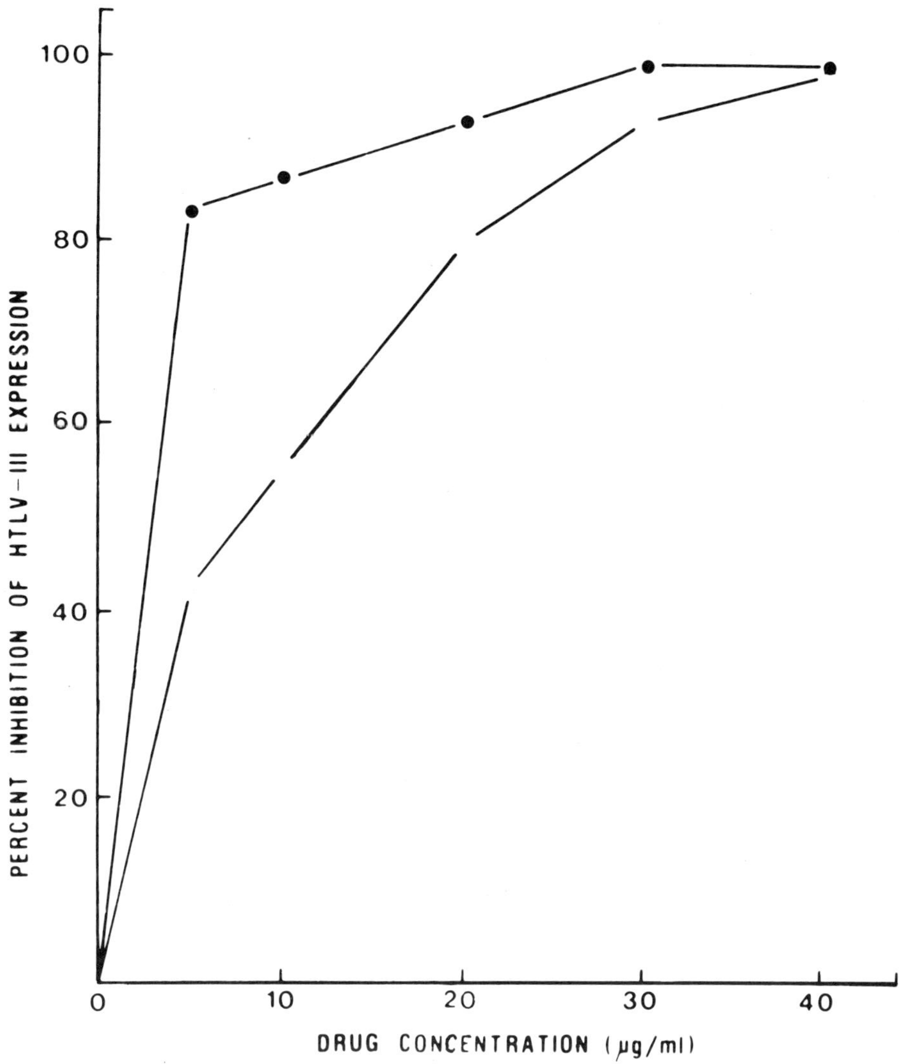

FIG. 3-8. Inhibition of HIV-1 virus expression by D- (— —) and L- (•••) penicillamine as measured by monoclonal antibodies to HIV-1 p17.

tomatic patients with generalized lymphadenopathy, D-penicillamine was given orally over a period of 6 weeks (Schulof et al., 1986). All patients had depressed T4/T8 ratios and impaired T-cell functioning. An escalating dose schedule was employed over 2–6 weeks, with doses ranging from 0.5–2.0 g/day. Ten patients treated for at least 2 weeks showed suppression of HIV-1 replication, and complete inhibition of virus expression occurred in 60% of the patients treated for 6 weeks. Two of these patients have remained virus-free for over 9 months (Sarin et al., 1987). A reversible decrease in lymph node size, absolute lymphocyte counts, and T-cell lympho-proliferative responses were observed in patients without change in baseline T4/T8 ratios. No significant toxicity was observed in these patients (Schulof et al., 1986; Parenti et al., 1987). In another clinical trial, seven asymptomatic patients with generalized lymphadenopathy were treated with D-penicillamine using dose schedules ranging from 0.6 to 1.8 g/day (Siedentopf & Chandra, 1988). In this study, vitamin B6 was given to all patients (40 mg/day) at least 2 hours before the first ingestion of D-penicillamine. Since D-penicillamine interacts with vitamin B6 to form a thiozolidine derivative, it should never be given together with B6. Two of these patients had antigenemia and could be monitored throughout the course of therapy by the p24 antigen-capture assay (Chandra, A., et al., 1987). Four of these patients became virus negative after 12 weeks of D-penicillamine treatment. The virus status was monitored by the co-cultivation

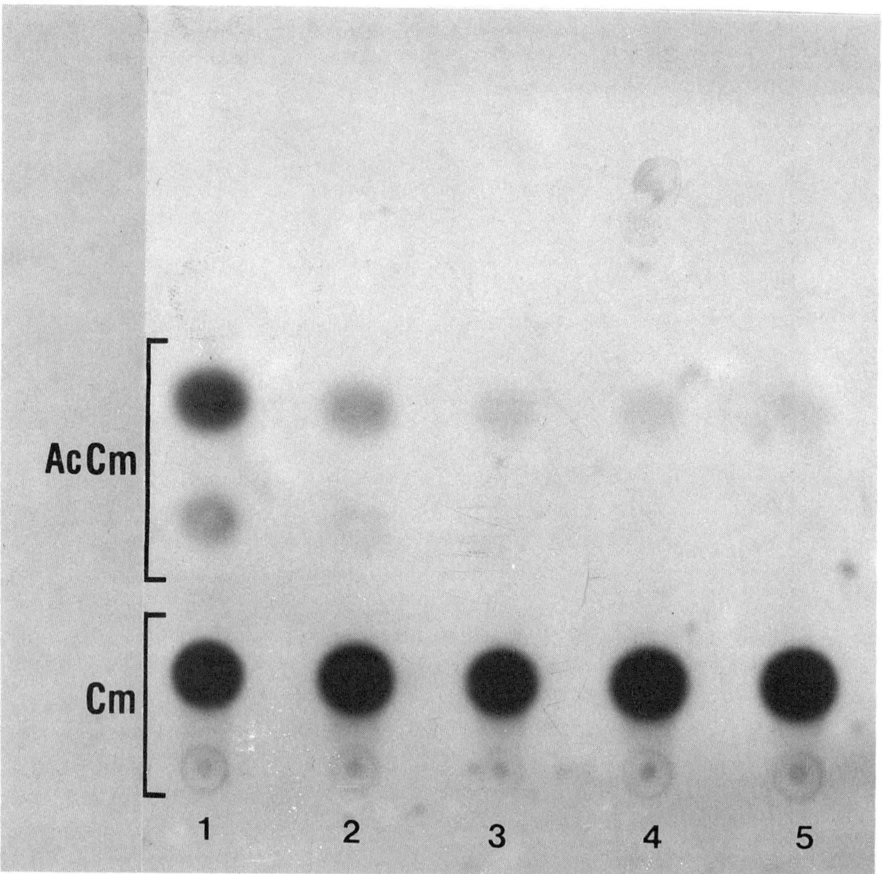

FIG. 3-9. Effect of D-penicillamine on the LTR (HIV-1)directed CAT expression catalyzed by the *tat*-protein. Lane 1: without D-penicillamine; lanes 2–5: with D-penicillamine (10, 20, 30, and 40 μg/ml).

assay, and in two cases also by the antigen-capture assay. The hematological records showed a transient rise in LDH activity in one of the patients. One of the patients developed a skin allergy in the fifth week of treatment, which was cured by local application of dexamethasone cream without interruption of the DPA therapy. No other side effects have been noted in these patients. The mode of action of D-penicillamine as an anti-HIV-1 drug has recently been studied in our laboratory. We have studied the effect of D-penicillamine on the transactivation of HIV-1 (LTR) by the **tat** protein. The studies were carried out in Jurkat cells which were co-transfected with plasmids containing HIV-1 (LTR) and **tat** gene sequences. For measuring transactivation, the HIV-1 LTR was fused to the indicator gene, chloramphenicol acetyltransferase (CAT). The transactivation of the LTR-linked CAT gene was measured by conversion of chloramphenicol to its acetylated forms by the enzyme synthesized in transfected cells. Jurkat cells transfected with plasmids pC15CAT (HIV-LTR-CAT) and pCV1 (**tat** gene) (Chandra, A., et al., 1988) express chloramphenicol acetyltransferase, as shown in Fig. 3-9 (lane 1). Cells incubated with different concentrations of D-penicillamine (10–40 μg/ml) exhibit a concentration-dependent inhibition of CAT expression (lanes 2–5).

Quantitative measurements have shown more than 90% inhibition of transactivation at 40 μg/ml D-penicillamine (Table 3-8).

These results suggest that inhibition of transactivation may be the molecular mechanism involved in the inhibition of HIV-1 replication by D-penicillamine.

TABLE 3-8. *Effect of D-Penicillamine on the LTR-(HIV-1)-Directed Expression Catalyzed by the* ***tat*** *Protein*

Experiment	Percentage conversion of chloramphenicol to acetylated forms
Without D-penicillamine (control)	23.33 ± 3.5 (100)
With D-penicillamine (μg/ml)	
10	2.9 ± 0.33 (12.4)
20	1.97 ± 0.29 (8.4)
30	1.46 ± 0.22 (6.25)
40	0.97 ± 0.15 (4.15)

The percentage conversion of chloramphenicol to acetylated forms was calculated by dividing the total number of counts in AcCm region (Fig. 3-9) with the total number of counts found in Cm and AcCm regions. This coefficient multiplied by 100 is depicted as the percentage value for the acetylated product. The values are mentioned as mean and standard deviation for three independent transfection experiments. The experimental procedures were same as under Fig. 3-9 and mentioned in the text. Figures in parentheses indicate the percent of control, with control taken as 100.

7. FUTURE PERSPECTIVES

The classical approach for developing inhibitors of reverse transcription should be very rewarding for two reasons: The reverse transcriptase of HIV-1 has some novel features (Chandra, P., et al., 1986; Chandra, A., et al., 1986a,b; Chandra, P., et al., 1987) and the knowledge of this subject is available from the past (Chandra, P., et al., 1979). However, these studies must be carried out carefully with purified enzymes and compared with homologous cellular enzymes. Without this type of comparative study, a reverse transcriptase inhibitor does not make any sense, and clinical trials with such compounds may end in a great disappointment. As we learn more about the pathogenic events at cellular and molecular levels induced or catalyzed by HIV-1, we can select potential targets for designing therapeutically active compounds. Based on existing knowledge, we can design some strategies to block HIV-1 replication chemically. For example, the self-regulatory mechanism of HIV-1 replication by the proteins coded by **tat** and **art/trs** genes is an attractive and novel target. *In vivo* modification of their gene products will abolish this control mechanism, resulting in the inhibition of virus replication. D-penicillamine is the first compound shown to inhibit virus replication at this level.

Acknowledgments—A part of this work was supported by the German Ministry of Research and Technology (BMFT, Grant No. FKZ II/02987) and the American Foundation for AIDS Research (Grant No. 000162). It is a great pleasure to acknowledge the skilled technical assistance of M. Dzwonkowski and G. Fischer. We are also grateful to Robert C. Gallo for useful discussions and we thank Günther Kahl and Dieter Hoffman for their help in the characterization of plasmids.

REFERENCES

Arya, S.K., Guo, C., Josephs S.F., and Wong-Staal, F. (1985) Transactivator gene of HIV-1 by the tat gene product. *Nature* **332**: 551.

Barre-Sinoussi, F., Cherman, J.C., Rey, F., Nugeyne, M.T., Charmaret, S., Gruest, J., Dauguet, C., Axler-Blin, C., Vennet-Brun, F., Rouzioux, W., Rozenbaum, W., and Montagnier, L. (1983) Isolation of a T-lymphotropic retrovirus from a patient at risk for acquired immune deficiency syndrome (AIDS). *Science* **220**: 868.

Berg, J.M. (1986) Potential metal-binding domains in nucleic acid–binding proteins. *Science* **232**: 485.

Broder, S., Yarchoan, R., Collins, J., and Lane, H.C. (1985) Effects of suramin on HTLV-III/LAV infection presenting as Kaposi's sarcoma or AIDS-related complex. Clinical pharmacology and suppression of virus replication *in vivo*. *Lancet* **2**: 627.

Chandra, A., Demirhan, I., Arya, S.K., and Chandra, P. (1988) D-Penicillamine inhibits transactivation of human immunodeficiency virus type 1 (HIV-1)-LTR. *FEBS Lett*. **236**: 282.

Chandra, A., Demirhan, I., Siedentopf, H.G., Behnken, L.J., Sun, D.K., Sarin, P.S., and Chandra, P. (1987) Antigen-capture assay in the modulation of antiviral chemotherapy of HIV infection by D-penicillamine. *AIDS Forsch*. **11**: 629.

Chandra, A., Gerber, T., and Chandra, P. (1986a). Biochemical heterogeneity of reverse transcriptase purified from AIDS virus, HTLV-III. *FEBS-Lett.* **197**: 84.

Chandra, A., Gerber, T., Kaul, S., Wolf, C., Demirhan, I., and Chandra, P. (1986b) Serological relationship between reverse transcriptases from human T-cell lymphotropic retroviruses, defined by monoclonal antibodies. *FEBS-Lett.* **200**: 327.

Chandra, P. (1979). Selective inhibition of oncornaviral functions (a molecular approach). In *Antimetabolites in biochemistry and biology and medicine*, J. Skoda, and P. Langen, eds., pp. 249–261. Oxford: Pergamon Press.

Chandra, P. (1974) Molecular approaches for designing antiviral and antitumor compounds. In *Topics in current chemistry*, Vol. 52, pp. 99–139. Heidelberg: Springer-Verlag.

Chandra, P., Chandra, A., Demirhan, I., and Gerber, T. (1987) Chemotherapeutic approaches in the control of the acquired immune deficiency syndrome. *AIDS Forsch.* **5**: 265.

Chandra, P., and Sarin, P.S. (1986) Selective inhibition of replication of the AIDS-associated virus, HTLV-III/LAV, by synthetic D-penicillamine. *Drug Res.* **36**: 184.

Chandra, P., Chandra, A., Demirhan, I., and Gerber, T. (1986) Antiviral approaches in the treatment of acquired immune deficiency syndrome. In *New experimental modalities in the control of neoplasia*, P. Chandra, ed., pp. 303–328. New York: Plenum Press.

Chandra, P., Vogel, A., and Gerber, T. (1985) Inhibitors of retroviral DNA polymerases: Their implication in the treatment of AIDS. *Cancer Res.* **45**: 4677.

Chandra, P., Demirhan, I., Ebener, U., and Kornhuber, B. (1984) Virus-associated DNA polymerizing activities: Their role in designing antiviral and antitumor drugs. In *Targets for the designing of antiviral agents*, E. DeClerque and R.T. Walker, eds., pp. 307–335. New York: Plenum Press.

Chandra, P., and Mildner, B. (1979a) Zur molekularen Wirkungsweise von Diamidinphenylindol (DAPI): I. Physikochemische Untersuchungen zur Charakterisierung von DAPI an Nukleinsäuren. *Cell. Mol. Biol.* **25**: 137.

Chandra, P., and Mildner, B. (1979b) Zur molekularen Wirkungsweise von Diamidinphenylindol (DAPI): III. Physikochemische Untersuchungen zur Bindung von DAPI-Derivaten an die DNA bzw. Polydesoxynukleotide und ihre Auswirkungen auf die Matrizenfunktion der Nukleinsäuren. *Cell. Mol. Biol.* **25**: 429.

Chandra, P., Steel, L.K., Ebener, U., Woltersdorf, M., Laube, H., Kornhuber, B., Mildner, B., and Götz, A. (1979) Chemical inhibitors of oncornaviral DNA polymerases: Biological implications and their mode of action. In *Inhibitors of DNA and RNA polymerases,* P.S. Sarin, and R.C. Gallo, eds., pp. 47–49. Oxford and New York: Pergamon Press.

Chandra, P., Steel, L.K., Ebener, U., Woltersdorf, M., Laube, H., Kornhuber, B., Mildner, B. and Götz, A. (1977a) Chemical inhibitors of oncornaviral DNA polymerases: Biological implications and their mode of action. *Pharmacol Ther A.* **1**: 231.

Chandra, P., Ebener, U., Bardos, T.J., Gericke, D., Kornhuber, B., and Götz, A. (1977b) Inhibition of viral reverse transcriptase by modified nucleic acids: Biological implications and their mode of action. In *Fogarty International Center Proceedings*, no. 28, pp. 169–186. Washington DC: U. S. Government Printing Office.

Chandra, P., Ebener, U., Steel, L.K., Laube, H., Gericke, D., Mildner, B., Bardos, T.J., Hoy, K., and Götz, A. (1977c) A molecular approach to inhibit oncogenesis by RNA tumor viruses. *Ann N.Y. Acad. Sci.* **284**: 444.

Chandra, P., and Koch, A. (1975) Die Toxizität von D- und L-Penicillamin bei akut toxischen und therapeutischen Dosen. In *Recent advances in D-penicillamine research,* J.C.P. Weber, and A.S.J. Dixon, eds, pp. 15–23. Karlsruhe: Verlag, G. Braun.

Chandra, P., Ebener, U., and Götz, A. (1975) Inhibition of oncornaviral DNA polymerase by 5-mercapto polycytidylic acid: Mode of action. *FEBS Lett.* **53**: 10.

Chandra, P., Will, G., Gericke, D., and Götz, A. (1974) Inhibition of DNA polymerases from RNA tumor viruses by tilorone and congeners: Site of action. *Biochem. Pharmacol.* **23**: 3259.

Chandra, P., and Bardos, T.J. (1972) Inhibition of DNA polymerases from RNA tumor viruses by novel template analogues: Partially thiolated polycytidylic acid. *Res. Commun. Chem. Phatol. Pharmacol.* **4**: 615.

Chandra, P., Zunino, F., Götz, A., Wacker, A., Gericke, D., DiMarco, A., Casazza, A.M., and Giuliani, F. (1972a) Template-specific inhibition of DNA polymerases from RNA tumor viruses by distamycin A and its structural analogues. *FEBS Lett.* **21**: 154.

Chandra, P., DiMarco, A., Zunino, F., Casazza, A.M., Gericke, D., Giuliani, F., Sorano, C., Thorbeck, R., Götz, A., Arcamone, F., and Thione, M. (1972b) The role of molecular structure on the inhibition of DNA polymerases from RNA tumor viruses, viral multiplication, and tumor growth by some antitumor antibiotics. *Naturwissenschaften* **59**: 448.

Chandra, P., Zunino, F., Götz, A., Gericke, D., Thorbeck, R., and DiMarco, A. (1972c) Specific inhibition of DNA polymerases from RNA tumor viruses by some daunomycin derivates. *FEBS Lett.* **21**: 264.

Chandra, P., Zunino, F., and Götz, A. (1972d) Bis-DEAE-fluorenone: A specific inhibitor of DNA polymerases from RNA tumor viruses. *FEBS Lett.* **22**: 161.

Chandra, P., Gericke, D., Zunino, F., and Kornhuber, B. (1972e) The role of chemical structure to cytostatic activity of some daunomycin derivates. *Pharmacol. Res. Commun.* **4**: 269.

Chandra, P., Ebener, U., and Gericke, D. (1972f) Molecular mechanisms for the control of RNA tumor viruses. In *Antiviral mechanisms in the control of neoplasia*, P. Chandra, ed., pp. 523–528. New York: Plenum Press.

Clapham, P.R., Whitby, D., Dagleish, A.G., Maddon, P., Axel, R., Sweet, R., and Weiss, R.A. (1988) Soluble CD4 neutralize infectivity and syncytia of HIV-1, HIV-2, and SIV. In *Abstract book I* from the IV International Conference of AIDS, June, Stockholm, p. 124.

Clements, J.E., and Naryano, O. (1981) A physical map of the linear unintegrated DNA of VISNA virus. *Virology* **113**: 494.

Davis, M.G., Kenny, S.C., Kamine, J., Pagano, J.S., and Huang, E.S. (1987) Immediate-early gene region of human cytomegalovirus trans-activates the promotor of human immunodeficiency virus. *Proc. Natl. Acad. Sci. USA* **84**: 8642.

Deen, K.C., McDougal, J.C., Inaker, R., Folena-Wasserman, G., Arthos, J., Rosenberg, J., Maddon, P.J., Axel, R., and Sweet, R.W. (1988) A soluble form of CD4 (T4) protein inhibits AIDS virus infection. *Nature* **331**: 82.

Ebener, U. (1977) Hemmung der viralen Reverse Transkriptase und Leukämogenese durch modifitzierte Nukleinsäuren. PhD. Dissertation, Johann Wolfgang von Goethe Universität zu Frankfurt am Main, BRD.

Emerman, M., Guydar, M., Montagnier, L., Baltimore, D., and Muesing, M.A. (1987) The specificity of the human immunodeficiency virus type 2 transactivator is different from that of human immunodeficiency virus type 1. *EMBO J.* **6**: 3755

Ehrlich, P., and Shiga, K. (1904) Über die anti trypanosomale Wirkung von Trypan Rot. *Klinische Wochenschrift* **41**: 329.

Feinberg, M.B., Jarret, R.F., Aldovini, A., Gallo, R.C., and Wong-Staal, F. (1986) Human T lymphotropic virus type III expression and production involve complex regulation at the level of splicing and translation of viral RNA. *Cell* **46**: 87

Felber, B.K., Paskalis, H., Kleinman-Ewing, C., Wong-Staal, F., and Pavlkis, G. (1985) The pX protein from human T cell leukemia virus type I is a transcriptional activator of its long terminal repeats. *Science* **229**: 675.

Feorino, P.M., Kalyanaraman, V.S., Haverkos, H.W., Carbradilla, D.T., Warefield, D.T., Faffe, H.W., Harrison, A.K., Gottlieb, M.S., Goldfinger, D., Cherman, J.C., Barre-Sinoussi, F., Speia, T.T., McDougal, J.S., Curran, J.W., Montagnier, L., Murphy, P.A., and Francis, D. (1984) Lymphadenopathy-associated virus infection of blood donor recipient pair with acquired immune deficiency syndrome. *Science* **225**: 69.

Fischl, M.A., Richman, D.D., Grieco, M.H., Gottlieb, M.S., Volberding, P.A., Laskin, O.L., Leedom, J.M., Groopman, J.E., Mildvan, D., Schooley, R.T., Jackson, G.G., Durack, D.T., King, D., and The AZT Collaborative Working Group. (1987) The efficacy of azidothymidine (AZT) in the treatment of patients with AIDS and AIDS-related complex: A double-blind, placebo-controlled trial. *New Eng. J. Med.* **317**: 185.

Fisher, A.G., Ensoli, B., Ivanoff, L., Chamberlain, M., Petway, S., Ratner, L., Gallo, R.C., and Wong-Staal, F. (1987) The *sor* gene of HIV-1 is required for efficient virus transmission *in vitro*. *Science* **237**: 888.

Fisher, R.A., Bertonis, J.M., Meier, W., Johnson, V.A., Costopopulos, D.S., Liu, T., Tizar, R., Walker, B.D., Hirsch, M.S., Schooley, R.T., and Flavell, A. (1988) HIV infection is blocked *in vitro* by recombinant soluble CD4. *Nature* **331**: 76.

Frankel, A.O., Bredt, D.S., and Pabo, C.O. (1988) Tat protein from human immunodeficiency virus forms metal-linked dimer. *Science* **240**: 70.

Gallo, R.C., Wong-Staal, F., Montagnier, L., Haseltine, W.A., and Yoshida, M. (1988) HIV/HTLV genome nomenclature. *Nature* **333**: 504.

Guy, M., Kieny, M.P., Riviere, Y., Le Peuch, C., Dott, K., Girad, M., Montagnier, L., and Lecoco, J.-P. (1987) HIV F/3′*orf* encodes a phosphorylated GTP-binding protein resembling an oncogene product. *Nature* **303**: 266.

Hahn, B.H., Shaw, G.M., Arya, S.K., Popovic, M., Gallo, R.C., and Wong-Staal, F. (1984) Molecular cloning and characterization of human T-cell leukemia-III virus associated with AIDS (acquired immune deficiency syndrome). *Nature* **312**: 166.

Haseltine, W.A. (1988) Replication and pathogenesis of the AIDS virus. In *Abstract book I* from the IV International Conference of AIDS, June, Stockholm, p. 107.

Hussey, R.E., Richardson, N.E., Kowalsky, M., Brown, N.R., Chang, H.C., Siciliano, R.F., Dorfman, T., Walker, B., Sodroski, J., and Reinherz, E.L. (1988) A soluble CD4 protein selectively inhibits HIV replication and syncytium formation. *Nature* **331**: 78.

Jones, K.A., Kadonga, J.T., Luciw, P.A. and Tijan, R. (1986) Activation of the acquired immune deficiency syndrome retrovirus promotor by cellular transcription factor. *Spl. Science* **232**: 755.

Keshet, E., and Temin, H.M. (1979) Cell killing by spleen necrosis virus is correlated with transient accumulation of spleen necrosis virus DNA. *J. Virol.* **31**: 376.

Levine, A.M., Gill, P.S., Cohen, J., Hawkins, S.C., Formenti, S.A., Meyer, P.R., Krailo, M., Parker, J., and Rasheed, S. (1986) Suramin antiviral therapy in the acquired immune deficiency syndrome: Clinical, immunologic, and virologic results. *Ann. Intern. Med.* **105**: 32.

Levy, J.A., Hoffmann, A.D., Kramer, S.M., Landis, J.A., and Shimabukuro, J.M. (1984) Isolation of lymphocytopathic retroviruses from San Francisco patients with AIDS. *Science* **225**: 840.

Maddon, P.J., Dagleish, A.G., and McDougal, J.S. (1987) The T4 gene encodes the AIDS virus receptor and is expressed in the immune system and in the brain. *Cell* **47**: 333.

Mildner, B., and Chandra, P. (1979) Zur molekularen Wirkungsweise von Diamidinphenylindol (DAPI) II. Einwirkung von DAPI auf die Martrizenfunktion der DNA bzw. Polydesoxynukleotide und ihre Auswirkung auf die Matrizenfunktion der Nukleinsäuren. *Cell. Mol. Biol.* **25**: 399.

Mitsuya, H., Popovic, M., Yarchoan, R., Matsushita, S., Gallo, R.C., and Broder, S. (1984) Suramin protection of T-cells *in vitro* against infectivity and cytopathic effect of human T-cell leukemia virus III. *Science* **226**: 172.

Montefiori, D.C., Robinson, W.E., Jr., and Mitchel, W.M. (1988) The role of N-glycosylation in HIV-1 pathogenesis in vitro. In *Abstract book I* from the IV International Conference of AIDS, June, Stockholm, p. 152.

Morbid Mortal Rep. (1981a) Pneumocystis pneumonia, **30**: 250.

Morbid Mortal Rep. (1981b) Kaposi's sarcoma and pneumocystis pneumonia among homosexual men—New York City and California, **30**: 305.

Muesing, M.A., Smith, D.H., and Capon, D.J. (1987) Regulation of mRNA accumulation by a human immunodeficiency virus *trans*-activation protein. *Cell* **48**: 691.

Nabel, G., and Baltimore, D. (1987) An inducible transcription-factor activates expression of human immunodeficiency virus in T-cells. *Nature* **326**: 711.

Okamoto, T., and Wong-Staal, F. (1986) Demonstration of virus specific transcriptional activator (s) in cells infected with HTLV-III by in vitro cell-free system. *Cell* **47**: 29.

Ostrove, J.M., Leonhard, J., Weck, K.E., Rabson, A.B., and Gendelman, H.E. (1987) Activation of the human immunodeficiency virus by herpes simplex virus. *J. Virol.* **61**: 3726.

Parenti, D.M., Scheib, R.G., Simon, G.L., Chandra, P., and Sarin, P.S. (1987) *Abstract* in 3rd International Conference on AIDS, p. 99.

Perno, C.F., Yarchoan, R., Cooney, D., Hao, Z., Gartner, S., Popovic, M., Hartman, N., Johns, D., and Broder, S. (1988) Protection of monocyte-macrophages (M/M) against HIV infection by dideoxynucleotisides *in vitro*. In *Abstract book I* from the IV International Conference of AIDS, June, Stockholm, p 220.

Perry, V.H., and Gordon, S. (1987) Modulation of CD4 antigen on macrophages and microglia in rat brain. *J. Expt. Med.* **166**: 1138.

Popovic, M., Sarangadharan, M.G., Reed, E., and Gallo, R.C. (1984) Detection, isolation, and continuous production of cytopathic human T-lymphotropic retrovirus (HTLV-III) from patients with AIDS and pre-AIDS. *Science* **224**: 497.

Planas-Bohne, F. (1981) Metabolism and pharmacokinetics of penicillamine in rats—an overview. *J. Rheumatol.* **8**: 35.

Ratner, L., Haseltine, W.A., Patarca, R., Livak, K.J., Starich, B., Josephs, F., Doran, E.R., Rafalsky, J.A., Whitehorn, E.A., Baumeister, K., Ivanoff, L., Petteway, S.R., Jr., Pearson, M.L., Lautenberger, J.A., Papas, T.S., Ghrayeb, J., Chang, N.T., Gallo, R.C., and Wong-Staal, F. (1985) Complete nucleotide sequence of the acquired immune deficiency virus, human T-cell leukemia virus type III. *Nature* **313**: 277.

Reza-Sadai, M., Benter, T., and Wong-Staal, F. (1988) Site directed mutagenesis of two trans-regulatory genes (*tat*-III, *trs*) of HIV-1. *Science* **239**: 910.

Rice, A.P., and Matthews, M.B. (1988) Transcriptional but not translational regulation of HIV-1 by the *tat* gene product. *Nature* **332**: 551.

Richman, D.D., Fischl, M.A., Grieco, M.H., Gottlieb, M.S., Volberding, P.A., Lascin, O.A., Groopman, J.E., and Mildvan, D. (1987) The toxicity of azido-thymidine (AZT) in the treatment of patients with AIDS and AIDS-related complex: A double-blind, placebo-controlled trial. *New Engl. J. Med.* **317**: 192.

Richman, D.D., Kornblut, R.S., and Carson, D.A. (1987) Failure of dideoxynucleosides to inhibit human immunodeficiency virus replication in cultured human macrophages. *J. Exptl. Med.* **166**: 1144.

Robert-Guroff, M., Brown, M., and Gallo, R.C. (1985) HTLV-III neutralizing antibody in patients with AIDS and ARC. *Nature* **316**: 72.

Rosen, C.A., Sodrosky, J.G., and Haseltine, W.A. (1985) The location of *cis*-acting regulatory sequences in the human T-cell lymphotropic virus type III long terminal repeat. *Cell* **41**: 813.

Rosen, C.A., Terwillinger, E., Dayton, A., Sodrosky, J.G., and Haseltine, W.A. (1988) Intragenic *cis*-acting art gene responsive sequences of the human immunodeficiency virus. *Proc. Natl. Acad. Sci. USA* **85**: 2071.

Sarin, P.S., Gallo, R.C., Sheer, D.I., Crews, F., and Lippa, A.S. (1985) Effect of a novel compound (AL 721) on HTLV-III infectivity *in vitro*. *New Engl. J. Med.* **313**: 1289.

Sarin, P.S., Sun, D., Civeira, M., Thornton, A., Schulof, R., and Chandra, P. (1987) Abstract. In 3rd International Conference on AIDS, p. 14.

Schuloff, R.S., Scheib, R.G., Parenti, D.M., Simon, D.M., DiGioia, G.L., Paxton, H.M., Sztein, M.B., Chandra, P., Courtless, J.W., Taguchi, Y.M., Sun, K.D., Goldstein, A.L., and Sarin, P.S. (1986) Treatment of HTLV-III/LAV-infected patients with D-penicillamine. *Drug Res.* **36**: 1531.

Siedentopf, H.G., and Chandra, P. (1988) Manuscript in preparation.

Siekevitz, M., Josefs, S.F., Dukovich, M., Pfeffer, N., Wong-Staal, F., and Green, W.C. (1987) Activation of the HIV-1 LTR by T-cell mitogens and the transactivator protein of HTLV-1. *Science* **238**: 1575.

Sodrosky, J., Goh, W.C., Rosen, C., Dayton, A., Terwillinger, E., and Haseltine, W. (1986) A second post-transcriptional trans-activator gene is required for HTLV-III replication. *Nature* **321**: 412.

Strebel, K., Daugherty, D., Clouse, K., Kolst, T., and Martin, M.A. (1987) The HIV "A" (*sor*) gene is essential for virus infectivity. *Nature* **328**: 728.

Traunecker, A., Lüke, W., and Karjalainen, K. (1988) Soluble CD4 molecules neutralize human immunodeficiency virus type 1. *Nature* **331**: 84.

Wacker, A., Heyl, E. and Chandra, P. (1966) Zum Wirkungsmechanismus von D- and L-Peniclliamin. *Drug Res.* **16**: 825.

Wacker, A., Heyl, E., and Chandra, P. (1971) Molekularbiologische Untersuchungen mit L-Penicillamin. *Drug Res.* **21**: 971.

Walshe, J.M. (1956) Wilson's disease, new oral therapy. *Lancet* **1**: 25.

Weller, S.K., Joy, A.E., and Temin, H.M. (1980) Correlation between cell killing and massive second superinfection by members of some subgroups of avian leukosis virus. *J. Virol.* **33**: 494.

Weiss, R.A. (1988) Receptor molecule blocks HIV. *Nature* **331**: 15.

Wong-Staal, F., Chanda, P.K., and Ghrayeb, J. (1987) Human immunodeficiency virus type III: The eight gene. *AIDS Res. Human Retrovir.* **3**: 33.

Yarchoan, R., and Broder, S. (1987) Development of antiviral therapy for the acquired immunodeficiency syndrome and related disorders: A progress report. *New Engl. J. Med.* **316**: 557.

CHAPTER 4

MOLECULAR ASPECTS IN THE DEVELOPMENT OF ANTHRACYCLINES AND OTHER ANTITUMOR ANTIBIOTICS

FEDERICO ARCAMONE
Menarini Ricerche Sud, Pomezia, Italy

Abstract—Most clinically useful anticancer drugs act through a mechanism involving an impairment of DNA synthesis and/or function. Among these are the antitumor anthracycline glycosides. Doxorubicin (Adriamycin) is well known because of its spectrum of activity against a variety of solid tumors in humans. New analogs have been developed that exhibit favorable pharmacological properties such as epirubicin (4′-epidoxorubicin), idarubicin (4-demethoxydaunorubicin), 4′-deoxy-4′-iododoxorubicin, 4′-tetrahydropyranyl-doxorubicin, and the biosynthetic compound aclacinomycin. Evidence is available that cell DNA is the main target of antitumor anthracyclines.

A new interesting objective in the field of compounds acting at the nucleic acid level is the identification of structural types endowed with selective DNA sequence specificity. The pyrrole amidine oligopeptide antibiotics, namely, distamycin and its congeners, bind according to a nonintercalative fashion in the minor groove of B-DNA and exhibit a high specificity for AT-rich sequences. Analogs possessing electrophilic reactive groups have been synthesized and studied. The compounds show noticeable antitumor properties. In the case of some derivatives in this series, the formation of covalent adducts could be demonstrated.

1. INTRODUCTION

More than 50 anticancer drugs have reached the clinical stage in the last 40 years. Essential drugs for cancer chemotherapy according to the World Health Organization are antibiotics such as bleomycin, dactinomycin, doxorubicin, metabolic inhibitors such as cytarabine, mercaptopurine, methotrexate, alkylating agents such as cyclophosphamide, procarbazine, cisplatin, plant products such as etoposide and vincristine, and hormones such as the corticosteroids, the estrogens, and the antiestrogen compound, tamoxifen. Although evidence of a cure or prolonged survival in a high proportion of patients is present for acute leukemias, lymphomas, testicular cancer, Ewing's sarcoma, soft tissue sarcomas, small-cell lung cancer, and Kaposi's sarcoma, and evidence of response is obtained in other tumors including breast cancer, no effective drugs are available in lung cancer except SCLC, in cancers of the oesophagus, colorectum, pancreas, cervix, penis, kidney, and malignant melanoma (Hansen et al., 1985). In addition, most anticancer agents presently in use are endowed with considerable side effects that limit both dose levels and duration of therapy. Therefore there is a great need of improved drugs with a larger spectrum of antitumor activity and lower toxicity, that is, a greater selectivity of action.

Practically all compounds mentioned interfere with DNA synthesis or function. The antibiotics bind to double-helical DNA by intercalation, the ultimate irreversible reactions being of different kinds, for example, DNA radical cleavage in the case of bleomycin and the formation of a cleavable tertiary complex with the enzyme topoisomerase II in that of doxorubicin. The antimetabolites inhibit proliferation through an impairment of the enzyme systems involved in DNA synthesis. The alkylating agents, the first anticancer drugs used in medical treatment of human tumors, react directly with the DNA target giving rise to covalent adducts. The natural products of plant origin interact with proteins relevant to DNA function, such as topoisomerase II or tubulin (Powis & Prough, 1987). The endocrinological agents, namely, the estrogens and the estrogen antagonist, also exert their pharmacological actions upon direct regulation of gene expression in human breast cancer. This occurs through the activation of specific transcriptional programs by the drug receptor complex (Dickson & Lippman, 1987).

In connection with the fact that many clinically useful anticancer drugs interact directly with the DNA molecule, it might be of interest to explore the pharmacology of DNA sequence-specific analogs. These might result in more selective antiproliferative agents were their affinity more pronounced toward base sequences involved in transcription processes for factors related with uncontrolled tumoral growth. A first step in this direction would be the evaluation of molecular requirements for base sequence specificity.

2. THE ANTHRACYCLINE GLYCOSIDES

2.1. The DNA Receptor

The anthracycline glycosides are of the greatest importance because of their spectrum of activity against a variety of hematological malignancies and of solid tumors in humans. Clinical usefulness has been established for different compounds in this series, the corresponding chemical structures being shown in Fig. 4-1. Evidence is available that cell DNA is the main biological target of antitumor anthracyclines (Fig. 4-2). This is deduced from a series of pharmacological and biochemical observations, and is in agreement with the high-affinity constant of doxorubicin and its clinically effective congeners for native double-stranded DNA (Arcamone, 1981, 1984). The crystal structure of the daunorubicin-d$(CGTACG)_2$ complex has been solved by X-ray diffraction analysis at atomic-level resolution by Wang et al. (1987). *Inter alia*, the structure of the intercalation complex shows that the 09 hydroxyl group of the antibiotic forms two hydrogen bonds with N3 and N2 of an adjacent guanine base, and the aminosugar lies in the minor groove without bonding to the DNA. The 3′-amino and 4′-hydroxyl groups are pointing away from the oligodeoxynucleotide and are possibly available for other interactions. This observation can be related with the established dependence of bioactivity on the orientation of the sugar substituents in the antitumor anthracycline glycosides (Arcamone & Penco, 1987).

Although the reversible intercalation mode is the generally accepted mechanism of DNA binding, anthracycline derivatives are known in which the formation of covalent adducts is apparently responsible for the biological effects. This is the case for 3′-deamino-3′-(2-cyanomorpholinyl)-doxorubicin whose binding onto DNA is irreversible and whose bioactivity is from two to three orders of magnitude higher than that of the clinically used anthracyclines. However, the compound has not been developed as an anticancer drug because of unfavorable pharmacological properties (Westendorf et al., 1985).

2.2. Base Specificity

The anthracyclines are now consistently considered, both on the basis of theoretical computations (Chen et al., 1985) and of experimental data (Chaires et al., 1987; Patel et al., 1981), as able to recognize specific DNA binding sites. The preferred sequence is represented by a triplet of bases containing two adjacent GC base pairs (the intercalation site) flanking an AT base pair positioned at the 5′ end of the said dinucleotide residues. The preference for the intercalation site would be due to the 9-hydroxy group because of hydrogen bonding interactions and that for the AT pair next to the intercalation site would be attributed to the repulsion between the daunosamine amino group and a guanine residue in that position. Changes in base preference were, however, recorded in anthracycline derivatives when these were compared with the parent antibiotic (Arcamone, 1988). A step forward toward improved selectivity would be the synthesis of derivatives endowed with recognition properties for base sequences longer than a mere triplet.

3. THE DISTAMYCIN DERIVATIVES

3.1. The DNA Complex

A group of compounds characterized by a strong and selective affinity for double-stranded B-DNA is represented by the antibiotics distamycin and netropsin, and by their natural or synthetic congeners (Fig. 4-3). Distamycin, an antiviral antibiotic active against

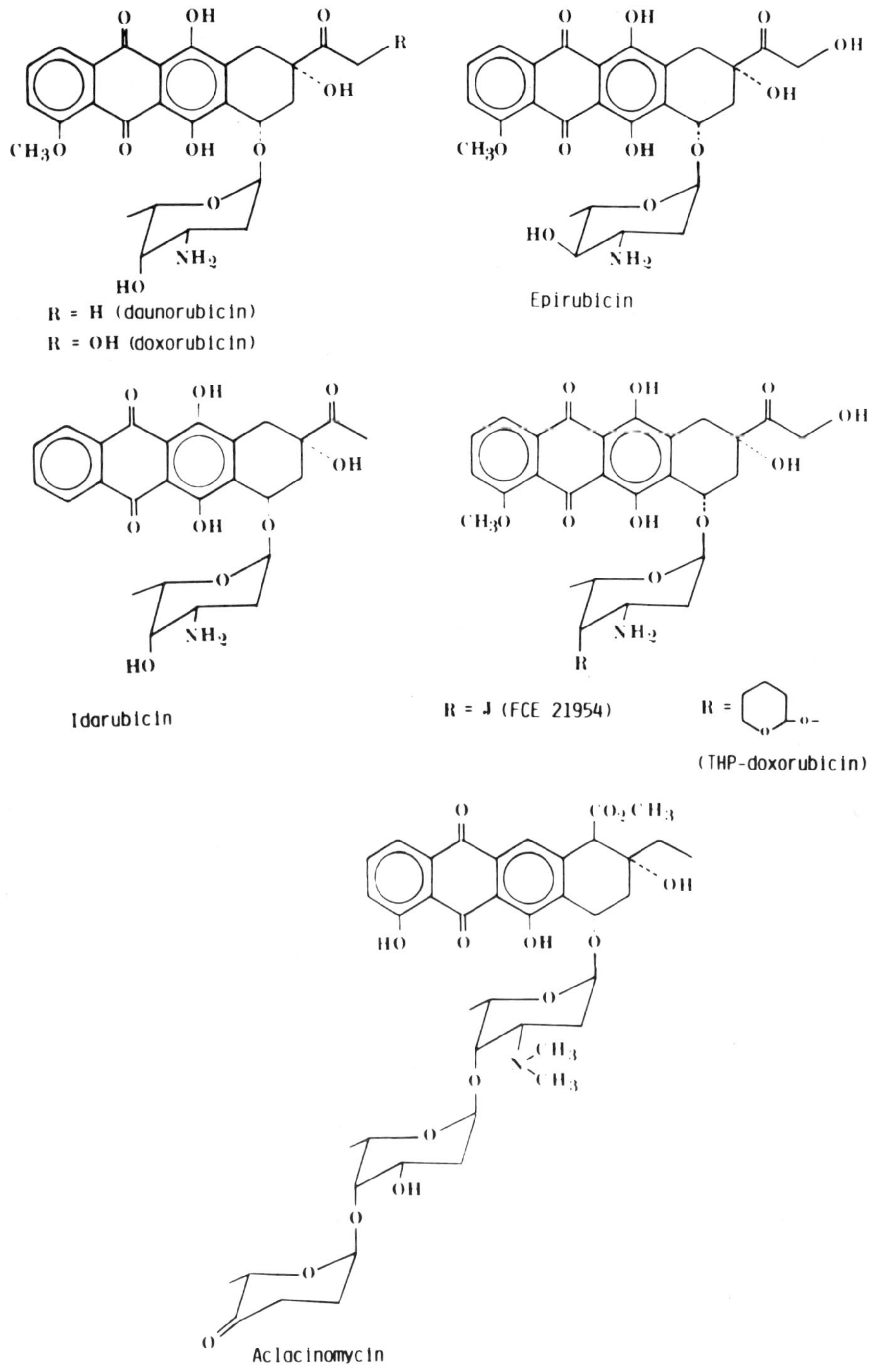

R = H (daunorubicin)
R = OH (doxorubicin)

Epirubicin

Idarubicin

R = I (FCE 21954)

(THP-doxorubicin)

Aclacinomycin

FIG. 4-1. Anthracycline glycosides of clinical interest.

human infections due to herpes simplex, herpes zoster, varicella, and poxvirus, was originally obtained from *Streptomyces distallicus* and also by total synthesis (Arcamone et al., 1964). The compound exhibits selective binding to AT-rich regions of double-helical DNA, a property that is at the base of current uses of distamycin in molecular biology and genetic analysis (for a comprehensive review, see Zimmer & Wähnert, 1986). A recent X-ray diffraction study has confirmed the structure formerly attributed to the DNA complex by elucidating the complex between the related netropsin and a B-DNA synthetic dodecamer

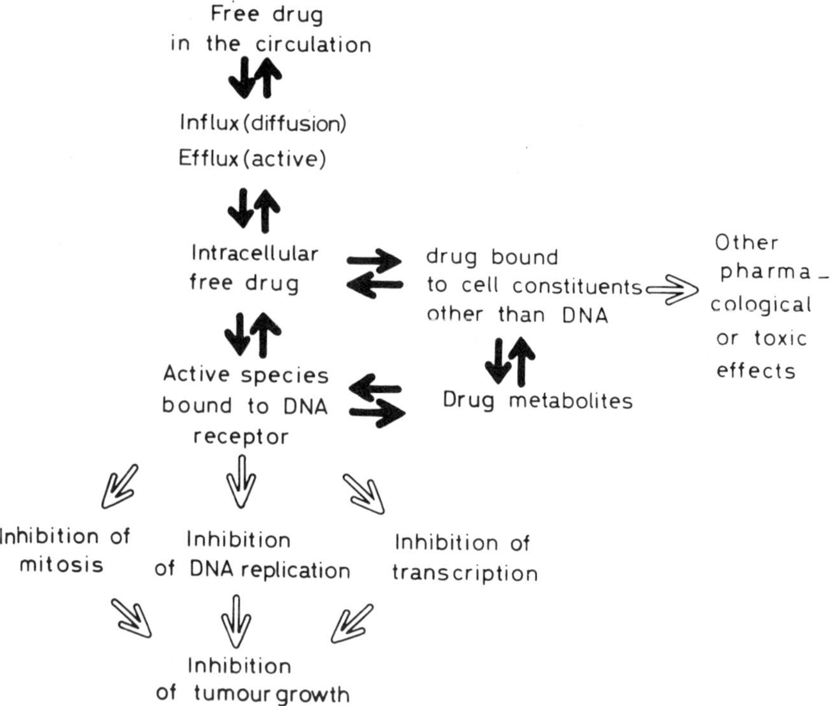

FIG. 4-2. Biochemical events related with cell pharmacology of antitumor anthracyclines.

(Kopka et al., 1985). The binding of the drugs as nonintercalating agents in the minor groove of the B-DNA double helix has been therefore definitely proved. According to theoretical computations that take into account the different components of the interaction energy, it has been deduced that, although hydrogen bonds between the carboxamido groups of the ligand and the proton accepting sites of the macromolecule (namely, N-3 of adenines and O-2 of thymines) contribute to the energy of binding, the favorable electronegative surface potentials generated by the AT sequences in minor groove are sufficient to allow stabilization of the complex (Pullman, 1987).

3.2. SEMISYNTHETIC DERIVATIVES

Former investigations involving the synthesis and biological evaluation of distamycin analogs indicated the favorable effect of increasing the number of the pyrrole units, the strict requirement of the N-formyl group, and the compatibility of different C-terminus side chains for antiviral activity (Arcamone, 1972). More recently, distamycinlike compounds in which a nonpyrrole ring was added with the same chemical arrangements on the left side of the molecule were synthesized and tested in cell cultures infected with herpes virus or with Moloney sarcoma virus. Compounds in which the added ring was a benzene ring or a thiophene ring showed remarkable antiviral properties and all compounds revealed the same strong preference for AT-rich sequences shown by the parent antibiotic (Arcamone et al., 1986).

To obtain potential cytotoxic derivatives in which the AT selective structures were associated with a chemically reactive function, compounds bearing electrophilic groups have been synthesized. A first type is represented by the nitrogen mustards presented in Fig. 4-4. These derivatives combine AT sequence specificity with alkylating properties and marked cytotoxic activity. In fact irreversibly bound adducts are formed upon incubation of the first compound of Fig. 4-4 with both calf thymus DNA and with poly d(A-T), but not with poly d(G-C). In the course of these investigations it was found that for nitrogen mustard

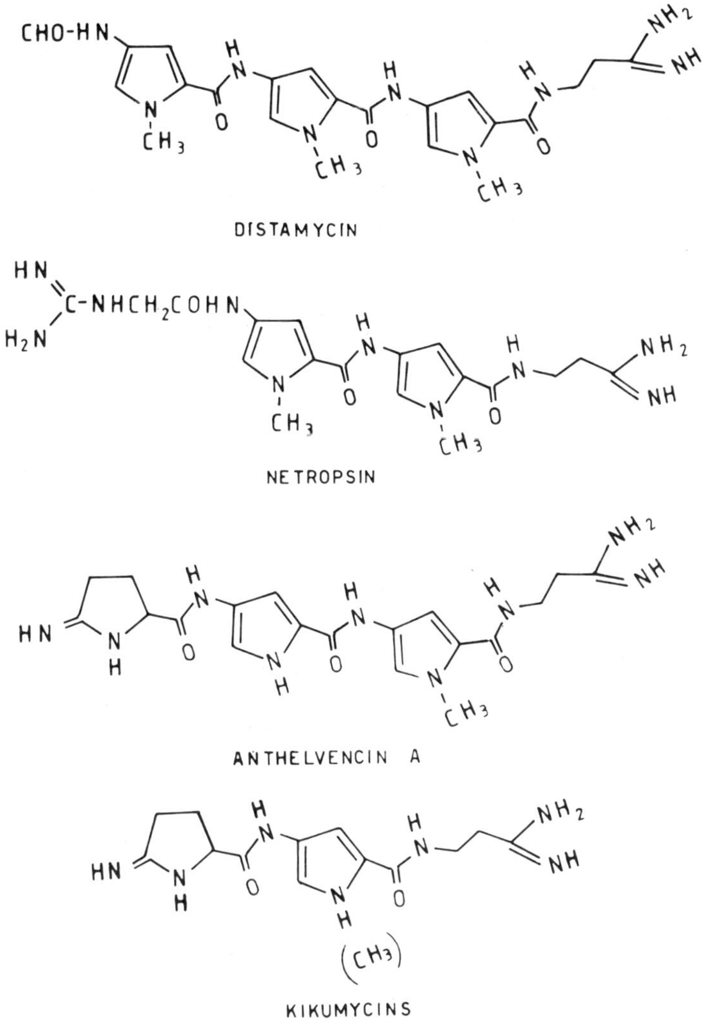

DISTAMYCIN

NETROPSIN

ANTHELVENCIN A

KIKUMYCINS

FIG. 4-3. The pyrroleamidine oligopeptide antibiotics.

derivatives in which the last ring on the left side was a benzene or a thiophene instead of a pyrrole (Fig. 4-4), the high selectivity for AT sequences was maintained but no alkylation of DNA was evidenced in the *in vitro* incubations. The compounds displayed, however, high cytotoxicity in cell cultures and remarkable antitumor activity in mice, allowing the deduction that instead of the formation of covalent adducts with DNA, alkylation of other molecules associated with AT-rich DNA sequences might be the pharmacologically relevant event responsible for the inhibition of cell viability (Arcamone et al., 1988).

4. CONCLUSION AND PERSPECTIVES

The DNA-binding antibiotics represent a group of compounds of considerable pharmacological importance, and some of them have been already used successfully in the medical treatment of cancer. Advancements in the knowledge of the chemical structure of their complexes with DNA have allowed better understanding of the molecular requirements for bioactivity and the synthesis of potentially effective new drugs. However, a jump toward an improved level of selectivity will be attained when the pharmacological consequences of different degrees of DNA sequence selectivity will be evaluated. As it has been recently shown, using distamycin (Bruzik et al., 1987), the possibility of specific regulation of gene

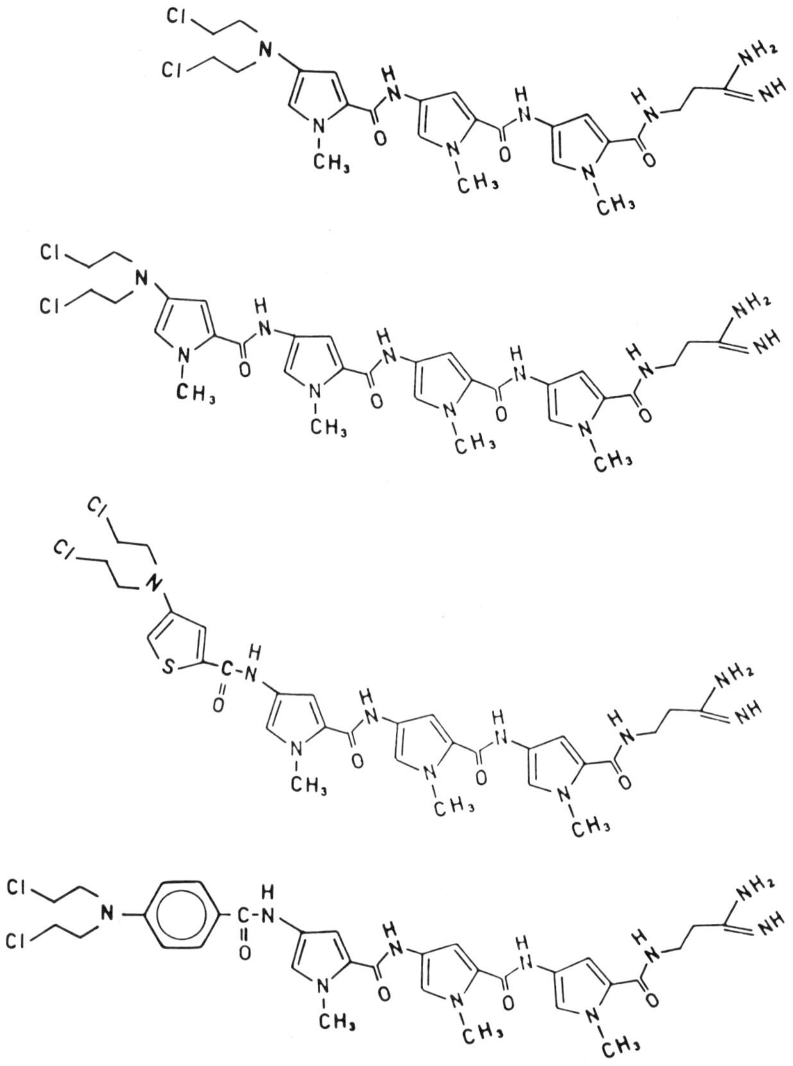

FIG. 4-4. Novel cancerostatic molecules derived from distamycin.

transcription with low-molecular sequence-selective DNA-binding compounds is real. This will provide to the medicinal chemist new approaches for the design of less toxic antiviral and anticancer drugs.

REFERENCES

Arcamone, F. (1988). Chemical approaches in anticancer drug development. *Cancer Treat. Rev.* **15**: 65–68.

Arcamone, F. (1984) Antitumor anthracyclines: Recent developments. *Med. Res. Rev.* **4**: 153–188.

Arcamone, F. (1981) *Doxorubicin, Medicinal chemistry series*, G. Stevens, ed., Vol. 17. New York: Academic Press.

Arcamone, F. (1972) On distamycin A and related compounds, selective antiviral agents. In *Medicinal chemistry*, P. Pratesi, ed., pp. 29–45. London: Butterworth.

Arcamone, F., Animati, F., Barbieri, B., Configliacchi, E., D'Alessio, R., Geroni, C., Giuliani, F. C., Lazzeri, E., Menozzi, M., Mongelli, N., Penco, S., and Verini, M. A. (1988) Synthesis, DNA-binding properties and antitumor activity of novel distamycin derivatives. *J. Med. Chem.*, in press.

Arcamone, F., and Penco, S. (1987). Chemical derivatives of anticancer antibiotics with different DNA binding properties. In *Molecular mechanism of carcinogenic and antitumor activity*, C. Chagas and B. Pullman, eds., pp. 225–241. Città del Vaticano: Pontificia Academia Scientiarum.

Arcamone, F., Lazzeri, E., Menozzi, M., Soranzo, C., and Verini, M. A. (1986) Synthesis, DNA binding, and antiviral activity of distamycin analogues containing different heterocyclic moieties. *Anti-Cancer Drug Design* **1**: 235–244.

Arcamone, F., Penco, S., Orezzi, P., Nicolella, V., and Pirelli, A. (1964) Structure and synthesis of distamycin A. *Nature* **203**: 1064–1065.

Bruzik, J. P., Auble, D. T., and de Haseth, P. L. (1987) Specific activation of transcription initiation by the sequence-specific DNA-binding agents distamycin A and netropsin. *Biochemistry* **26**: 950–956.

Chaires, J. B., Fox, K. R., Herrera, J. E., Britt, M., and Waring, M. J. (1987) Site and sequence specificity of the daunomycin–DNA interaction. *Biochemistry* **26**: 8227–8236.

Chen, K., Gresh, N., and Pullman, B. (1985) A theoretical study of the comparative binding affinities of daunomycin derivatives to a double-stranded oligomeric DNA. Proposal for new high-affinity derivatives. *J. Biomol. Struct. Dynam.* **3**: 445–466.

Dickson, R. B., and Lippman, M. E. (1987). Estrogenic regulation of growth and polypeptide growth factor secretion in human breast carcinoma. *Endocrine Reviews* **8**: 29–43.

Hansen, H. H., Hoth, H. D., Lira Puerto, V., Olweny, C. L., and Tattersall, M. (1985) Essential drugs for cancer chemotherapy: Memorandum from a WHO meeting. *Bull. WHO* **63**: 999–1002

Kopka, M. L., Yoon, C., Goddsell, D., Pijura, P., and Dickerson, R. E. (1985) The molecular origin of DNA–drug specificity in netropsin and distamycin. *Proc. Natl. Acad. Sci. USA* **82**: 1376–1380.

Patel, D. J., Kozlowski, S. A., and Rice, J. A. (1981) Hydrogen bonding, overlap geometry, and sequence specificity in anthracycline antitumor–DNA complexes in solution. *Proc. Natl. Acad. Sci. USA* **78**: 3333–3337.

Powis, G., and Prough, R. A. (eds.). (1987) *Metabolism and action of anti-cancer drugs.* London: Taylor & Francis.

Pullman, B. (1987) Introductory lecture: Carcinogens, antitumor agents and DNA. In *Molecular mechanisms of carcinogenic and antitumor activity*, C. Chagas and B. Pullman, eds., pp. 3–31. Città del Vaticano: Pontificia Academia Scientiarum.

Wang, A. H., Ughetto, G., Higley, G. J., and Rich, A. (1987) Interactions between an anthracycline antibiotic and DNA: Molecular structure of daunomycin complex to d(CpGpTpApCpG) at 1.2-Å resolution. *Biochemistry* **26**: 1152–1163.

Westendorf, J., Groth, G., Steinheider, G., and Marquardt, H. (1985) Formation of DNA-adducts and induction of DNA crosslinks and chromosomal aberrations by the new potent anthracycline antitumor antibiotics: Morpholinodaunomycin, cyanomorpholinodaunomycin, and cyanomorpholinoadriamycin. *Cell Biol. Toxicol.* **1**: 87–101.

Zimmer, C., and Wähnert, V. (1986) Nonintercalating DNA-binding ligands: Specificity of interaction and their use as tools in biophysical, biochemical and biological investigations of the genetic material. *Prog. Biophys. Molec. Biol.* **47**: 31–112.

CHAPTER 5

NEW CONCEPTS FOR THE DEVELOPMENT OF SELECTIVE ANTICANCER DRUGS

LUTZ F. TIETZE

Institute of Organic Chemistry, University of Göttingen, Göttingen, Federal Republic of Germany

Abstract—Based on the findings that the pH in tumors can be decreased to even 5.2 by stimulation of the tumor cell glycolysis through hyperglycemia, a new concept was developed for more selective anticancer agents. Thus, nontoxic prodrugs of aldophosphamide—the active metabolite of cyclophosphamide—and other cytotoxic aldehydes were synthesized, from which the cytotoxic agent is preferentially liberated at lower pH by proton-catalyzed or enzymatic hydrolysis. For example, application of the 2-hexenopyranoside of aldophosphamide 10 in cell cultures causes a decrease of the survival fraction by 10^4 at pH 5.6 compared to the pH in the serum of 7.4.

1. INTRODUCTION

Today, a quarter of all deaths are connected to malignant tumors (McKay, 1982; Miller & McKay, 1984). Yet the treatment of cancer is extremely difficult, considering the more than 100 different types of cancer that are known. Also, our knowledge of the pathogenesis of malignant tumors is still highly limited, so we can assume that the prevention of cancer by immunization or a change of life-style will not occur in the near future. However, when a direct connection between toxins and cancer can be identified, prevention is feasible—as for the so-called "asbestos"-, "aniline"-, and "arsenic"-induced cancers. Eventually this may also be possible for smoking-induced cancer (Cairns, 1986).

The main methods for the treatment of cancer are based on radiology, surgery, and chemotherapy (Tanneberger, 1980; Bruhn, 1980; Schmähl, 1981; Brunner & Nagel, 1985; Brade & Niemeyer, 1987); surgery, although more successful than other methods, often reaches its limits, since malignant tumors have an invasive character and are difficult to delimitate. In this respect chemotherapy should provide the solution, since it works at the molecular level.

2. BIOCHEMICAL DIFFERENCES OF MALIGNANT AND NORMAL CELL POPULATIONS

All known cytotoxic agents used for the treatment of cancer display strong side effects, which very often result in the discontinuation of their application. Thus chemotherapy of cancer is discussed in a very controversial way today (Frei & Canellos, 1980; Evans et al., 1986). Different types of cytotoxic compounds are known such as alkylating compounds, antimetabolites, antibiotics, antimitotic drugs, and metal complexes (Fig. 5-1.). These compounds have different sites of attack, but in all cases the differentiation between normal and malignant cells is based only on the difference in the amount of proliferating cells in the tumor and the normal cell population. This means that all rapidly proliferating normal cells, for example, the gonads, the intestinal membranes, and the roots of hairs, are also damaged by the application of these chemotherapeutic agents.

The main goal in the development of new antitumor agents is therefore not to find substances of higher activity, but to increase their therapeutic index. There are some new approaches, for example, activation of the immunosystem; however, a breakthrough in this area has not been obtained so far.

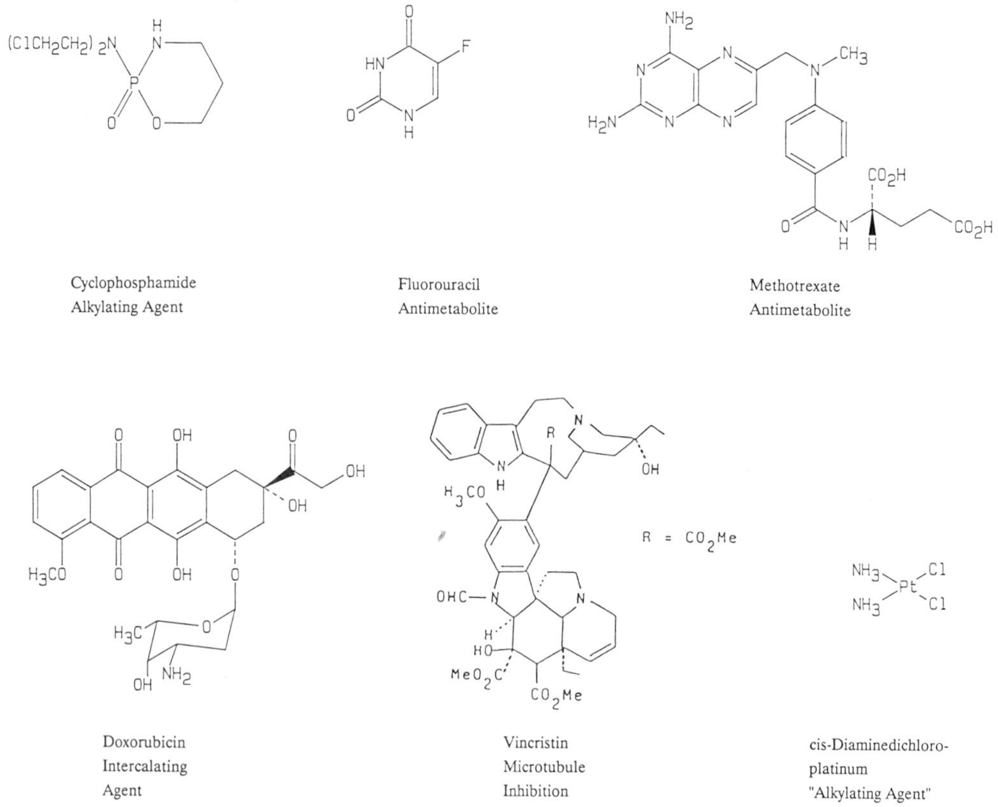

Cyclophosphamide
Alkylating Agent

Fluorouracil
Antimetabolite

Methotrexate
Antimetabolite

Doxorubicin
Intercalating
Agent

Vincristin
Microtubule
Inhibition

R = CO_2Me

cis-Diaminedichloro-
platinum
"Alkylating Agent"

FIG. 5-1. Different types of cancer chemotherapeutic agents

For the development of more selective cytostatic agents, it is necessary to utilize biochemical differences at the molecular level of malignant and normal cell populations; the differences may be situated in the structure of the cell membrane (Unger et al., 1987) or in the metabolism of the cells (Bodansky, 1975). A few examples of such differences are known already (Gros et al., 1981); thus a higher content of glucuronidase and potassium cations, a lower content of calcium cations, and the lack of asparagine synthetase in malignant cells have been observed. Also, in some cases of leukemia, an RNA-dependent DNA polymerase is found. However, these differences cannot be used for a general chemotherapy since they are not common for all malignant tumors. But there is one main difference in metabolism between normal and malignant cell population which is common for nearly all known types of cancer; this is an increase of the rate of glycolysis.

Warburg (1930) showed, in *in vitro* experiments, that normal cells do not in general produce lactic acid in the presence of glucose and oxygen. Under the same conditions a large amount of lactic acid was formed in malignant cell populations. Previously, Cori and Cori (1925a,b) found that infusion of glucose to mice with a mammary carcinoma causes the formation of lactic acid in the tumor. Recently Jähde and Rajewsky (1982) have established a quantitative correlation between the blood-sugar level and the pH in a tumor. At a concentration of 50 mM, an average of pH 6 was found, and in necrotic areas even pH 5.2. These findings have been confirmed by other authors (Wike-Hooley et al., 1984) by different and independent methods. Some (Osinskii et al., 1987) assume that the average pH may be even lower. In all cases it has been shown that the pH in normal cells is not or almost not influenced by the glucose infusion, an average pH of 7 being measured in brain and the kidneys.

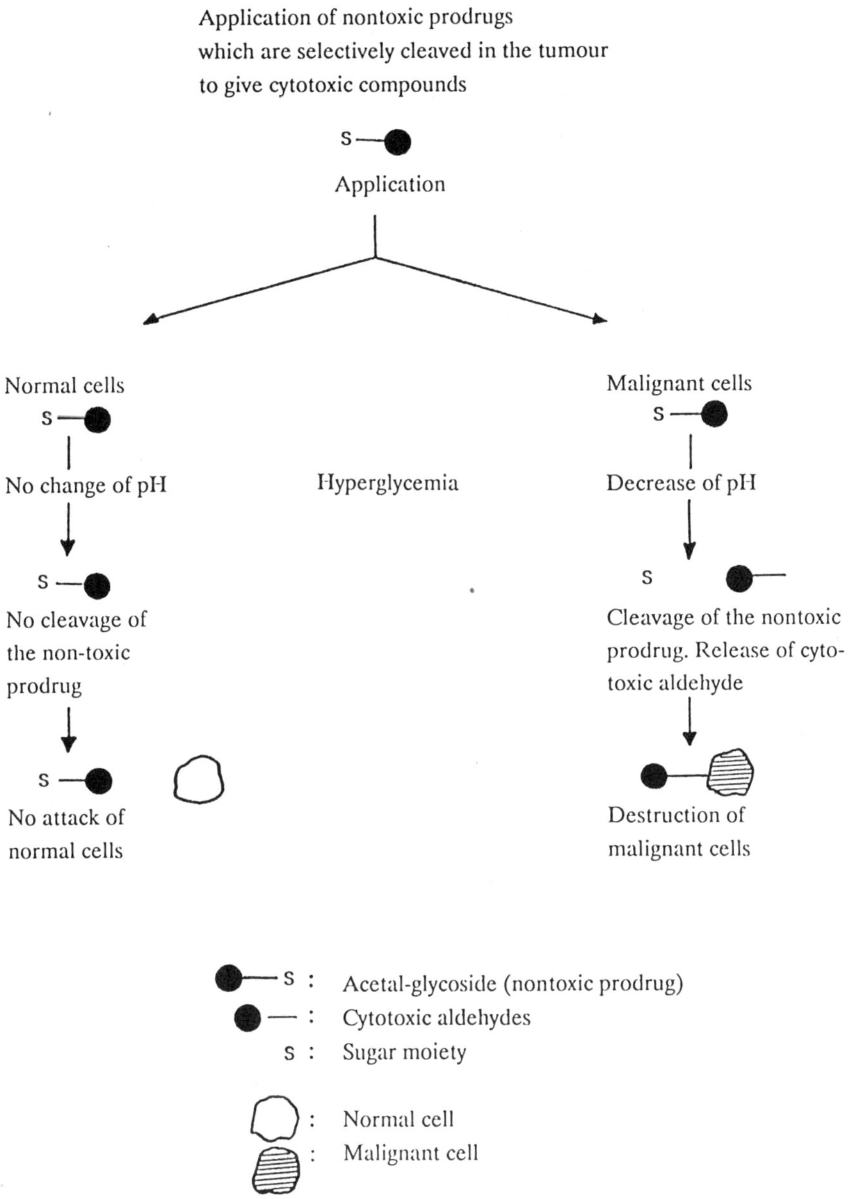

Application of nontoxic prodrugs
which are selectively cleaved in the tumour
to give cytotoxic compounds

S—●
Application

Normal cells
S—●
No change of pH
↓
S—●
No cleavage of the non-toxic prodrug
↓
S—●
No attack of normal cells

Hyperglycemia

Malignant cells
S—●
Decrease of pH
↓
S ●—
Cleavage of the nontoxic prodrug. Release of cytotoxic aldehyde
↓
Destruction of malignant cells

●—S : Acetal-glycoside (nontoxic prodrug)
●— : Cytotoxic aldehydes
S : Sugar moiety

: Normal cell
: Malignant cell

FIG. 5-2. Systematic description of concept I.

3. THE CONCEPT*

Our concept for the development of more selective anticancer drugs is based on the difference of pH in normal and malignant cell populations† (Figs. 5-2 and 5-3):

1. Development of a prodrug which is nontoxic per se, but which can be cleaved selectively in the tumor to give a highly cytotoxic compound. The cleavage can be accomplished

*This project is being carried out in cooperation with M. F. Rajewsky and K.-H. Glüsenkamp, Institut für Zellbiologie (Tumorforschung), Universität Essen, and E. Jähde, Universität Tübingen.

†There are some earlier experiments based on a similar concept (Schulze & Horn, 1970; von Ardenne & Reitnauer, 1975); however, none of these approaches was successful since the compounds employed did not meet the necessary requirements.

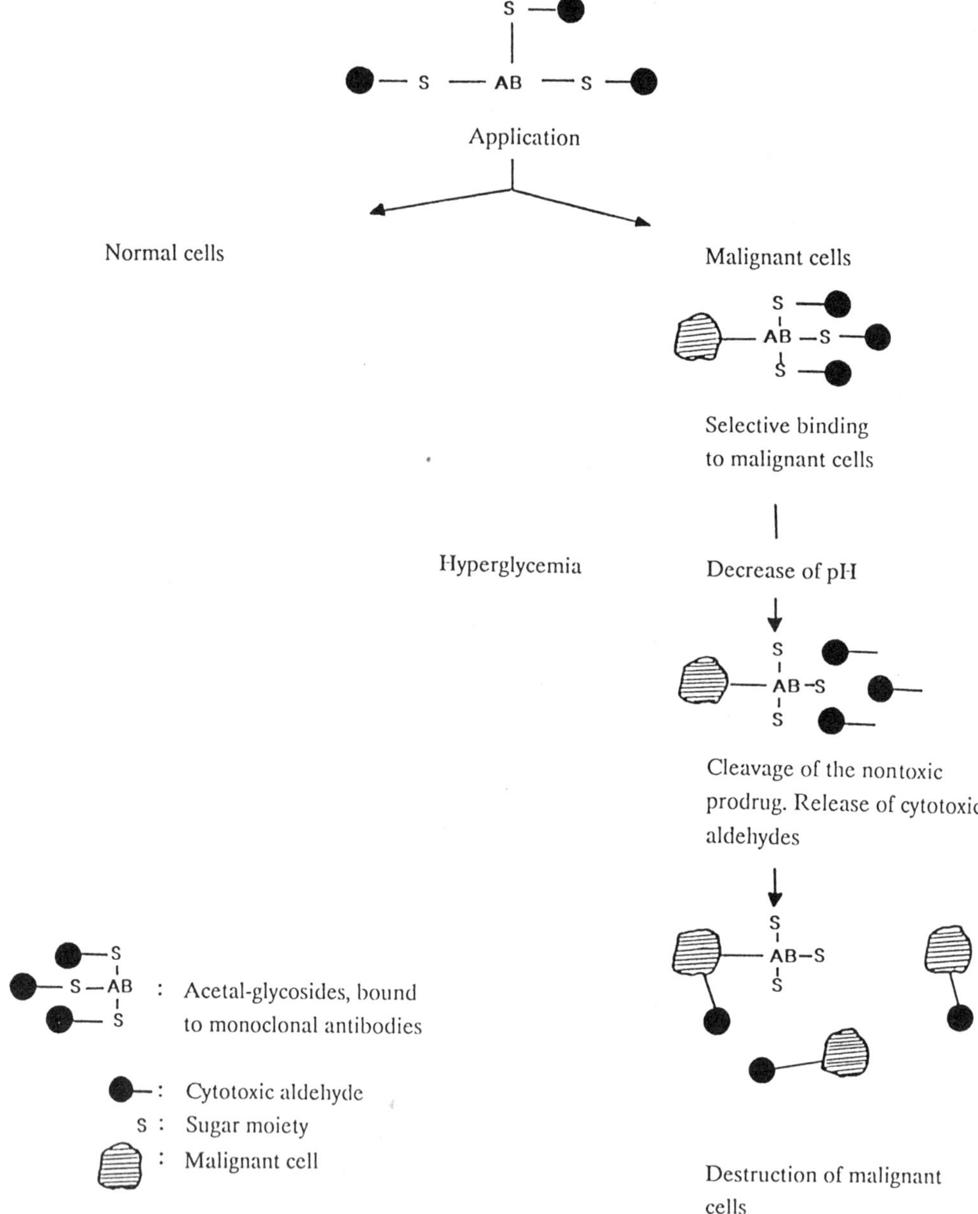

FIG. 5-3. Systematic description of concept II.

by acid-catalyzed hydrolysis at pH 5–6 or by enzymatic hydrolysis with enzymes which have their optimum activity at pH 5–6. The enzymes can be endogenous or can be injected additionally.

2. The selectivity of these compounds can be increased by linking to a monoclonal antibody, which binds to surface antigens of the malignant cells.

3. The enzyme which catalyzes the cleavage of the prodrug can also be linked to an antibody.

For the realization of this concept, all known cytostatic agents which can be blocked to give a nontoxic prodrug could be used. At the moment our interest centers on the use of aldehydes and mustard derivatives. In general, free aldehydes cannot be applied for cancer therapy, since they have a high general toxicity and they are deactivated quite rapidly after intravenous application through reaction with serum proteins and glutathione or by reaction with aldehyde dehydrogenase (Schauenstein et al., 1977).

A few aldehydes, for example, phenylglyoxal and methylglyoxal, have been used in cancer therapy, although with little success (Wolstenholme et al., 1979). *In vitro*, aldehydes exhibit a strong inhibition of DNA synthesis (Tables 5-1 and 5-2).

Another compound which shows a high cytostatic effect is aldophosphamide (Brade & Niemeyer, 1987; Slordal & Aarbakke, 1987). This compound is an intermediate in the metabolism of cyclophosphamide which is in itself inactive. Thus this drug is activated through oxidation in the liver by the hepatic mixed function oxidase system to give the 4-hydroxycyclophosphamide, which is in equilibrium with aldophosphamide (Boyd et al., 1986). A fast elimination of acrolein yields phosphoramide mustard, which forms the aziridinium salt probably as the ultimate cytotoxic compound which reacts with DNA (Fig. 5-4).

4. SELECTION OF ACID-LABILE OR ENZYMATIC CLEAVABLE CHEMICAL MOIETIES

4.1. Synthesis and Toxicity of Acetal-glycosides of Cytotoxic Aldehydes

There are many acid-labile moieties known that could be used for blocking an aldehyde or other cytotoxic compounds to form a nontoxic prodrug. However, the functionality which best meets the requirements is that of an acetal. Since these compounds are not water soluble, and since they cannot be cleaved by enzymes, usually we have designed a new type of compound which consists of a sugar moiety, an aldehyde, and an alcohol.

For the synthesis of these so-called acetal-glycosides (Tietze & Fischer, 1981a,b; Tietze et al., 1987a,b), an acetal of nearly any aldehyde is treated with a protected trimethylsilyl glycoside in the presence of a catalytic amount of trimethylsilyl trifluoromethanesulfonate (TMS-triflate) (Fig. 5-5).

The method is highly selective; thus trimethylsilyl α-glycosides lead to acetal-α-glycosides and the use of trimethylsilyl-β-glycosides gives access to acetal-β-glycosides and, indeed, even the acetal-β-mannosides (L. F. Tietze, R. Seele, and B. Leiting, unpublished results) can be obtained with an anomeric ratio of $> 95:5$. In this reaction it is also possible to use the free aldehydes instead of the acetals; in this case, an alkyl trimethylsilyl ether has to be added.

The toxicity of some of these compounds has been tested *in vivo* (L. F. Tietze and H. D. Schlumberger, unpublished results) and *in vitro* using mice and neuroectodermal cells of

Table 5-1. *Toxicity and Inhibition of DNA Synthesis by Unsaturated Aldehydes*

Compound	Toxicity: mice (LD50) i.p. (mM/kg body weight)	Inhibition of DNA synthesis 10–8 mol per 106EATC, (50% inhibition of thymidine incorporation)
Acrolein	0.103	0.25
2-Butenal	2.3	6.0
2-Hexenal	3.0	8.75
4-Hydroxy-2-pentenal	1.0	4.8
4-Hydroxy-2-heptenal	1.2	5.6

From Schauenstein et al. (1977).

TABLE 5-2. *Effects of Aliphatic Aldehydes on Oxygen Consumption and Leucine Incorporation into Protein in Liver Slices and Yoshida AH130 Ascites Hepatoma Cells in vitro* (concn. 5 mM)

	Inhibition (%) liver slice		Inhibition (%) hepatoma cells	
Aldehyde	oxygen consumption	leucine incorporation	oxygen consumption	leucine incorporation
Acetaldehyde	—	—	0.2	51
Propionaldehyde	0	78	—	37
Butyraldehyde	0	87	0	38
Isobutyraldehyde	4	98	0	48
Crotonaldehyde	5	58	0	31
Lactaldehyde	14	88	7	66
Glyceraldehyde	11	77	15	57
α-Hydroxybutyraldehyde	0	36	12	75
β-Hydroxybutyraldehyde	25	78	36	99
α,β-Dihydroxybutyraldehyde	10	55	5	91

From Perin et al. (1972).

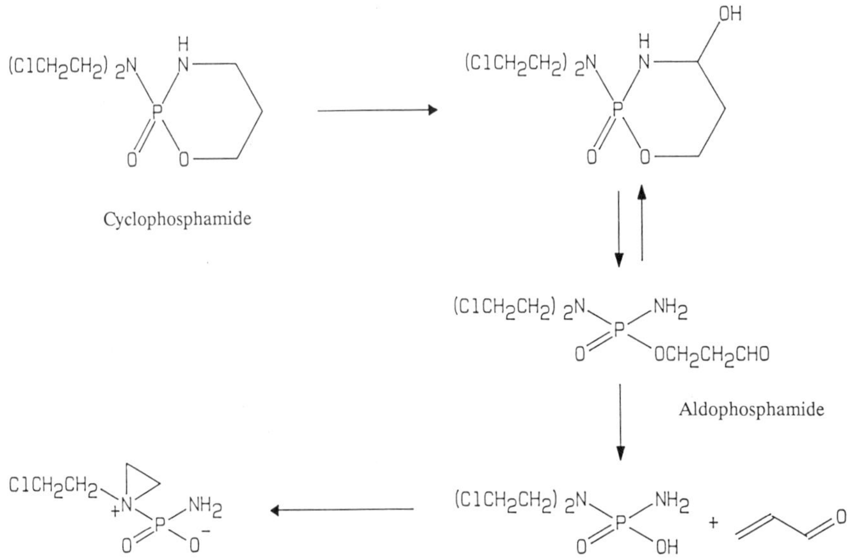

FIG. 5-4. Aldophosphamide: Intermediate in the mode of activation of cyclophosphamide.

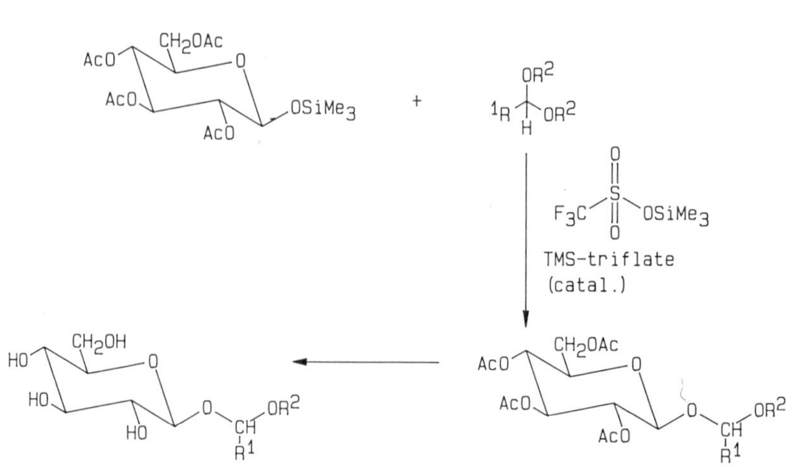

FIG. 5-5. Synthesis of acetal-glycosides: Nontoxic, water-soluble acid-sensitive prodrugs.

BDIX rats on BT1C and TV1C tumors (L. F. Tietze and E. Jähde, unpublished results). The systemic toxicity of these compounds is extremely low, and the LD_{50} could not be determined. By intraperitoneal application of a dose of even 1000 mg/kg body weight, all animals survived; in contrast, using the same dose of cyclophosphamide, all animals died. Also, in cell cultures the acetal-glycosides did not show any cytotoxicity (L. F. Tietze and E. Jähde, unpublished results). Thus, these compounds are nontoxic prodrugs of highly toxic compounds.

4.2. Enzymatic Cleavage and Cytotoxic Action of Acetal-glycosides

The cytotoxic principle of these prodrugs can be released by acid-catalyzed as well as enzymatic hydrolysis (Fig. 5-6). For the enzymatic cleavage of the acetal-glycosides, glycoside hydrolases such as α-glucosidase, α-mannosidase, β-glucosidase, and β-glucuronidase can be applied in accord with the used sugar. The combination of the acetal-β-glucoside of bromoacetaldehyde and β-D-glucosidase, as well as of the acetal-α-glucoside of bromoacetaldehyde with α-D-glucosidase, shows a strong inhibition of cell growth of neuroectodermal cells of the BDIX rat even in a 10^{-5} molar solution; the enzymes themselves were proven to be nontoxic (L. F. Tietze, M. F. Rajewsky, and E. Jähde, unpublished results). Surprisingly, the acetal-glucosides of formaldehyde and 5-hydroxy-2-methoxydihydrofuran did not influence cell growth after addition of the appropriate enzymes. Since it is known that some glycoside hydrolases are found in malignant cells in a higher concentration, for example, β-D-glucuronidase (Conchie & Levvy, 1957; Fishman, 1955; Whitaker, 1960), a selective cleavage in the tumor of appropriate acetal-glycosides should be possible even without a decrease of the pH. However, many glycoside hydrolases show a pronounced dependence of activity on the pH of the medium. Thus β-D-glucosidase, α-D-mannosidase, and β-D-glucuronidase have their rate maxima between pH 5 and 6 and their minima at pH 7. In contrast α-D-glucosidase has its maximum activity at pH 6.5 (Figs. 5-7 and 5-8). The enzymatic hydrolysis rate of the acetal-β-glucoside of bromoacetaldehyde was 10 times more rapid at pH 5.5 than at pH 7.5. An even higher selectivity was obtained with the acetal-α-mannosides. The rate ratio at pH 7 and pH 6 was 1:9.5 for the formaldehyde derivative and 1:15 for the bromoacetaldehyde derivative (Fig. 5-9).

The *in vitro* investigations of these compounds were not only in accord with the measured kinetics but showed even a much higher effect than expected. At pH 7.4 the acetal-β-glucoside and acetal-α-mannoside of bromoacetaldehyde had almost no effect on the growth of the tumor cells, whereas at pH 6.2 a *complete remission* was obtained (Figs. 5-10

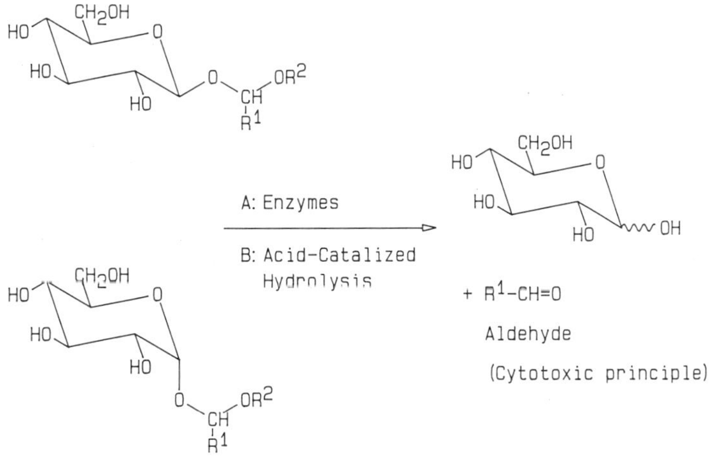

Fig. 5-6. Cleavage of acetal-glycosides.

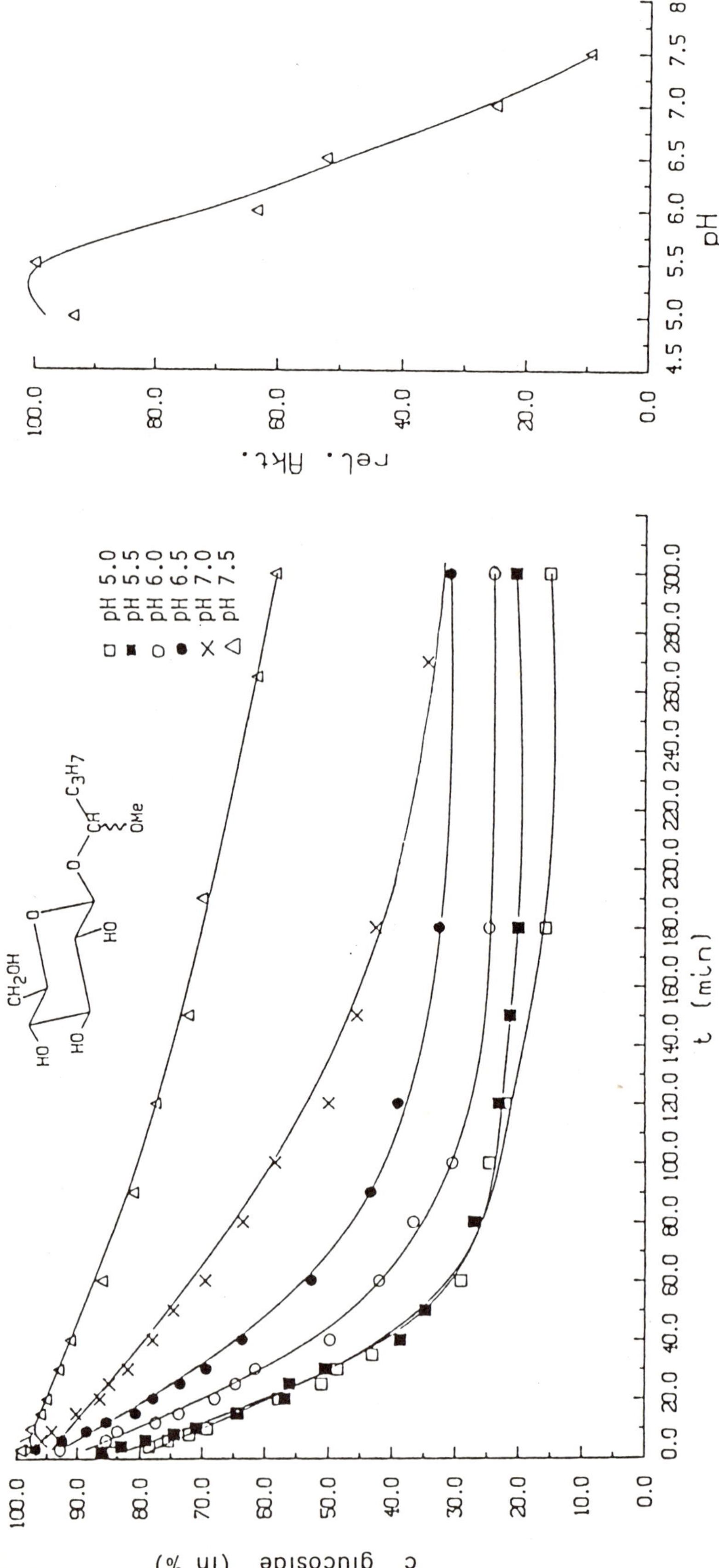

FIG. 5-7. Enzymatic cleavage of acetal-β-glucosides with β-glucosidase at different pH.

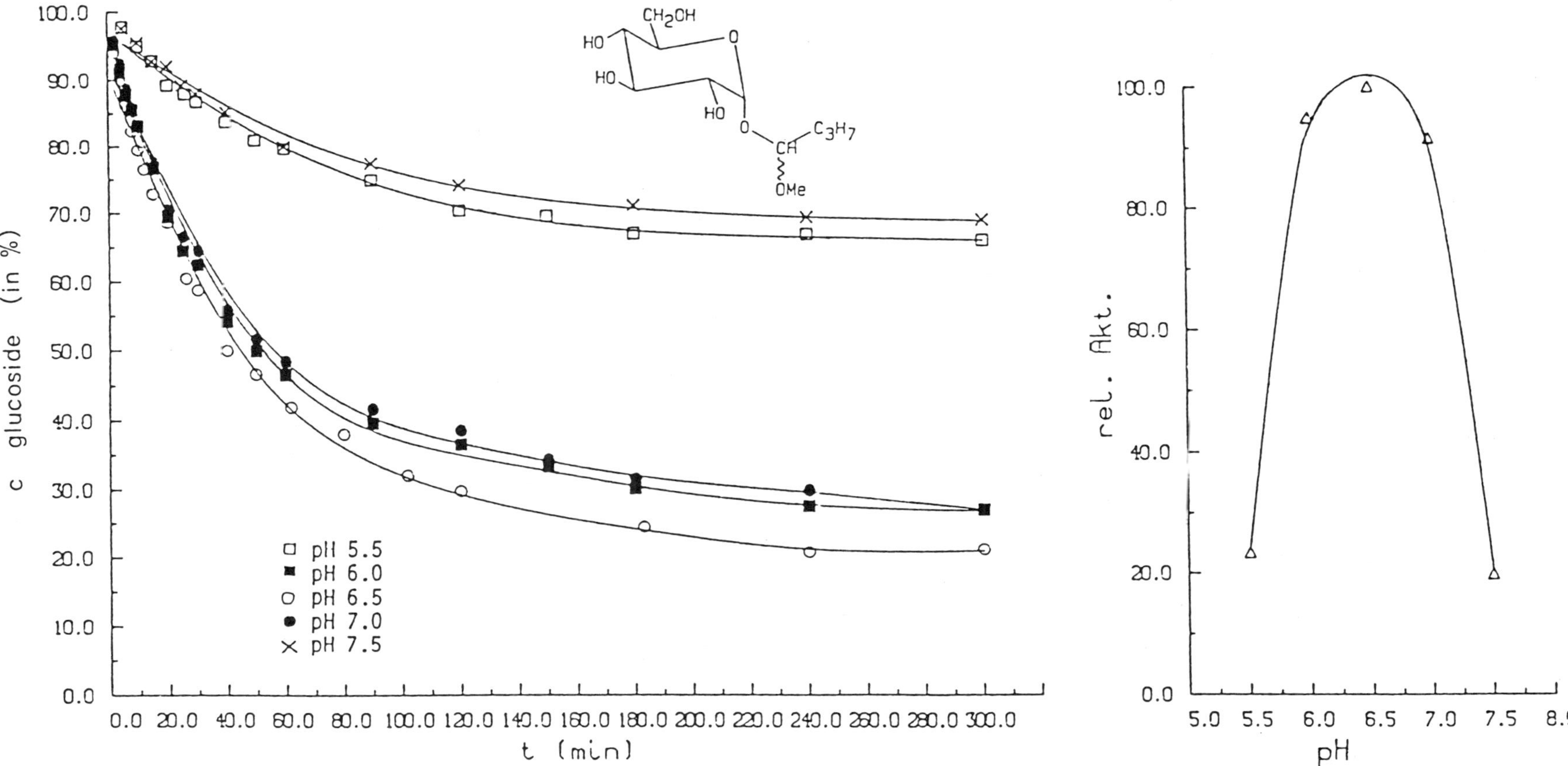

FIG. 5-8. Enzymatic cleavage of acetal-α-glucosides with α-glucosidase at different pH.

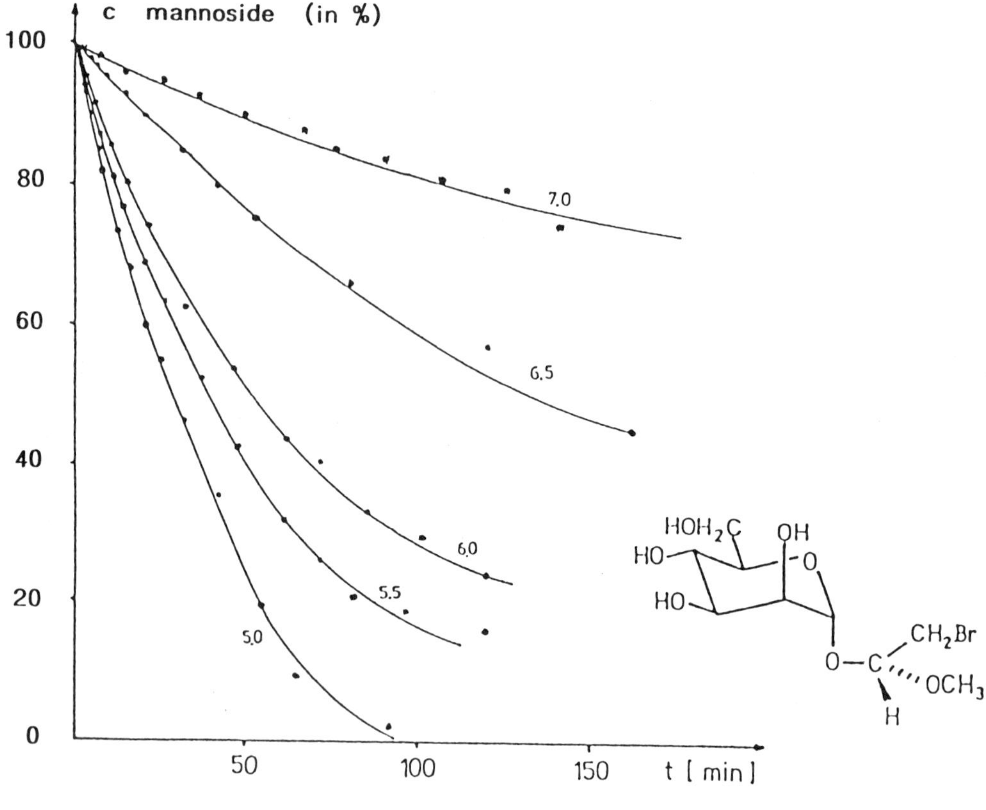

rate constants		factor of selectivity
pH 6.0	pH 7.0	
$8.95 \cdot 10^{-3}$ min^{-1}	$5.98 \cdot 10^{-4}$ min^{-1}	15.0

FIG. 5-9. Enzymatic cleavage of acetal-α-mannoside of bromoacetaldehyde with α-mannosidase at different pH.

and 5-11). Control experiments have clearly proven that this high selectivity is not due to direct damage of the tumors by the hydronium ion concentration.

4.3. Synthesis of Acid-labile Acetal-glycosides of Cytotoxic Aldehydes

Hydrolysis of glycosides, acetals, and similar compounds requires protonation at an oxygen, cleavage of two carbon–oxygen bonds, and the addition of water as well as proton transfer. The reaction is described by the equation (1). It is well established for simple acetals that the rupture of the carbon–oxygen bond leads to a carboxonium ion as an intermediate.

$$R^1R^2C(OR)_2 + H^+ \underset{+ROH}{\overset{-ROH}{\rightleftharpoons}} R^1R^2C^+{-}OR \underset{-H_2O}{\overset{+H_2O}{\rightleftharpoons}} R^1R^2C(OR)(OH) + H^+ \rightleftharpoons R^1R^2C{=}O + ROH + H^+ \quad (1)$$

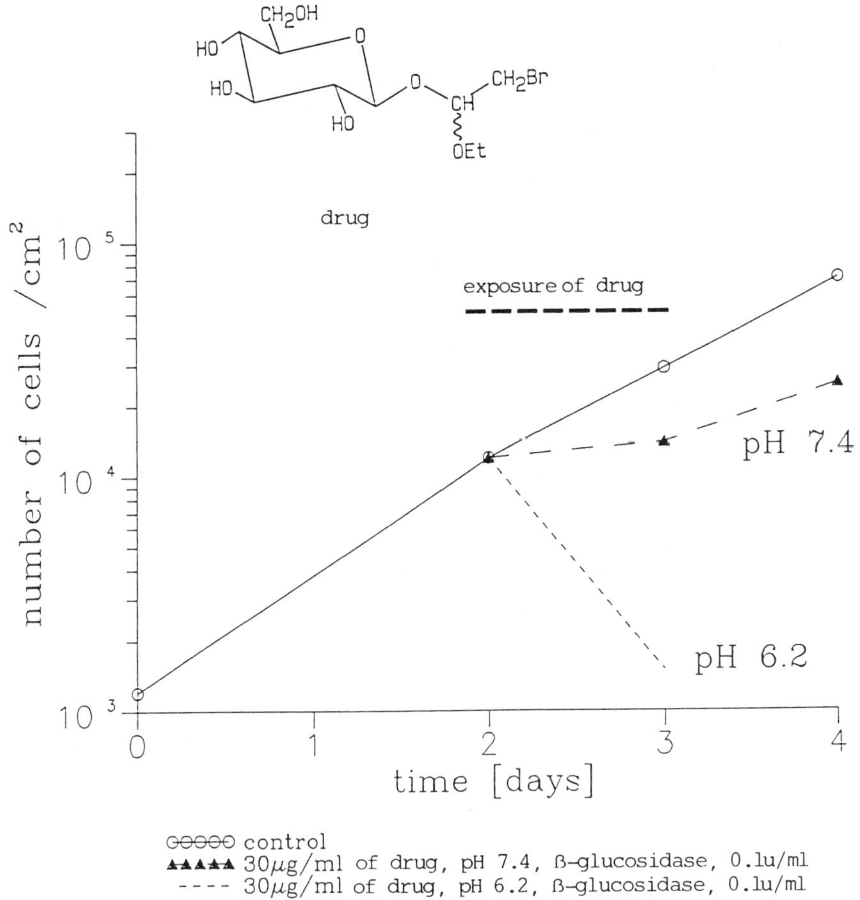

FIG. 5-10. Growth rate of M1R cells in the presence of acetal-glycosides at different pH with application of enzymes.

Mechanistic studies on the acid-catalyzed hydrolysis of glycosides have shown that protonation usually occurs at the *exo*-oxygen of the glycoside, followed by cleavage of the glycosyl–oxygen bond to give a glycosyl cation (Szejtli, 1976; BeMiller, 1967; Capon, 1969). The rate-determining step in the hydrolysis is the formation of the glycosyl cation; therefore, any substituents at the sugar moiety which stabilize the cation should increase the rate of hydrolysis. Thus, acetal-glycosides of glucose (**1** in Fig. 5-12) show an acid lability which is not sufficient to allow cleavage in a tumor under hyperglycemic conditions by proton-catalyzed hydrolysis. At pH 2, a rate constant of $(9.5 \pm 2.3) \cdot 10^{-4}\ s^{-1}$ and at pH 3 of $(6.9 \pm 0.9) \cdot 10^{-5}\ s^{-1}$ was found. At pH 4, hydrolysis could not be detected anymore within 48 hr (L. F. Tietze, A. Goerlach, F. Krach, and B. Leiting, unpublished results). However, acetal-glycosides from 2-deoxy-α-D-arabino-hexopyranose and 2,6-dideoxy-α-L-arabino-hexopyranose (**2** and **3** in Fig. 5-12) show an increase in acid lability. The best results so far were obtained with acetal-glycosides of 2,3-dideoxy-D-erythro-2-hexenopyranose (**4** in Fig. 5-12). These compounds show a fast cleavage at pH 5 to give the corresponding aldehyde and 2,3-dideoxy-D-erythro-2-hexenopyranose. For the synthesis (Fig. 5-13) of the acid-labile acetal-glycoside of aldophosphamide, trimethylsilyl 4,6-diacetyl-2,3-dideoxy-D-erythro-2-hexenopyranoside, **5** was used. Reaction of **5** with the diethylacetal of 3-(p-methoxybenzyloxy)propanal **6** in the presence of catalytic amounts of trimethylsilyl trifluoromethanesulfonate afforded the acetal-glycoside **7**. Oxidative debenzylation of **7** afforded the alcohol **8**, which gave the phosphoric acid amide monochloride **11** by reac-

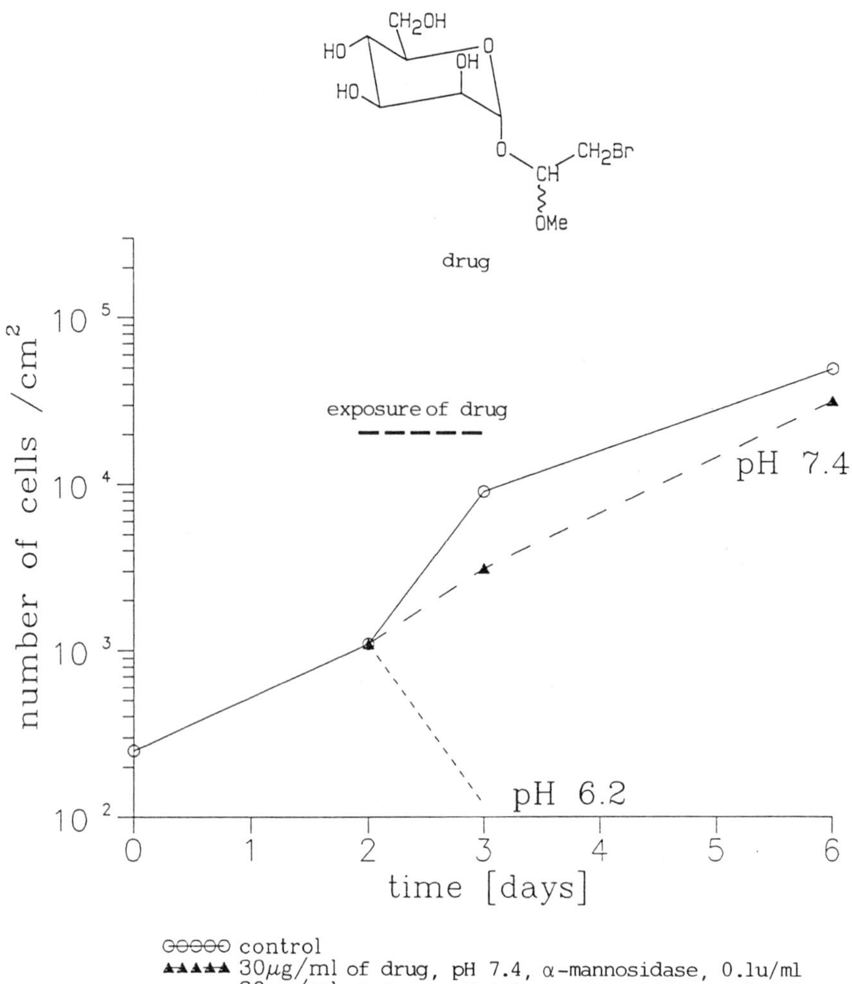

FIG. 5-11. Growth rate of M1R cells in the presence of acetal-glycosides at different pH with application of enzymes.

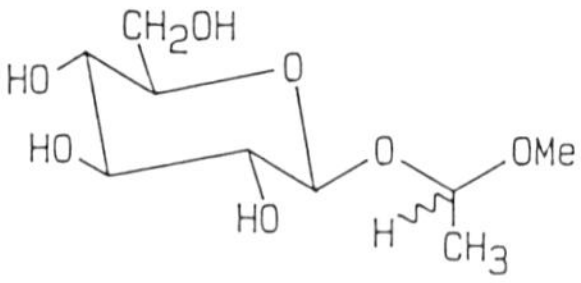

1

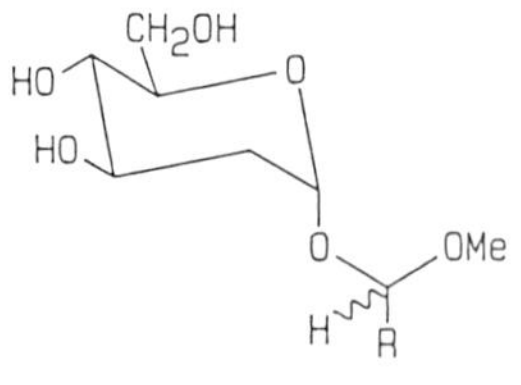

2 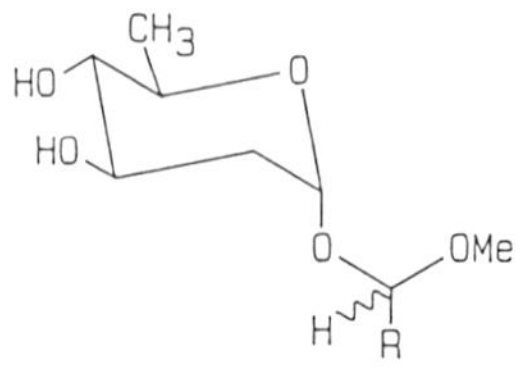 3 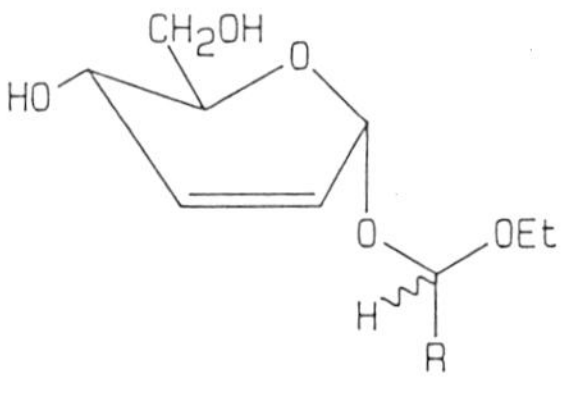 4

FIG. 5-12. Acid-labile acetal-glycosides.

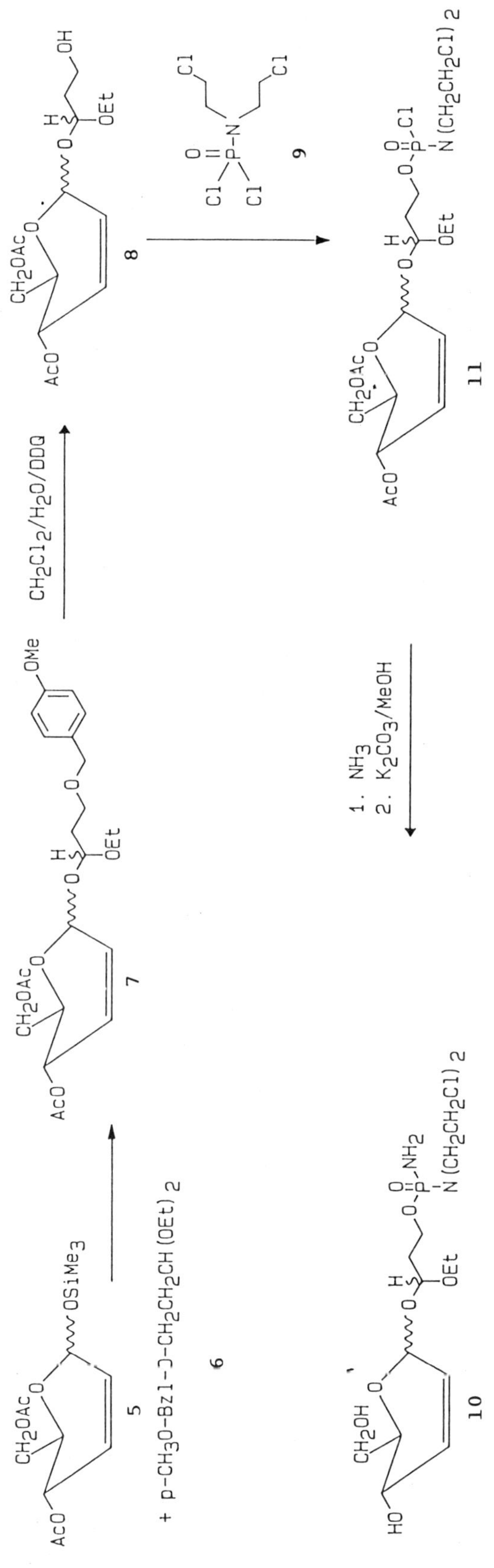

FIG. 5-13. Synthesis of aldophosphamide derivative.

tion with the phosphoric amide dichloride **9**. The latter compound is easily obtainable by mixing N,N-bis(2-chloroethyl)amine hydrochloride and phosphorous oxychloride. The monochloride **11** is not stable; after formation, however, it can be transformed to the desired amide **10** *in situ* by reaction with ammonia (L. F. Tietze, R. Fischer, M. Neumann, M. Beller, and T. Moellers, unpublished results).

4.4. Systemic Toxicity and Cytotoxic Action of Acid-labile Acetal-2-hexenopyranoside of Aldophosphamide

The acute toxicity of the acetal-2-hexenopyranoside of aldophosphamide is low. Intraperitoneal application in mice with concentrations of 1000 mg/kg body weight did not cause any mortality. Using the same dose of cyclophosphamide, all animals died. The cytotoxic action of the aldophosphamide derivative was measured *in vitro* with M1R rat mammary carcinoma cells within 24 to 48 hr exposure time. At physiological pH (7.4), the cytotoxic action of **10** (Fig. 5-13) evaluated by survival of colony-forming cells after treatment, was low.

Application of **10** at a concentration of 100 μg/ml for 24 hr caused only a decrease of the surviving fraction of M1R cells by a factor of 0.65 compared to untreated controls. With prolonged exposure time, the picture nearly did not change. However, in an acidic environment, a strong cytotoxic action of **10** was observed. At pH 6.2 and an exposure time of 24 hr the enhancement was moderate, because of the small rate of hydrolysis of **10** at this pH. As expected, prolonged exposure time, as well as a lower pH, increased the cytotoxic action of **10** dramatically. Application of 100 μg/ml of **10** for 48 hr at pH 6.2 in the culture medium of M1R cells caused a decrease of the survival fraction to 4×10^{-5}. This is an increase of selectivity by the factor of $\approx 10^4$. At lower pH, for example, pH 5.6, this value can also be obtained in malignant tumors by stimulation of the tumor cell glycolysis—the exposure time can be shorter. Application of **10** at a concentration of 100 μg/ml at pH 5.6 for 24 hr caused a decrease of the surviving fraction of M1R cells to 10^{-5}. Again, the selectivity is increased by the factor of $>10^4$.

4.5. Connection of Acetal-glycosides with Monoclonal Antibodies

The main problem in using monoclonal antibody–toxin conjugates which bind to antigens on the surface of malignant cells (Greten & Klapdor, 1986; Smyth et al., 1986) is the occurrence of cross-selectivity. In addition, there is always a fraction of tumor cells to which the added monoclonal antibodies will not bind. Since this fraction will not be destroyed by the monoclonal antibody–toxin conjugate, complete remission of the tumor is not possible. However, in our concept the monoclonal antibody is only used as a carrier to increase the concentration of the nontoxic prodrug in the tumor. Proton-catalyzed hydrolysis of the monoclonal antibody–acetal-glycoside conjugate will liberate the toxin. Using this concept, cross-selectivity of the monoclonal antibody will not be of great importance. In addition also those malignant cells can be destroyed to which the monoclonal antibody–toxin conjugate did not bind.

5. CONCLUDING REMARKS

It seems to be well established that a decrease of the pH in malignant tumors because of their higher rate of glycolysis can be obtained by an increase of the blood sugar level. Since the pH of normal cell populations is almost not affected, this can be used as a basis for the development of more selective anticancer agents. In a rational drug design new types of compounds, called acetal-glycosides, were synthesized, which consist of a sugar moiety, an alcohol, and an aldehyde. These compounds are prodrugs with very little toxicity, but they can be cleaved selectively in the tumor either by proton-catalyzed or by enzymatic hydrolysis to give a cytotoxic compound. *In vitro* experiments with these compounds, using cell cultures of malignant tumors, show a strong difference in cytotoxicity in the enzymatic as well as in the proton-catalyzed cleavage at pH 7.4 and pH 6.2. In some cases the ratio of the rates of survival at pH 7.4 and 6.2 exceeds the factor of 10^4. These results are very promising, and we expect that our concept will enable us to increase the selectivity and thus decrease the negative side effects in some aspects of anticancer chemotherapy.

Acknowledgment—The work is generously supported by the Bundesminister für Forschung und Technologie (Förderkennzeichen 03189-52A9) and the Fonds der Chemischen Industrie.

REFERENCES

BeMiller, J. N. (1967) Acid-catalyzed hydrolysis of glycosides. *Adv. Carbohydr. Chem.* **2**: 25–108.
Bodansky, O. (1975) *Biochemistry of human cancer.* New York: Academic Press.
Boyd, V. L., Robbins, J. D., Egan, W., and Ludeman, S. M. (1986) ^{31}P Nuclear magnetic resonance spectroscopic observation of the intracellular transformations of oncostatic cyclophosphamide metabolites. *J. Med. Chem.* **29**: 1206–1210.
Brade, W. P., and Niemeyer, U. (1987) Antitumormittel. In *Arzneimittel*, A. Kleemann, E. Lindner, and J. Engel, eds., pp. 1240–1366. Weinheim: Verlag Chemie.
Bruhn, H. D. (1980) *Zytostatika-Fibel.* Stuttgart, New York: Schattauer.
Brunner, K. W., and Nagel, G. A. (eds.). (1985) *Internistische Krebstherapie.* Berlin: Springer-Verlag.
Cairns, J. (1986) Der Kampf gegen Krebs. *Spektrum der Wissenschaft* **1**: 38–51.
Capon, B. (1969) Mechanism in carbohydrate chemistry. *Chem. Rev.* **69**: 407–498.
Conchie, J., and Levvy, G. A. (1957) Comparison of different glycosidase activities in conditions of cancer. *Brit. J. Cancer* **11**: 487–493.
Cori, C. F., and Cori, G. T. (1925a) The carbohydrate metabolism of tumors. I. *J. Biol. Chem.* **64**: 11–22.
Cori, C. F., and Cori, G. T. (1925b) The carbohydrate metabolism of tumors. II. *J. Biol. Chem.* **65**: 397–405.
Evans, W. E., Crom, W. R., Abromowitch, M., Dodge, R., Look, A. T., Bowman, W. P., George, S. L., and Pui, C. H. (1986) Clinical pharmacodynamics of high-dose methotrexate in acute lymphocytic leukemia. *N. Engl. J. Med.* **314**: 471–477.
Fishman, W. H. (1955) Beta-glucuronidase. *Adv. Enzymol.* **16**: 361–409.
Frei, E., and Canellos, G. P. (1980) Dose: A critical factor in cancer chemotherapy. *Amer. J. Med.* **69**: 585–594.
Greten, H., and Klapdor, R. (eds.) (1986) *New Tumor-Associated Antigens.* Stuttgart: Thieme Verlag.
Gros, L., Ringsdorf, H., and Schupp, H. (1981) Polymere Antitumormittel auf molekularer und zellulärer Basis. *Angew. Chem.* **93**: 311–332; *Angew. Chem. Int. Ed. Engl.* **20**: 305–326.
Jähde, E., and Rajewsky, M. F. (1982) Tumor-selective modification of cellular microenvironment *in vivo*: Effect of glucose infusion on the pH in normal and malignant rat tissues. *Cancer Res.* **42**: 1505–1512.
Jähde, E., Rajewsky, M. F., and Baumgärtl, H. (1982) pH-Distributions in transplanted neural tumors and normal tissues of BD IX rats as measured with pH-microelectrodes. *Cancer Res.* **42**:1498–1504.
McKay, F. W. (1982) Cancer mortality in the United States 1950–1977. In *National Cancer Department Monograph*, Vol. 59. Washington, DC: U.S. Government Printing Office.
Miller, R. W., and McKay, F. W. (1984) Decline in U.S. childhood cancer mortality. *J. Am. Med. Ass.* **251**: 1567–1570.
Osinskii, S. P., Bubnovskaya, L. N., and Sergienko, T. (1987) Tumor pH under induced hyperglycemia and efficacy of chemotherapy. *Anticancer Res.* **7**: 199–201.
Perin, A., Sessa, A., Scalabrino, G., Arnaboldi, A., and Ciaranfi, E. (1972) Preferential inhibition of protein synthesis in normal or neoplastic tissues in relation to molecular structure. *Europ. J. Cancer* **8**: 111–119.
Schauenstein, E., Esterbauer, H., and Zollner, H. (1977) *Aldehydes in biological systems.* London: Pion-Academic Press.
Schmähl, D. (ed.) (1981) *Maligne Tumoren. Entstehung, Wachstum, Chemotherapie.* Aulendorf: Editio Cantor.
Schulze, W., and Horn, G. (1970) Zusammenhänge zwischen chemischer Struktur und biologischer Wirksamkeit bei Azomethinen mit Stickstofflost-Gruppen am Ehrlich-Ascitestumor der weissen Maus. *Arzneim.-Forsch.* **20**: 329–335.
Slordal, L., and Aarbakke, J. (1987) Effect of anticancer drugs on drug metabolism. *Pharmac. Ther.* **35**: 217–226.
Smyth, M. J., Pietersz, G. A., and McKenzie, I. F. C. (1986) Potentiation of the *in vitro* cytotoxicity of chlorambucil by monoclonal antibodies. *J. Immunol.* **137**: 3361–3366.
Szejtli, J. (1976) *Säurehydrolyse glycosidischer Bindungen.* Leipzig: Akadémiai Kiadó, VEB Fachbuchverlag.
Tanneberger, S. (ed.) (1980) *Allgemeine und spezielle Tumor-Chemotherapie.* Stuttgart, New York: G. Fischer Verlag.
Tietze, L. F., Fischer, R., Guder, H. J., Goerlach, A., Neumann, M., and Krach, T. (1987a) Synthesis of acetal-α-glucosides. A stereoselective entry into a new class of compounds. *Carbohydr. Res.* **164**: 177–194.
Tietze, L. F., Fischer, R., Guder, H. J., and Neumann, M. (1987b) Development of selective cytostatica for cancer therapy. Synthesis of acetal-β-glucosides from cytotoxic aldehydes. *Liebigs Ann. Chem.* 847–856.

Tietze, L. F., and Fischer, R. (1981a) Stereoselektive Synthese von β-Glucosiden mit 1,1′-Diacetal-Struktur. *Angew. Chem.* **93**: 1002; *Angew. Chem. Int. Ed. Engl.* **20**: 969.

Tietze, L. F., and Fischer, R. (1981b) Stereoselektive Synthese von α-Glucosiden mit 1,1′-Diacetal-Struktur. *Tetrahedron Lett.* **22**: 3239–3242.

Unger, C., Eibl, H., and Nagel, G. A. (eds.) (1987) *Die Zellmembran als Angriffspunkt der Tumortherapie*. Zuckschwerdt Verlag.

Von Ardenne, M., and Reitnauer, P. G. (1975) Bedingungsmatrix für die Konzeption neuer Kanzerostatika mit Aktivierung in optimiert übersäuerten Krebsgeweben. *Arch. Geschwulstforsch.* **45**: 34–39.

Warburg, O. (1930) *The metabolism of tumours*. London: Constable.

Whitaker, B. L. (1960) Plasma-β-glucuronidase levels in breast cancer. *Brit. J. Cancer* **14**: 471–477.

Wike-Hooley, J. L., Haveman, J., and Reinhold, J. S. (1984) The relevance of tumor pH to the treatment of malignant disease. *Radiother. Oncol.* **2**: 343–366.

Wolstenholme, G. E. W., Fitzsimons, D. W., and Whelan, J. (eds.) (1979) *Submolecular biology and cancer. Ciba Foundation Symposium 67*. Amsterdam: Excerpta Medica.

CHAPTER 6

MOLECULAR ASPECTS OF THE ANTITUMOR AND CARCINOGENIC ACTION IN TRIAZENE COMPOUNDS: A CHEMIST'S VIEWPOINT

G. F. Kolar

Institute of Toxicology and Chemotherapy, German Cancer Research Center, Heidelberg, Federal Republic of Germany

Abstract—The activity mechanism of the antitumor and carcinogenic dialkyl aryltriazenes [Ar—N=N—N(CH_3)$_2$] depends on metabolic transformation to reactive intermediates by oxidation at the dimethylamino terminus. *N*-Hydroxymethyltriazenes [Ar—N=N—N(CH_3)CH_2OH] seem to be important cornerstone metabolites, and their *in vivo* generation, synthesis, and reactivity became our major research topic. Their preparation can be achieved either (1) by a direct condensation of monomethyltriazenes with formaldehyde or (2) by *N*-azo coupling with methylamine-formaldehyde mixture. The latter route affords several simple and complex products whose structures (by MS and NMR) offer a plausible mechanistic explanation for the dual biological activity of 1-aryl-3,3-dimethyltriazenes.

1. INTRODUCTION

The beginnings of triazene chemistry are closely linked with the discovery of aromatic diazonium salts and dye intermediates (Griess, 1858) in the second half of the last century. The diazo coupling at nucleophilic carbon was soon extended to substrates containing nucleophilic nitrogen, and Griess (1862) was the first to report a triazene synthesis.

The generic name "triazene" [—N=N—N⟨] implies that this class of compounds is derived from a monounsaturated open-chain unit of three nitrogen atoms by a progressive substitution of terminal valencies with a variety of aliphatic, aromatic, or heterocyclic groups. The number and nature of substituents introduced at the N atoms provide a rational basis for the subdivision and reactivity of two series of related structures:

1. 1,3,3-trisubstituted diazoimino compounds [X—N=N—N—(Y,X)], represented by the formula of 3,3-dimethyl-1-phenyltriazene (Fig. 6-1). These compounds themselves are probably not biologically active but require enzymatic activation by mixed function oxidases to yield biologically reactive intermediates.
2. 1,3-disubstituted diazoamino compounds [X—N=N—NH—Y], the directly methylating monoalkyl triazenes that undergo tautomerism by a prototropic shift. These have been shown to arise by enzymatic dealkylation from the corresponding dialkyl precursors.

3,3-Dialkyl-1-aryltriazenes represent the most important group because of their varied biological activity. Individual compounds are potent carcinogens and mutagens, whereas the related heterocyclic (imidazole) derivatives are useful anticancer agents. The chemical and biological aspects of triazene compounds have been reviewed (Wilman & Connors, 1983; Kolar, 1984; Spassova & Golovinsky, 1985; Kolar, 1986; Wilman, 1986; Gescher & Threadgill, 1987; Newell et al., 1987).

Dialkyl aryltriazenes were developed first after World War II in England and the United States. The earliest account of their antineoplastic activity was the demonstration more than 30 years ago (Clarke et al., 1955; Burchenal et al., 1956) that dimethyl phenyltriazene and derivatives inhibited the growth of rodent tumors.

The therapeutic use of triazene anticancer drugs originated from an attempt to design antagonists of 5-aminoimidazole-4-carboxamide (AIC), the ribotide of which is a precursor in purine biosynthesis. These efforts resulted in the synthesis of dacarbazine, 5-(3,3-dimethyl-1-triazeno)imidazole-4-carboxamide (Fig. 6.2) (Shealy et al., 1962a), which is used

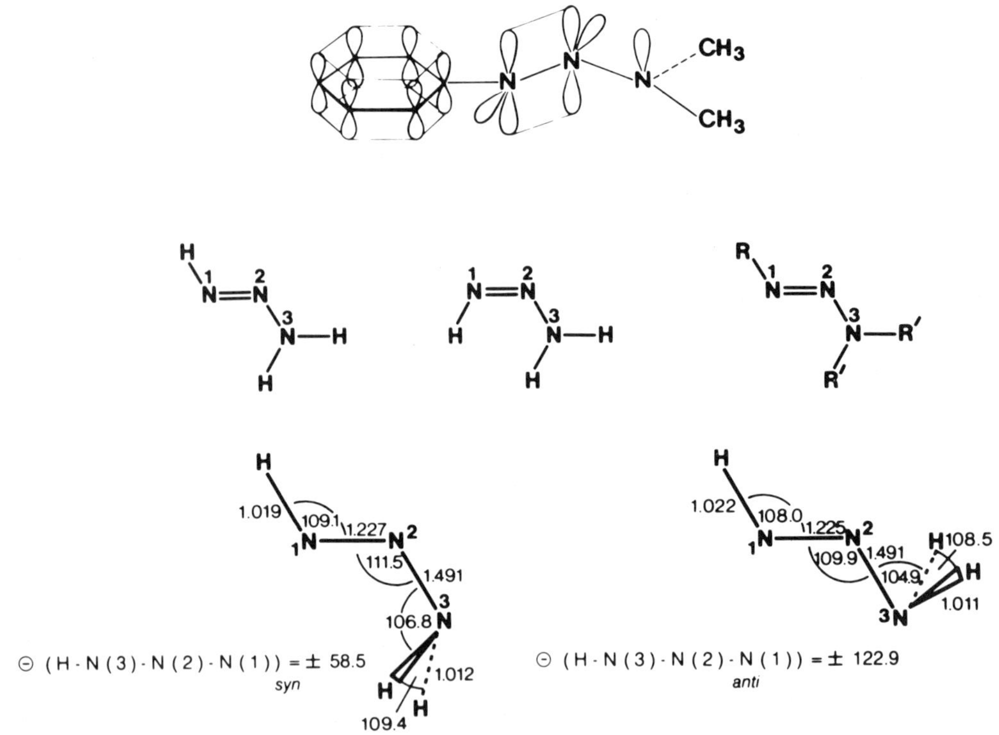

Fig. 6-1. Molecular orbital formula and bond angles of 3,3-dimethyl-1-phenyltriazene.

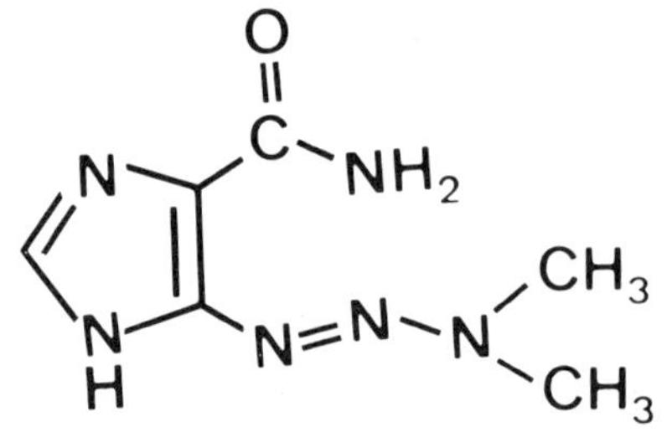

Fig. 6-2. 5-(3,3-Dimethyl-1-triazeno)imidazole-4-carboxamide (DTIC, NSC-45388).

in the treatment of malignant melanoma and other human cancers (Lucas & Huang, 1982). Dacarbazine has marked inhibitory activity against L1210 leukemia and other rodent neoplasms (Shealy et al., 1962b; Montgomery, 1976). Clinically, it appears to have optimal activity in advanced melanoma and in combination therapy for refractory Hodgkin's disease (Comis, 1976; Dorr & Fritz, 1980). Its activity is, however, considered to be weak, and while approximately 20% of patients respond to therapy, there has been no demonstrated prolongation of life.

2. MECHANISMS OF ACTION, METABOLISM, AND DETOXIFICATION

The mechanisms by which dimethyltriazene compounds act as carcinogens or inhibit tumors are not clearly understood; nevertheless there is convincing evidence that metabolic activation by the host is required and the important oxidative transformation occurs at the terminal dimethylamino group of the triazene side chain.

More than a decade ago, Connors and colleagues (1976) deduced that only those triazene derivatives display antitumor activity that can be metabolized to the corresponding monomethyl analogs. Since the monomethyltriazenes had been shown to be direct alkylating agents both *in vitro* (Preussmann & von Hodenberg, 1969) and *in vivo* (Preussmann et al., 1969), the authors suggested that tumor growth was inhibited mainly by methylation of crucial nucleophilic sites in cellular biopolymers. However, despite intensive effort, no correlation was found between microsomal demethylation *in vitro* and the antitumor activity *in vivo*. Moreover, there was no satisfactory explanation for the antitumor activity of 1-(4-methoxyphenyl)-3,3-dimethyltriazene ($t_{0.5}$ = 11 min; Kolar & Preussmann, 1971). These findings cast serious doubt as to the validity of the proposed methylation hypothesis and to the finding that the monomethyltriazenes proved to be less effective antitumor agents than the corresponding dimethyltriazenes.

With evidence obtained from combined *in vivo/in vitro* test systems, Hickman (1978) concluded that hepatic activation of dimethyltriazenes generated additional intermediary metabolites which were responsible for the selective tumor inhibition *in vivo*.

As our early *in vivo* experiments with 3,3-dimethyl-1-phenyltriazene showed the excretion of several labile metabolites (Kolar & Schlesiger, 1975), we selected 1-(4-chlorophenyl)-3,3-dimethyltriazene (Kolar & Schlesiger, 1976a,b) and the ring-halogenated 3,3-dimethyl-1-(2,4,6-trichlorophenyl)triazene (DM-2,4,6 Cl_3-PT) for our metabolic studies. Blocking of all three *ortho* and *para* positions with chlorine not only prevented ring hydroxylation but also stabilized the $N_2—N_3$ bond against hydrolytic cleavage. After administration of the trichlorinated triazene to rats, only one metabolite with an intact triazene structure was detected on thin layer chromatograms. The structure of the metabolite (Kolar & Carubelli, 1979a,b) was elucidated by NMR spectroscopy (Fig. 6-3) and mass spectrometry (Fig. 6-4) as [1-methyl-3-(2,4,6-trichlorophenyl-2-triazeno]-methyl-β-D-glucopyranoside uronate, M1. Since the isolated M1 accounted for no more than about 20% of the administered dose, we examined alternative detoxification modes and searched for additional metabolites.

In more recent studies, we found that M1 was also effectively excreted in the bile of rats and, more important, that two additional N-glucopyranoside uronates could be isolated from the bile (M2) and from the urine (M3) of the treated animals.

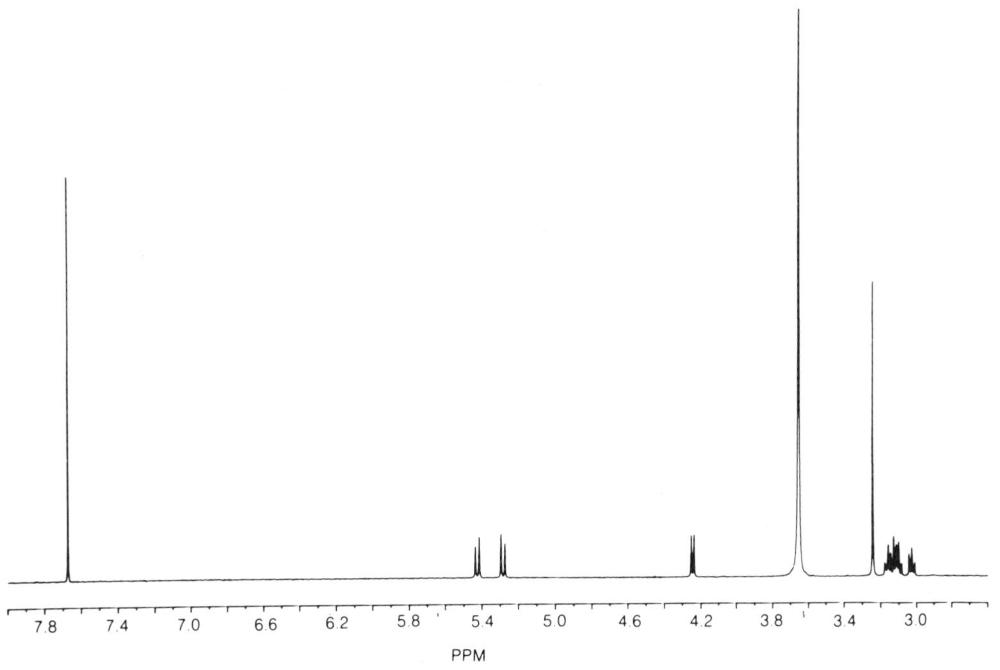

FIG. 6-3. NMR spectrum of [1-methyl-3-(2,4,6-trichlorophenyl-2-triazeno]methyl-β-D-glucopyranoside uronate, M1.

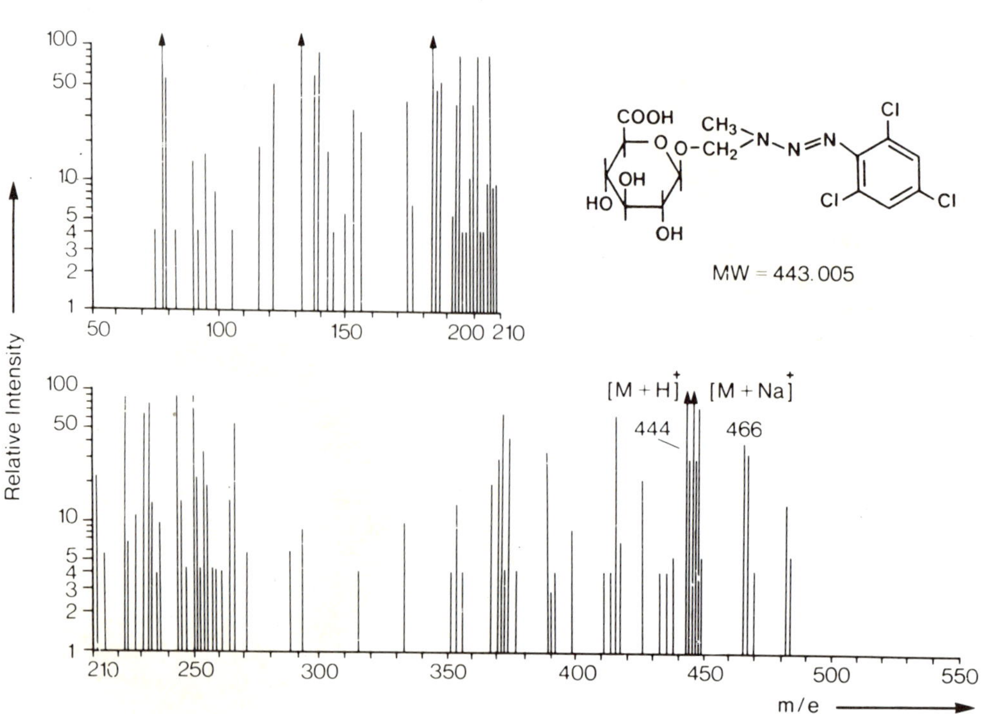

Fig. 6-4. Field desorption mass spectrum and structure of [1-methyl-3-(2,4,6-trichlorophenyl)-2-triazeno]methyl-β-D-glucopyranoside uronate, M1.

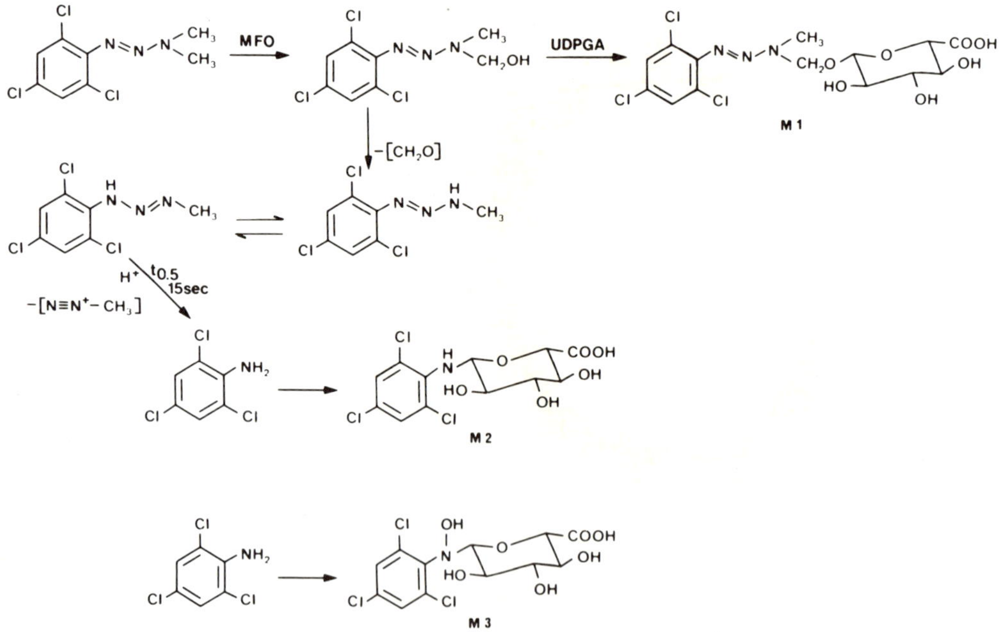

Fig. 6-5. Metabolic activation and detoxification of 3,3-dimethyl-1-(2,4,6-trichlorophenyl)-triazene.

The structures of all three metabolites, M1, the biliary 1-deoxy-1-(2,4,6-trichlorophenylamino)-β-D-glucopyranoside uronate (M2), and of the related urinary 1-deoxy-1-(2,4,6-trichlorophenylhydroxylamino)-β-D-glucopyranoside uronate (M3), are shown in Fig. 6.5. Since neither M2 nor M3 contained a triazene substructure but were conjugates of the catabolically released 2,4,6-trichloroaniline, we investigated the transformation by a direct administration of trichlorinated aniline itself.

The studies on metabolism were extended by comparative chronic tests of biological activity: The carcinogenicity assays were performed at low equimolar dose levels (20 × 0.1 mmol/kg/week; rat), using both 4- and 2,4,6-chlorinated and -brominated analogs (Kolar & Habs, 1984). Similar assays with the same protocol and dose level were carried out with the corresponding ring-halogenated monomethyltriazenes (Berger & Kolar, 1986). The results indicated that 3,3-dimethyl-1-phenyltriazene and 3-methyl-1-phenyltriazene were the strongest carcinogens in each series, respectively, and that the carcinogenic potency in both series decreased with progressive ring halogenation.

In addition, the halogenated 3,3-dimethyl-1-phenyltriazenes were tested for tumor-inhibiting activity against TLX5 lymphoma and PC6 plasmocytoma in tumor-bearing female CBA mice (K. R. Harrap and G. F. Kolar, unpublished data).

The comparative tests showed that 4-Cl/Br and especially the 2,4,6-Cl_3/Br_3 phenyl-3,3-dimethyltriazene were the more effective antitumor agents compared to the respective unhalogenated compound. From these results, one can conclude that the carcinogenic and tumor inhibitory effects of the individual triazenes are not positively correlated.

In subsequent metabolic studies of the clinically used dacarbazine (Fig. 6.2), Kolar and colleagues (1980) detected a structurally related urinary product with lower mobility than the parent DTIC. The metabolite was not retained on an anionic exchanger, which fact indicated the absence of the expected covalent binding of the drug to endogenic anionic substrates (glucuronic acid). Presumably, the lower R_f of the compound was due to an enzymatic introduction of a polar, but nonacidic, oxygen function into the terminal dimethylamino group of the side chain. The labile DTIC metabolite was identified as 5-(3-hydroxymethyl-3-methyl-1-triazeno)imidazole-4-carboxamide (HMIC) by comparison with an authentic sample, synthesized by condensation of 5-(3-methyl-1-triazeno)imidazole-4-carboxamide (MTIC) with excess formaldehyde in anhydrous methanol. The structure of HMIC was established by NMR spectroscopy (a doublet at δ 5.10 of the N_3 methylene; J = 7 Hz) and confirmed by FD mass spectrometry (M^+ 198).

The structures of both conjugated and free metabolites provide not only direct proof for the formation of stable hydroxymethyltriazenes *in vivo*, but have also stimulated intensive research into their chemistry and antitumor activity.

3. SYNTHESIS AND REACTIVITY OF N-HYDROXYMETHYLTRIAZENES

Attempts to synthesize N-hydroxymethyltriazenes are not new. In 1973, prompted by the elimination of formaldehyde from enzymatically generated α-hydroxymethyl intermediates, we reversed the reaction and condensed 3-methyl-1-phenyltriazene with methanolic formaldehyde to obtain the corresponding hydroxymethyl derivative. The mass spectrum of the product showed a molecular ion at m/z 165 and a base peak at m/z 105. Loss of 60 mass units, CH_3NCH_2OH, was analogous to fragmentation of 3,3-dimethyl-1-phenyltriazene (Kolar, 1984).

An important advance in the synthesis of N-hydroxymethyltriazenes was reported by Gescher and colleagues (1978) who introduced a one-pot N-azo coupling of (−M)-substituted arenediazonium salts with methylamine–formaldehyde mixture. Subsequent experience from several laboratories (Cheng et al., 1983; Lafrance et al., 1983) showed that the structures and proportions of products depend not only on the nature of substituents but also on the ratio of reactants, the temperature, and pH. The complex reaction is versatile and can be modulated, as shown by a few examples.

In an attempt to prepare a hydroxymethyltriazene bearing a powerful (−M)-substituent, we coupled 4-trifluoromethylbenzenediazonium chloride with methylamine–formaldhyde and acidified the cool mixture to pH 1. Standing at 4°C transformed the intermediary hydroxymethyl triazene to a heterocycle, 3,7-bis-(4-trifluoromethylphenyl)-1,5,3,7 dioxadiazocane (Fig. 6-6). Additional 3,7-bis(4-X-aryl)-1,5,3,7-dioxadiazocanes, substituted with

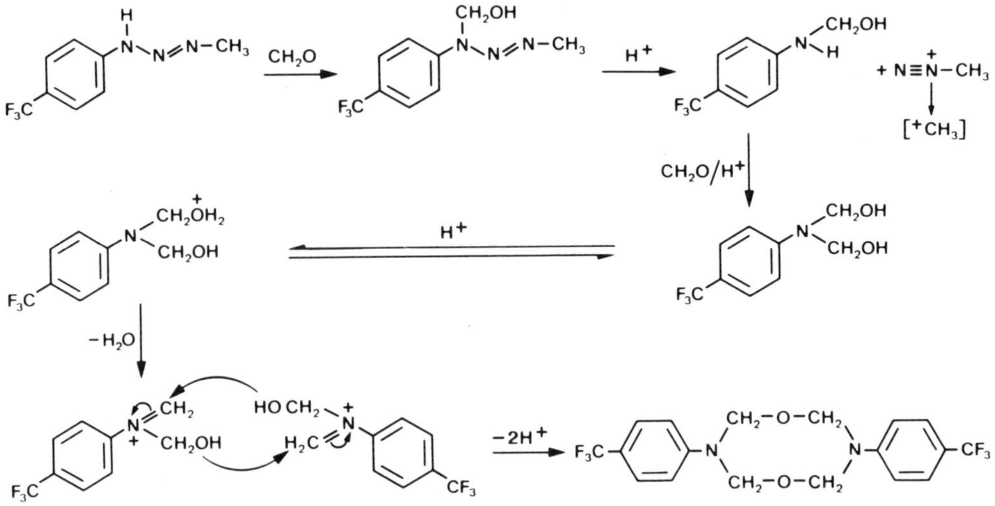

FIG. 6-6. Proposed mechanism of 3,7-bis-(4-trifluoromethylphenyl)-1,5,3,7-dioxadiazocane formation.

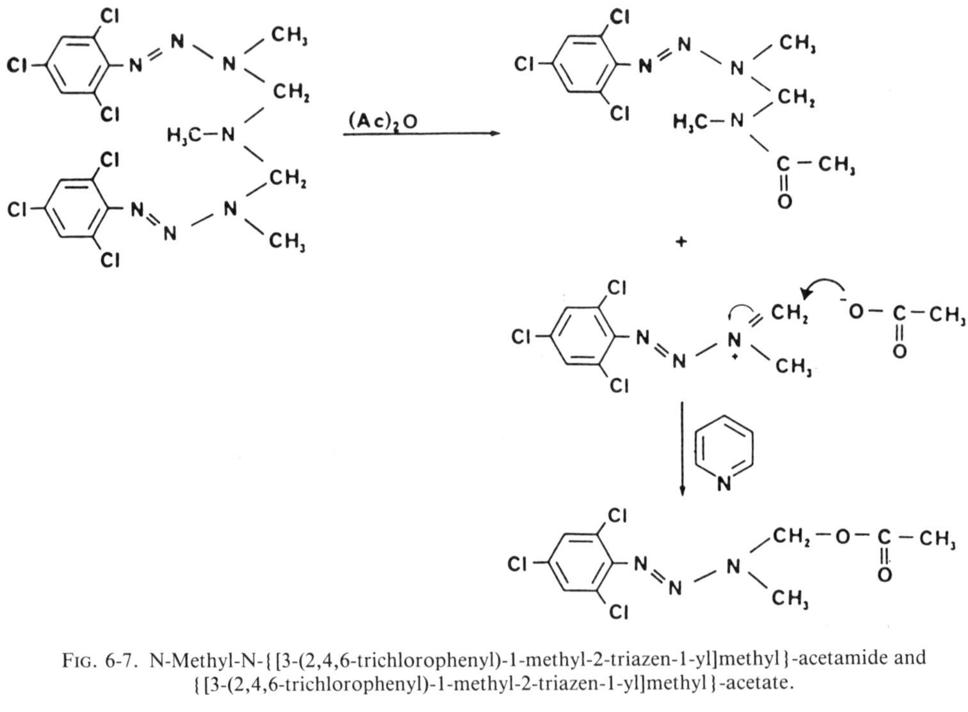

FIG. 6-7. N-Methyl-N-{[3-(2,4,6-trichlorophenyl)-1-methyl-2-triazen-1-yl]methyl}-acetamide and {[3-(2,4,6-trichlorophenyl)-1-methyl-2-triazen-1-yl]methyl}-acetate.

CH_3OOC-, $NC-$, and O_2N-, were prepared by analogous methods (Kolar & Schendzielorz, 1985).

Because of general interest in the O-glucuronoside of 3-hydroxymethyl-3-methyl-1-(2,4,6-trichlorophenyl)-triazene, M1 (Fig. 6-5), attempts were made in several laboratories to prepare the unconjugated triazene methylol. Although our coupling experiments led to the isolation of a crystalline minor product, the viscous extract decomposed during column chromatography. Therefore, the crude residue was stabilized by acetylation, yielding N-methyl-N-{[3-(2,4,6-trichlorophenyl)-1-methyl-2-triazen-1-yl]-methyl}-acetamide and {[3-(2,4,6-trichlorophenyl)-1-methyl-2-triazen-1-yl]-methyl}-acetate (Fig. 6-7), as major products (Kolar & Schendzielorz, 1986).

In the same way, 3-pyridinediazonium-, 2-chloro-5-pyridinediazonium-, and 2-methoxy-5-pyridinediazonium ions reacted with an excess of deeply cooled (−10°C) methylamine–formaldehyde premix which was neutralized to pH 6. In each case the reaction led to crystalline heterocyclic hydroxymethyl derivatives which were characterized by NMR spectroscopy and mass spectrometry.

3-Hydroxymethyl-3-methyl-1-(3-pyridyl)-triazene and 3-hydroxymethyl-3-methyl-1-(2-chloro-5-pyridyl)-triazene and their derivatives were tested for their cytotoxic effects against S180 cells *in vitro* and compared with those of the corresponding monomethyl- and dimethyltriazenes (Fig. 6-8). The hydroxymethyltriazenes were found to be one to two orders of magnitude more cytotoxic than the corresponding dimethyl analogs. The effects of 3-hydroxymethyl-3-methyl-1-(3-pyridyl)-triazene were assessed by cell growth, colony forming, and macromolecular synthesis assays (Fig. 6-9). Comparable effects were observed with the related monomethyltriazenes, indicating that the activity of hydroxymethyltriazenes could result, at least in part, from the release of monomethyl derivatives.

Although the majority of aryl hydroxymethyltriazenes, or their derivatives, are substituted with (−M) 4-X groups, an unexpected adduct was isolated from the coupling of 4-methoxybenzenediazonium chloride with premixed methylamine–formaldehyde. After a conventional diazotization of 4-anisidine, the unreacted nitrous acid was destroyed with an excess of urea. Nevertheless, the presence of this weak nuclophile in the mixture affected the course of the reaction and thereby the nature of the product.

The isolated compound had an M^+ 469, and peak matching established its molecular formula as $C_{22}H_{31}N_9O_3$, which was confirmed by an elemental analysis.

A proton NMR spectrum (Fig. 6-10) shows the characteristic doublet of doublets (AA′BB′ pattern) of p,p′-disubstituted benzene around δ 5.67–5.16 (d and c) and five sharp singlets (g, h, a, f, i) which are indicative of a highly symmetrical structure. Due to lack of coupling, it appeared that the proton signals ($-CH_2$, $-CH_3$) were located at carbon atoms that were flanked by identical or dissimilar hetero atoms. Since the adduct released two equivalents of 4-methoxybenzenediazonium ion, the combined analytical evidence could be rationalized as a bis-triazenyl structure, built around one of two central heterocycles:

1. 3,5-Bis{[3-(4-methoxyphenyl)-1-methyl-2-triazenyl]-methyl}-N-methyl-1,3,5-oxadiazinane-4-imine, or the isomeric
2. 1,3-Bis{[3-(4-methoxyphenyl)-1-methyl-2-triazenyl]-methyl}-5-methyl-hexahydro-1,3,5-triazinan-2-one.

No.	Structure	Half-life (min)	No.	Structure	Half-life (min)
I	3-pyridyl–N=N–N(CH_3)CH_3	6×10^5	IV	Cl-pyridyl–N=N–N(CH_3)CH_3	stable*
II	3-pyridyl–N=N–N(CH_3)H	40.5	V	Cl-pyridyl–N=N–N(CH_3)H	55.4
III	3-pyridyl–N=N–N(CH_3)CH_2OH	36.3	VI	Cl-pyridyl–N=N–N(CH_3)CH_2OH	64.1
			VII	Cl-pyridyl–N=N–N(CH_3)$CH_2OC(=O)-CH_3$	61.8

* No decrease in absorption after two weeks incubation

FIG. 6-8. Structures and half-lives of 3-pyridyltriazenes.

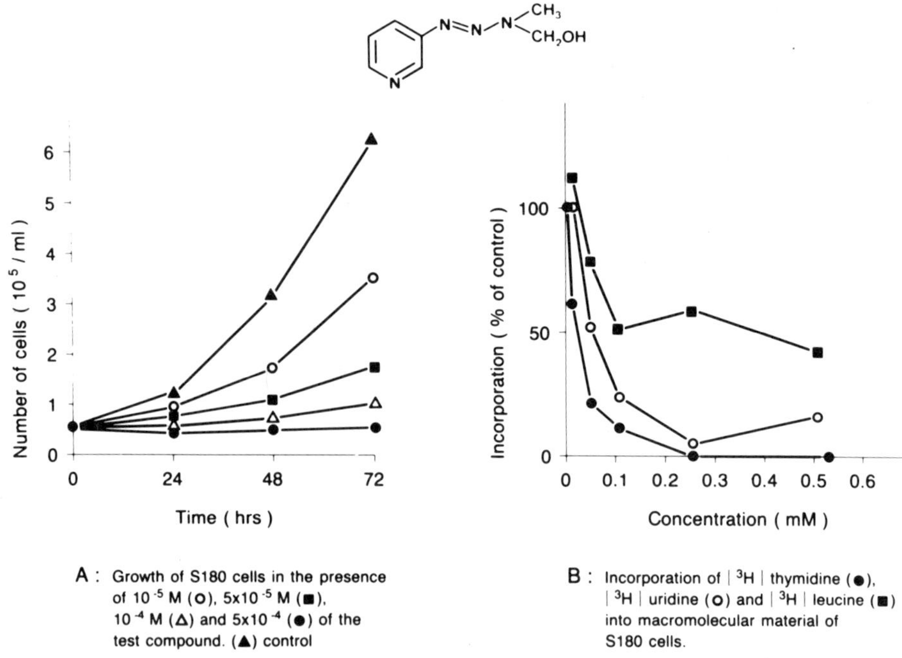

FIG. 6-9. Cytotoxic effects of 3-hydroxymethyl-3-methyl-1-(3-pyridyl)-triazene.

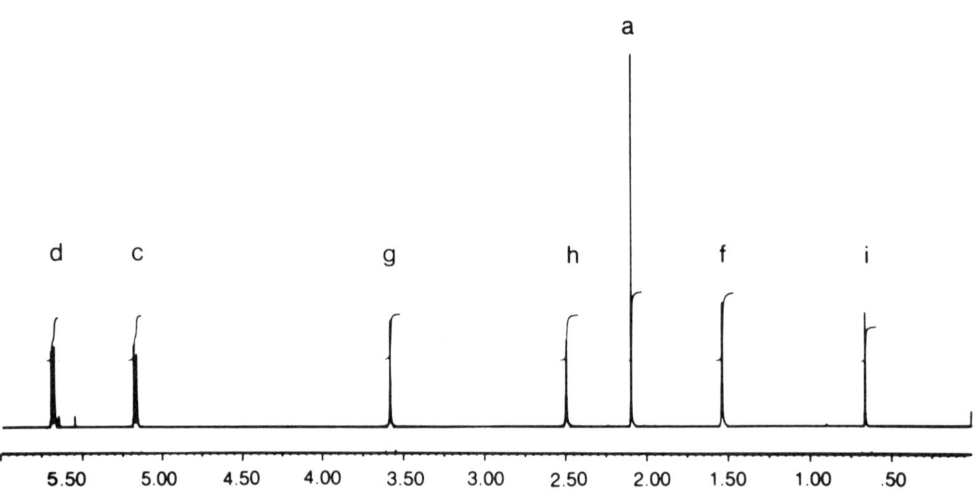

FIG. 6-10. ^{1}H-NMR spectrum of 1,3-bis{[3-(4-methoxyphenyl)-1-methyl-2-triazen-1-yl]methyl}-5-methyl-1,3,5-triazinan-2-one.

Unequivocal differentiation between the two isomeric $C_{22}H_{31}N_9O_3$ structures 1 and 2 was achieved by long-range proton decoupled experiments since such an assignment is absolute and independent of arguments based on chemical shifts.

The key to the problem was to distinguish between the unsaturated N-methyl amino group ($CH_3{-}N{=}C\langle$) in 1 and the tertiary N-methyl amino group plus $\rangle C{=}O$ in 2 with their surrounding magnetic environments, respectively. The answer was obtained from three-bond proton decoupled $^1H{-}^{13}C$ measurements which confirmed the bis-triazenyl substituted 1,3,5-hexahydro-triazinan-2-one structure 2 (Fig. 6-11).

Since no such heterocyclic structure has been reported, the isolation of 1,3-bis{[3-(4-methoxyphenyl)-1-methyl-2-triazenyl]-methyl}-5 methyl-hexahydro-1,3,5-triazinan-2-one

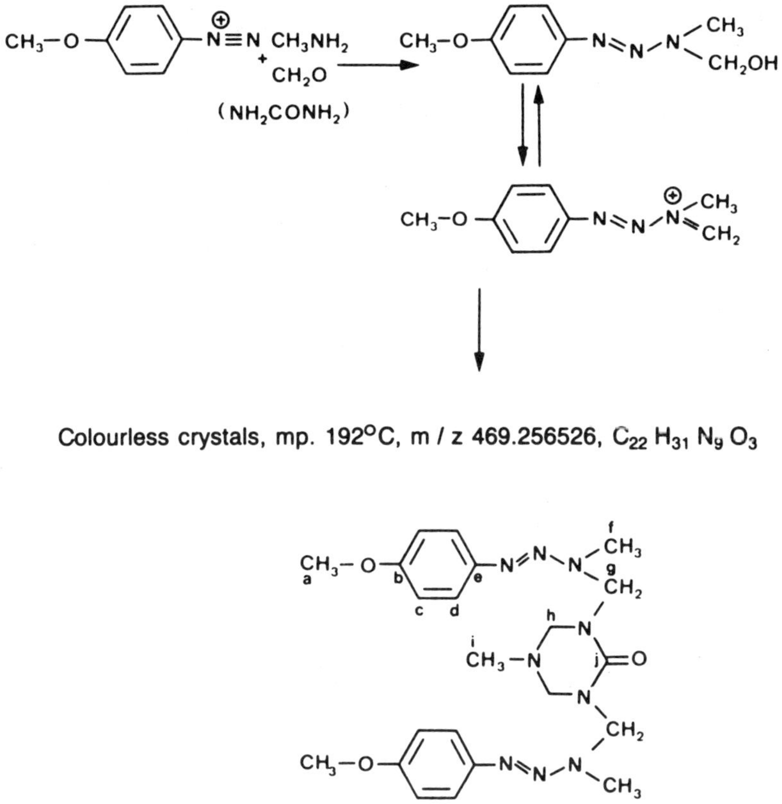

Colourless crystals, mp. 192°C, m / z 469.256526, $C_{22}H_{31}N_9O_3$

FIG. 6-11. 1,3-Bis-{[3-(4-methoxyphenyl)-1-methyl-2-triazenyl]methyl}-5-methyl-hexahydro-1,3,5-triazinan-2-one.

could only arise by a direct reactivity of the (+M)-substituted 3-hydroxymethyl-3-methyl-1-(4-methoxyphenyl)-triazene, which was in equilibrium with its triazenium (iminium) species. Moreover, the formation of this adduct is reproducible (yield 15–20%), provided that urea has been added to the reaction. Therefore, the adduct may serve as a plausible model for a similar reaction of hydroxymethyltriazenes with nucleophilic sites in cellular biopolymers. It is tempting to speculate whether the release of 4-methoxybenzenetriazenium ion, or related iminium species, participates in tumor inhibition by dimethyltriazenes.

4. RECENT DEVELOPMENTS

Metabolism of the tumor inhibitory and carcinogenic 3,3-dimethyl-triazenes, initiated by the cytochrome P-450–mediated oxidation of the terminal N-methyl group, represents the first step toward the generation of reactive intermediates. The process may be either a prelude to formaldehyde release, or it may give rise to a relatively stable N-hydroxymethyltriazene.

During the last decade, the chemistry, reactivity, and fate of the hydroxymethyltriazenes, in equilibrium with the corresponding iminium (triazenium) cation, became an area of extensive research. There is little doubt that the ability of hydroxymethyltriazenes to form such reactive iminium species depends on the presence of (+M) 4-X aryl substituent and the basicity of the terminal N_3 (Overton et al., 1985). Although an example of direct reaction of 3-hydroxymethyl-3-methyl-1-(4-methoxyphenyl)-triazene was recently demonstrated (Fig. 6-11), the urea adduct may represent a unique case.

Hemens and colleagues (1984) presented evidence that iminium-type intermediates are only rarely formed because of the poor leaving group character of the hydroxide ion. However, the authors further showed that the hydroxymethyltriazenes must be conjugated with a suitable leaving group, such as acetate, which activates an otherwise unreactive N-hydroxymethyl compound. The 3-acetoxy methyltriazenes were found to undergo methanolysis to the N-(methoxy-methyl)triazenes, probably via the intermediate iminium ion, whereas the unconjugated hydroxymethyltriazene did not generate iminium ions under the same conditions.

In this context, Iley and colleagues (1987) reported that the methylol-O-ether derivatives can be synthesized directly in excellent yields from hydroxymethyltriazenes that react readily with a variety of alcohols in the presence of HCl under anhydrous conditions. Similarly, the thiols (EtSH, Pr^iSH, and Bu^tSH) were also found suitable media for the synthesis of thioether derivatives. Unfortunately, the reaction did not succeed with amines or aminoalcohols.

Recent progress in hydroxymethyltriazene chemistry includes the synthesis of three azidomethyltriazenes and the biomimetic synthesis of N-alkyl-N-formyltriazenes.

3-Acetoxymethyl-3-methyl-1-aryltriazenes were found to react with a large molar excess of sodium azide in aqueous acetone to afford a high yield of 3-azidomethyl-3-methyl-1-aryltriazenes (Vaughan et al., 1987). These important derivatives undergo hydrolysis in aqueous solution with kinetic parameters analogous to those of acetoxymethyltriazenes and hydroxymethyltriazenes. Therefore, the azidomethyltriazenes are capable of generating an alkylating species *in situ*, and, more important, they can do so without the need for a metabolic oxidation. The α-substituted azidomethyltriazenes represent an additional prodrug form of a cytotoxic electrophilic species. In fact, the azidomethyltriazenes show comparable antitumor activity against the P388 and PC6 tumors, as the related triazene derivatives. From the limited series of compounds known, it appears that a correlation may exist between a cleavage of an α-substituted triazene and its antitumor activity.

Another significant development concerns an improved synthesis of N-formyltriazenes which have been implicated as possible metabolites or as antitumor agents themselves (Lassiani et al., 1980). Very recently, Iley and Ruecroft (1988) described a biomimetic synthesis of N-alkyl-N-formyltriazenes by the oxidation of the corresponding N-alkyl-N-methyl-, N-alkyl-N-hydroxymethyl-, and N-alkyl-N-methoxymethyltriazenes. The method makes use of the cytochrome P-450 model oxygenase system, using tetraphenylporphyrinatomanganese (III) chloride-iodosobenzene ($TPPMn^{III}$ PhIO).

The relevance of the N-formyltriazenes to the cytotoxic activity of dimethyltriazenes is reflected by their reaction with nitrogen nucleophiles. Thus, methylamine, morpholine, and piperidine react rapidly with formyltriazenes to form the N-formylated amines and the cytotoxic monomethyltriazenes, already proposed as the ultimate metabolites of the dimethyltriazene prodrugs.

5. CONCLUSIONS

3,3-Dimethyltriazene (diazoimino) compounds, including dacarbazine, DTIC, are an important group of antitumor agents whose mode of action complements other categories of drugs used in the therapy of human cancers. Although no secondary malignancies have been observed in patients treated with DTIC, the imidazole triazene was demonstrated to be carcinogenic in laboratory animals.

Oxidative metabolism of dimethyltriazenes, initiated by the generation of N-hydroxymethyl intermediates, represents the universal pathway for the expression of the biological activity of this class. The cytochrome P-450–mediated process leads to either

1. A loss of formaldehyde and subsequent release of the directly alkylating monomethyltriazene, which is a known proximate carcinogen, or
2. The generation of a stabilized hydroxymethyltriazene, existing in equilibrium with the corresponding triazenium species. The latter intermediate appears to be responsible for the tumor inhibition.

The hydroxymethyltriazenes have been recognized as cornerstone metabolites, and their synthesis, reactivity, conjugation, and cytotoxic activity are emphasized in this chapter.

The structure of the isolated 1,3-bis{[3-(4-methoxyphenyl)-1-methyl-2-triazenyl]-methyl}-5-methyl-hexahydro-1,3,5-triazinan-2-one could be accounted for by a direct condensation of the (+M) 4-methoxybenzenetriazenium ion with urea nitrogen; nevertheless, the available evidence indicates that the majority of (−M)-substituted hydroxymethyltriazenes must be activated by a suitable leaving group (e.g., acetate) to favor the generation of such iminium species.

DTIC and related dimethyltriazenes undergo, basically, the same metabolic route *in vitro* and in laboratory animals. Although the triazenes are active against experimental rodent tumors, their chemotherapeutic potency against human malignancies is often low. Whether the limited clinical activity of the dimethyltriazene prodrugs is a consequence of their poor activation or of some other biological event remains to be clarified.

If the lower metabolic potential of the human liver is indeed the limiting factor, then the development and use of second-generation diazoimino drugs with an effective α-substituted leaving group (e.g., azide or another as yet unknown group) may lead to an improved therapeutic efficacy against human cancer.

REFERENCES

Berger, M. R., and Kolar, G. F. (1986) Comparative carcinogenicity of ring-halogenated 3-methyl-1-phenyltriazenes and their 3,3-dimethyl analogs at equimolar dose levels in male Sprague-Dawley rats. *J. Cancer Res. Clin. Oncol.* **111**: 129–132.

Burchenal, J. H., Dagg, M. K., Beyer, M., and Stock, C. C. (1956) Triazenes as antitumor agents. *Proc. Soc. Exp. Biol. Med.* **91**: 398–403.

Cheng, S. C., de S. Fernandez, M. L., Iley, J., and Rosa, M. E. N. (1983) Triazenes: A reinvestigation of the coupling reaction between methylamine–formaldehyde mixtures. *J. Chem. Research* **(S)**: 108–109.

Clark, D. A., Barclay, R. K., Stock, C. C., and Rondestvedt, C. S. (1955) Triazenes as inhibitors of mouse sarcoma 180. *Proc. Soc. Exp. Biol. Med.* **90**: 484–489.

Comis, R. L. (1976) DTIC (NSC-45388) in malignant melanoma: A perspective. *Cancer Treat. Rep.* **60**: 165–176.

Connors, T. A., Goddard, P. M., Merai, K., Ross, W. C. J., and Wilman, D. E. V. (1976) Tumor inhibitory triazenes: Structural requirements for an active metabolite. *Biochem. Pharmac.* **25**: 241–246.

Dorr, R. T., and Fritz, W. L. (1980) *Cancer chemotherapy handbook.* New York: Elsevier.

Gescher, A., and Threadgill, M. D. (1987) The metabolism of triazene antitumor drugs. *Pharmac. Ther.* **32**: 191–205.

Gescher, A., Hickman, J. A., Simmonds, R. J., Stevens, M. F. G., and Vaughan, K. (1978) α-Hydroxylated derivatives of antitumor dimethyltriazenes. *Tetrahedron Lett.*: 5041–5044.

Griess, P. (1862) Über eine neue Klasse organischer Verbindungen, in denen Wasserstoff durch Stickstoff vertreten ist. *Liebigs Ann. Chem.* **121**: 257–280.

Griess, P. (1858) Vorläufige Notiz über die Einwirkung von salpetrige Säure auf Aminonitro- und Aminotrophenylsäure. *Liebigs Ann. Chem.* **106**: 123–125.

Hemens, C. M., Manning, H. W., Vaughan, K., Lafrance, R. J., and Tang, Y. (1984) Open chain nitrogen compounds. V. Hydroxymethyltriazenes: Synthesis of some new homologues of the antitumor 3-methyl-3-hydroxymethyltriazenes and preparation of the derived acetoxymethyl, benzoyloxymethyl, and methoxymethyltriazenes. *Can. J. Chem.* **62**: 741–748.

Hickman, J. A. (1978) Investigation of the mechanism of action of antitumor dimethyltriazenes. *Biochemie* **60**: 997–1002.

Iley, J., and Ruecroft, G. (1988) Triazene drug metabolites. Part 7.1: A biomimetic synthesis of N-alkyl-N-formyltriazenes. *J. Chem. Research* **(S)**: 24–25.

Iley, J., Rosa, E., and Fernandez, L. (1987) Triazene drug metabolites. Part 5.1: A simple direct synthesis of 3-alkoxymethyl and 3-alkylthiomethyl-1-aryl-3-alkyl-triazenes from 1-aryl-3-hydroxy-methyl-3-alkyltriazenes. *J. Chem. Research* **(S)**: 264–265.

Kolar, G. F. (1986) Carcinogenicity of cytostatic triazenes. In *Carcinogenicity of alkylating cytostatic drugs*, pp. 111–126 (IARC Scientific Publications No. 78).

Kolar, G. F. (1984a) Triazenes. *Chemical carcinogens* **2**: 869–914.

Kolar, G. F.(1984b) *American Chemical Society Monograph* **182**: 869–914.

Kolar, G. F., and Schendzielorz, M. (1986) Reactions of substituted arenediazonium chlorides with methylamine–formaldehyde premix revisited: Reactivity and transformations of methylolamine intermediates and their biological significance. *Z. für Naturforsch.* **42c**: 41–46.

Kolar, G. F., and Schendzielorz, M. (1985) 3,7-Bis-(4-trifluormethylphenyl)-1,5,3,7-dioxadiazocine: A novel cyclic product from a reaction of 4-trifluoromethylbenzenediazonium chloride and methylamine-formaldehyde. *Tetrahedron Lett.* **26**: 1043–1044.

Kolar, G. F., and Habs, M. (1984) Comparative metabolism and carcinogenicity of ring-halogenated 3,3-dimethyl-1-phenyltriazenes. *J. Cancer Res. Clin. Oncol.* **108**: 71–75.

Kolar, G. F., Maurer, M., and Wildschütte, M. (1980) 5-(3-Hydroxymethyl-3-methyltriazeno)imidazole-4-carboxamide (DIC, DTIC, NSC 45388). *Cancer Lett.* **10**: 241–253.

Kolar, G. F., and Carubelli, R. (1979a) [1-Methyl-3-(2,4,6-trichlorophenyl)-2-triazeno]methyl-β-D-glucopyranosiduronic acid is a novel metabolite of 1-(2,4,6-trichlorophenyl)-3,3-dimethyltriazene. In *Glycoconjugates*,

Proceedings of the Fifth International Symposium, Kiel, pp. 656–657, edited by R. Schauer, P. Boer, E. Buddecke, M. F. Kramer, J. F. G. Vliegenthart, and H. Wiegandt. Stuttgart: George Thieme.

Kolar, G. F., and Carubelli, R. (1979b) Urinary metabolites of 1-(2,4,6-trichlorophenyl)-3,3-dimethyltriazene with an intact diazoamino structure. *Cancer Lett.* **7**: 209–214.

Kolar, G. F., and Schlesiger, J. (1976a) Metabolism of the tumor-inhibitory 3,3-dimethyl-1-phenyltriazene and its 4-chlorophenyl analogue. In *Chemotherapy*, K. Hellman and T. A. Connors, eds., Vol. 8, pp. 91–96. New York: Plenum Press.

Kolar, G. F. and Schlesiger, J. (1976b) Urinary metabolites of 3,3-dimethyl-1-phenyltriazene. *Chem. Biol. Interact.* **14**: 301–311.

Kolar, G. F., and Schlesiger, J. (1975) Biotransformation of 1-(4-chlorophenyl)-3,3-dimethyltriazene into 3-chloro-4-hydroxyaniline. Intramolecular hydroxylation-induced chlorine migration during a catabolic degradation of a chemical carcinogen. *Cancer Lett.* **1**: 43–47.

Kolar, G. F., and Preussmann, R. (1971) Validity of a linear Hammett plot for the stability of some carcinogenic 1-aryl-3,3-dimethyl-triazenes in an aqueous system. *Zeitschrift für Naturforschung* **26b**: 950–953.

Lafrance, R. I., Tang, Y., Vaughan, K., and Hooper, D. L. (1983) N,N-Bis-(1-aryl-3-methyltriazene-3-yl-methyl)methylamines (1,9-diaryl-3,5,7-trimethyl-1,2,3,5,7,8,9-hepta-azanona-1,8-dienes): Novel coupling products from the reaction of arenediazonium ions with methylamine and formaldehyde. *J. Chem. Soc. Chem. Commun.* **13**: 721–722.

Lassiani, L., Nisi, C., Sigon, F., Sava, G., and Giraldi, T. (1980) Synthesis of 1-aryl-3-formyl-3-methyltriazenes, potential metabolites of 1-aryl-3,3-dimethyltriazenes. *J. Pharmaceutical Sciences* **69**: 1098–1099.

Lucas, V. S., and Huang, A. T. (1982) Chemotherapy of melanoma. In *Clinical management of melanoma*, A. Seigler, ed., pp. 381–404. The Hague: Martinus Nijhoff.

Montgomery, J. A. (1976) Experimental studies at Southern Research Institute with DTIC (NSC 45388). *Cancer Treat. Rep.* **60**: 125–134.

Newell, D., Gescher, A., Harland, S., Ross, D., and Rutty, C. (1987) N-Methyl antitumor agents. *Cancer Chemother. Pharmacol.* **19**: 91–102.

Overton, M., Hickman, J. A., Threadgill, M. D., Vaughan, K., and Gescher, A. (1985) The generation of potentially toxic, reactive iminium ions from the oxidative metabolism of xenobiotic N-alkyl compounds. *Biochem. Pharmac.* **34**: 2055–2061.

Preussmann, R., and von Hodenberg, A. (1969) Mechanism of carcinogenesis of 1-aryl-3,3-dialkyltriazenes. Enzymatic dealkylation by rat liver microsomal fraction *in vitro*. *Biochem. Pharmac.* **18**: 1–13.

Preussmann, R., Druckrey, H., Ivankovic, S., and von Hodenberg, A. (1969) Chemical structure and carcinogenicity of aliphatic hydrazo, azo, and azoxy compounds and of triazenes, potential *in vivo* alkylating agents. *Ann. N.Y. Acad. Sci.* **163**: 697–714.

Shealy, Y. F., Krauth, C. A., and Montgomery, J. A. (1962a) Imidazoles. I. Coupling reactions of 5-diazo-imidazole-4-carboxamide. *J. Org. Chem.* **27**: 2150–2154.

Shealy, Y. F., Montgomery, J. A., and Laster, W. R., Jr. (1962b) Antitumor activity of triazenoimidazoles. *Biochem. Pharmacol.* **11**: 674–676.

Spassova, M. K., and Golovinksy, E. V. (1985) Pharmacobiochemistry of arylalkyltriazenes and their application in cancer chemotherapy. *Pharmac. Ther.* **27**: 333–352.

Vaughan, K., Gamage Nicholas, K. U. K., Singer, R. D., Roy, M., and Gibson, N. W. (1987) Triazene metabolism. VI. 3-Azidomethyl-3-alkyl-1-aryltriazenes, a new class of antitumor triazene with potential prodrug application. *Anti-Cancer Drug Design* **2**: 279–287.

Wilman, D. E. V. (1988) The development of a second-generation triazene. *Cancer Treatment Reviews* **15**: 69–72.

Wilman, D. E. V. (1986) Prodrugs in cancer chemotherapy. *Biochemical Society Transactions* **14**: 375–382.

Wilman, D. E. V., and Connors, T. A. (1983) Molecular structure and antiumor activity of alkylating agents. In *Molecular aspects of anti-cancer drug action*, S. Neidle and N. J. Waring, eds., Vol. 8, pp. 233–282. Weinheim: Verlag Chemie.

CHAPTER 7

INTERSTRAND DNA CROSS-LINKING IN TUMOR CELLS BY 1-NITROACRIDINES, ANTHRACYCLINES, AND AMINOANTHRAQUINONES

JERZY KONOPA

Department of Pharmaceutical Technology and Biochemistry, Technical University of Gdańsk, Gdańsk, Poland

Abstract—Potent anticancer 1-nitro-9-aminoacridine derivatives, including Nitracrine, anthracyclines (adriamycin, daunomycin, rubidazon, epirubicin, aclacinomycin A, marcellomycin, and cinerubin A), and aminoanthraquinones are able to induce covalent interstrand cross-links in DNA of tumor cells, as was shown by mild procedures developed to detect interstrand DNA cross-links. Metabolic activation is a prerequisite for interstrand DNA cross-linking by these antitumor agents. Some data which indicate the importance of cross-linking potency of 1-nitro-9-aminoacridines, anthracyclines, and aminoanthraquinones for their biological activity are also presented.

1. INTRODUCTION

Studies on antitumor activity of acridine derivatives conducted by the late Zygmunt Ledóchowski and Andrzej Ledóchowski in the Department of Pharmaceutical Technology and Biochemistry, Technical University of Gdańsk, led to the development of a group of potent, antitumor 1-nitro-9-aminoacridine derivatives. One of these acridine derivatives (Fig. 7-1) has been accepted under the name of Ledakrin (WHO recommended the name Nitracrine) as an antitumor drug in Poland.

1-Nitro-9-aminoacridines exhibit exceptionally high cytotoxic activity (Konopa et al., 1969; Pawlak et al., 1984) and potent antitumor activity (Hrabowska et al., 1982). It is important to note that 2-, 3-, and 4-nitro isomers of 9-aminoacridine, which differ from the very active 1-nitro isomers only in the position of a nitro group, are biologically inactive (Konopa et al., 1969).

2. NITRO-9-AMINOACRIDINES BINDING TO DNA

Comparative biochemical studies of a group of 1-, 2-, 3-, and 4-nitro-9-aminoacridines, including Ledakrin, which differ in the position of a nitro group and the number of methylene groups in the side chain, were performed to elucidate the role of intercalation to DNA in biological activity of this class of compounds. Thermal denaturation–renaturation

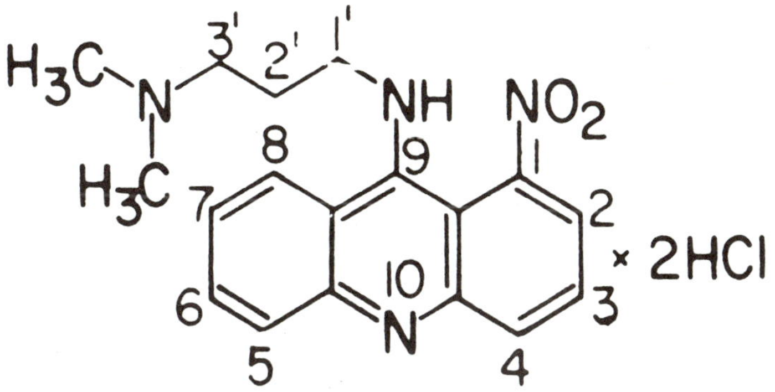

FIG. 7-1. Structure of Ledakrin (Nitracrine), 1-nitro-9-(3′-dimethylaminopropylamino)acridine dihydrochloride.

studies of DNA complexes with these nitroacridine isomers showed that 2-, 3-, and 4-nitro-9-aminoacridine derivatives increase the temperature of DNA denaturation, thus stabilizing the secondary DNA structure to a greater extent than 1-nitro-9-amino derivatives. Moreover, the cytotoxic activities of the nitro isomers tested do not correlate with either affinity to DNA, expressed as association constants, or the number of binding sites in DNA.

Among all nitro-9-aminoacridines examined, Ledakrin and other 1-nitro-9-aminoacridines are the weakest inhibitors of DNA polymerase reactions. This finding allows us to conclude that intercalation into DNA, and other types of physicochemical binding of 1-nitro-9-aminoacridines to DNA, including Ledakrin, cannot be considered as a basis for the exceptionally high biological activity of 1-nitro derivatives (Pawlak, K., et al., 1983).

The existing correlation between activity of 1-nitro-9-aminoacridines and their ability to inhibit biosynthesis of macromolecules (DNA, RNA, and proteins) in tumor cells, suggests that these derivatives may undergo intracellular metabolic activation (Pawlak, K., et al., 1983).

Initially, the possibility of reduction of the 1-nitro group to an N-hydroxylamino group, which is able to bind covalently to DNA, was considered and experimentally demonstrated. Radiolabeled Ledakrin very effectively binds covalently to DNA and other cellular macromolecules both in tumor cells (HeLa, Ehrlich ascites carcinoma) as well as in the presence of microsomes (Konopa et al., 1976, Pawlak & Konopa, 1979, Pawlak, K., et al., 1983). Of the total amount of Ledakrin covalently bound to macromolecules in HeLa cells, only 15% is bound to DNA. At optimal conditions, 1 Ledakrin residue binds per 400 and 50 base pairs in HeLa cells and in *B. subtilis* SB 1058, respectively. The ^{32}P-postlabeling assay shows that similarly high levels of covalent binding to DNA in tumor cells occurs also for other 1-nitroacridines (Bartoszek & Konopa, 1989). Metabolic activation, which will be discussed in detail shortly, is a prerequisite for covalent binding of Ledakrin to DNA in bacterial and tumor cells (Pawlak, K., et al., 1983). It is interesting that high levels of covalent binding of Ledakrin to DNA were observed also under reducing conditions provoked by the presence of dithiothreitol (Szmigiero & Gniazdowski, 1981). Biologically inactive 2-, 3-, and 4-nitro-9-aminoacridines do not bind covalently to DNA in tumor cells, as demonstrated by ^{32}P-postlabeling assay (Bartoszek & Konopa, 1987).

Fractionation of the enzymatic digest of DNA, isolated from Ehrlich ascites tumor cells treated with radiolabeled Ledakrin, led to separation of a fraction of modified nucleosides, which were not present in the digest of DNA of control cells. Field desorption mass spectrometry revealed that this fraction contained five Ledakrin nucleoside adducts, and that the mass ion of some of these adducts corresponded to the molecular weight of adducts formed by one Ledakrin residue and two nucleosides. Such adducts could be formed as a result of DNA cross-linking by Ledakrin (Pawlak, J. W., et al., 1983).

3. COVALENT INTERSTRAND DNA CROSS-LINKING

3.1. 1-NITRO-9-AMINOACRIDINES

Formation of covalent interstrand cross-links in DNA of HeLa cells in culture, Ehrlich ascites tumor-bearing mice, and *Bacillus subtilis* SB 1058 was demonstrated by three independent procedures, namely, thermal denaturation–renaturation curve analysis, hydroxylapatite column chromatography, and partitioning in a dextran–polyethylene glycol 600 biphasic system of DNA isolated from cells treated with nitroacridines (Konopa et al., 1976, 1983; Pawlak, K., et al., 1984). An example of the thermal denaturation–renaturation curves obtained for DNA isolated from HeLa cells treated with Ledakrin is shown in Fig. 7-2. The denatured DNA from cells treated with Ledakrin (Figs. 7-2B, 7-2C) after cooling renatured to the native, double-stranded form to a greater extent than did DNA from nontreated HeLa cells (Fig. 7-2A). With a second cycle of heating, DNA from cells treated with Ledakrin melted cooperatively within a sharp transition region at a T_m very close to the value observed during the first heating cycle (Figs. 7-2B, 7-2C). In the case of

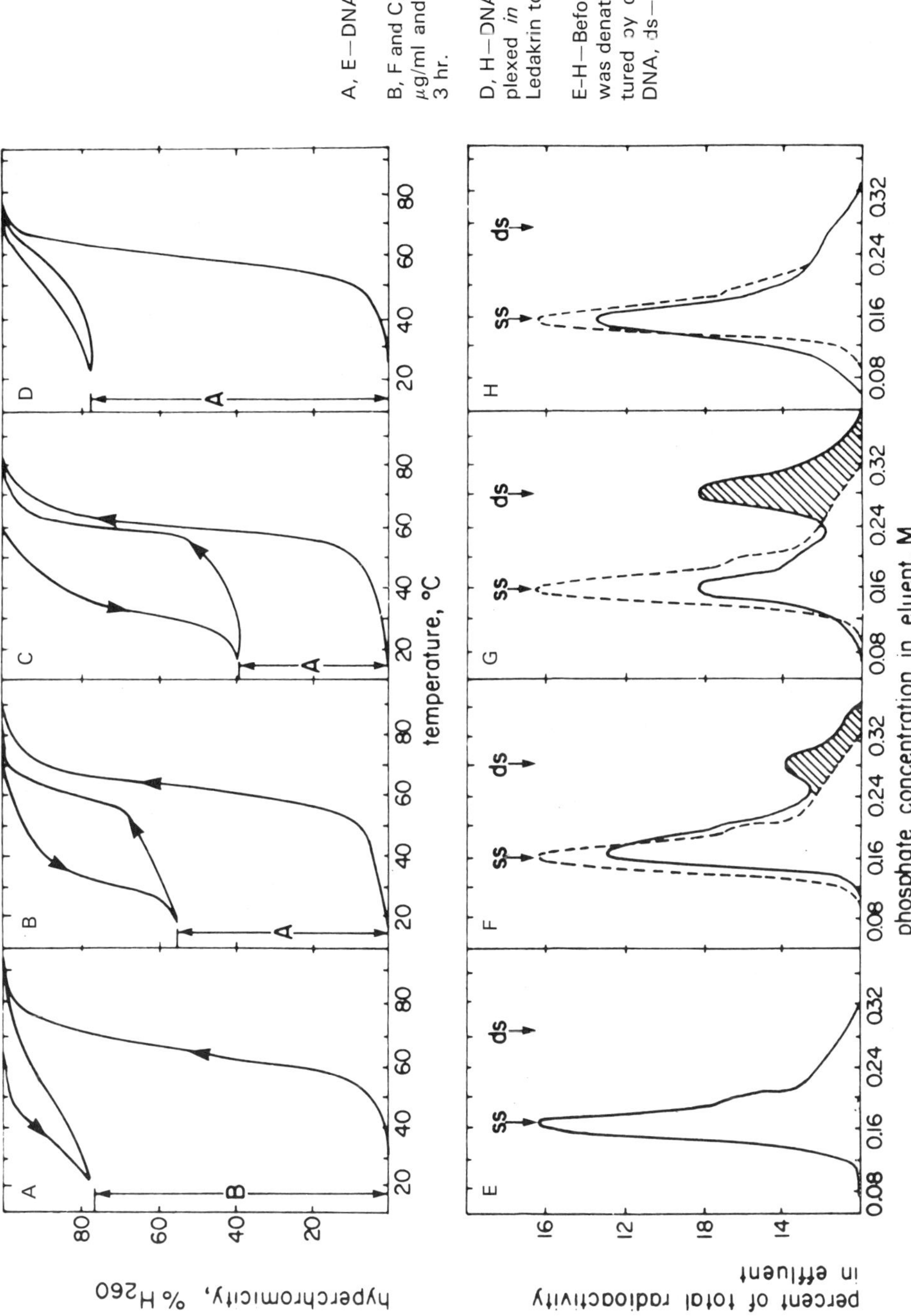

A, E—DNA from nontreated HeLa cells.

B, F and C, G—DNA from HeLa cells treated with 0.5 μg/ml and 1.5 μg/ml of Ledakrin, respectively, for 3 hr.

D, H—DNA isolated from nontreated HeLa cells complexed *in vitro* with Ledakrin, molecular ratio of Ledakrin to DNA 1:100.

E-H—Before chromatography on hydroxylapatite, DNA was denatured by heating (100°C, 6 min) and renatured by cooling in ice water. ss—single-stranded DNA, ds—double-stranded DNA.

Fig. 7-2. Thermal denaturation–renaturation studies (A–D) and chromatographic separation on hydroxylapatite (E–H) of DNA isolated from HeLa cells treated with Ledakrin, and DNA from HeLa cells complexed *in vitro* with Ledakrin. (From Konopa et al. (1983).)

DNA from nontreated HeLa cells, only a small fraction of the DNA renatured, perhaps due to spontaneous pairing of bases, as could be concluded from the nonsigmoidal shape of a "second heating" curve (Fig. 7-2A). When DNA from control nontreated HeLa cells was complexed *in vitro* with Ledakrin, the shape of the thermal denaturation–renaturation curve (Fig. 7-2D) was similar to that of control DNA (Fig. 7-2A).

It follows that Ledakrin forms interstrand cross-links in DNA not directly, but must be preceded by metabolic activation. When DNA samples from either nontreated or Ledakrin-treated HeLa cells, after denaturation and renaturation, were fractionated using hydroxylapatite, fractions of renatured double-stranded DNA in samples derived from treated cells appeared (Fig. 7-2F, 7-2G). This suggests that Ledakrin is a DNA interstrand cross-linking agent. The absence of fractions of renatured DNA in the case of complexing isolated DNA *in vitro* with Ledakrin (Fig. 7-2H) additionally proves that Ledakrin is able to form interstrand DNA cross-links after metabolic activation (Konopa et al., 1983). Formation of interstrand cross-links in DNA of L1210 cells by Ledakrin (Filipski et al., 1977), as well as *in vitro* covalent interstrand cross-linking of DNA by this drug in the presence of dithiothreitol (Gniazdowski et al., 1981) was also observed. When compared with mitomycin C, Ledakrin is 10-fold more potent in inducing interstrand cross-links in DNA of *B. subtilis* (Fig. 7-3), but biological activity of Ledakrin in this system is also 10 times higher than is that of mitomycin C (Konopa et al., 1983). It has been estimated that Ledakrin, under optimal conditions, forms one covalent interstrand cross-link per approximately 2.0×10^4 (*B. subtilis*), 5.6×10^4 (HeLa), and 8.0×10^4 (Ehrlich ascites) DNA base pairs (Konopa et al., 1983). Biologically inactive 2-, 3-, and 4-nitro-9-aminoacridines are unable to induce interstrand DNA cross-links (Konopa et al., 1983).

As mentioned earlier, metabolic activation of Ledakrin and other 1-nitro-9-aminoacridines is a prerequisite for their covalent binding to DNA, thus for interstrand DNA cross-linking. The proposed pathways of metabolic activation of Ledakrin are shown in Fig. 7-4. The most important pathways, probably responsible for the formation of covalent inter-

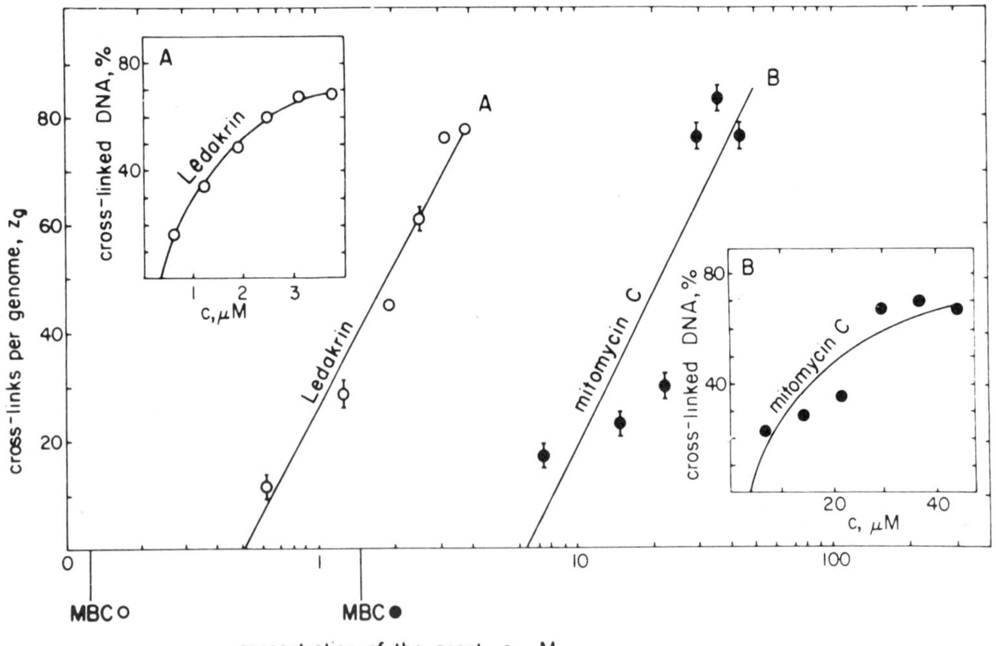

Fig. 7-3. Average number of induced cross-links per single *Bacillus subtilis* SB 1058 cell genome after incubation of the cells with either Ledakrin or mitomycin C, as determined by thermal denaturation-renaturation curve analysis. MBC—minimal bacteriostatic concentration. (From Konopa et al. (1983).)

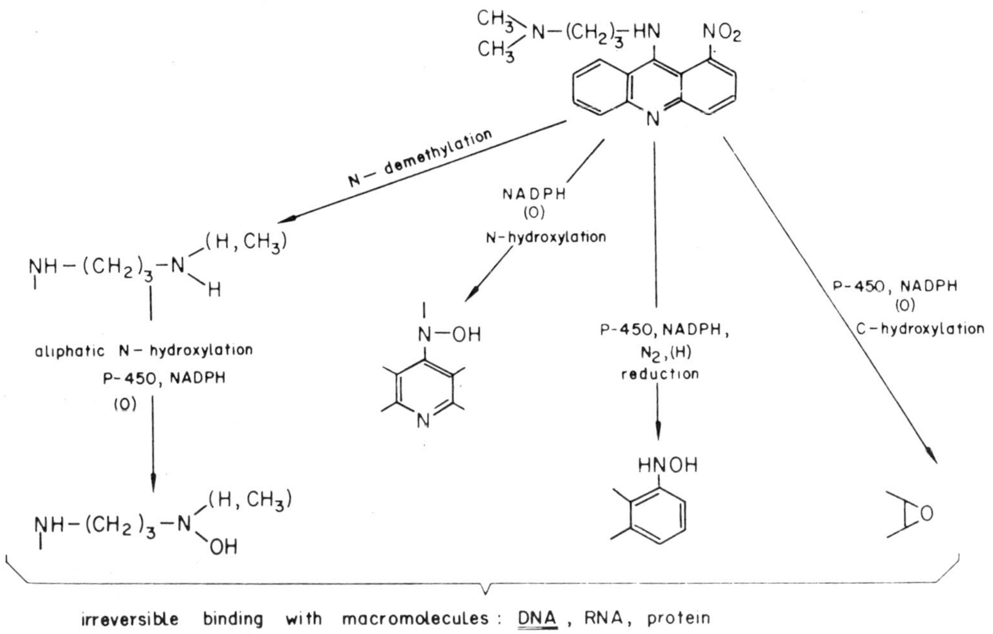

FIG. 7-4. Possible pathways of metabolic activation of Ledakrin. (From Pawlak and Konopa (1977).)

strand cross-links by Ledakrin and other 1-nitroacridines, are the reduction of a nitro group to a hydroxylamino group, and the oxidation of an amino group in the position 9 to a hydroxylamino group. Such metabolic activation is unique, because 1-nitro-9-amino-acridines are activated simultaneously by two types of reaction: reduction and oxidation. Other DNA cross-linking agents are activated by only one type of reaction, for example, mitomycin C by reduction and cyclophosphamide by oxidation.

These unique properties of 1-nitro-9-aminoacridines result from their chemical structure. The fused-ring system of Ledakrin is not planar but has a butterflylike shape, in contrast to other derivatives of acridine. The nitro group is twisted out of the plane of the three-ring acridine system, and the typical properties of the aromatic nitro group are lost. The amino group in position 9 exists rather as an amino group and the central ring is not aromatic (Dauter et al., 1975, 1976).

3.1.1. *Relevance to Biological Activity*

After the demonstration that 1-nitroacridines are potent interstrand DNA cross-linking agents the question about relevance of this phenomenon to the biological activity of 1-nitro-9-aminoacridines is pertinent. The inability of biologically inactive 2-, 3-, and 4-nitro-9-aminoacridine derivatives to induce interstrand DNA cross-links (Konopa et al., 1983) suggests that this lesion represents the crucial event responsible for biological activity of 1-nitroacridines. This was supported additionally by studies on the correlation between biological activity and DNA cross-linking potency of 1-nitro-9-aminoacridines. The ability to induce covalent interstrand cross-links in DNA of HeLa S_3 cells for a series of 1-nitroacridines (Table 7-1) is presented in Fig. 7-5. The derivatives studied differed in the structure of the side chain and exhibited divergent cytotoxic activity against this cell line. For each acridine it was possible to estimate by extrapolation a concentration C_0 at which the first cross-link could be detected. The difference between C_0 values of the most, and least, active 1-nitro-9-aminoacridines is about 150, similar to the difference between cytotoxic activities of these compounds. Statistical analysis of these results showed that a significant correlation exists between *in vitro* interstrand DNA cross-linking potency of 1-nitroacri-

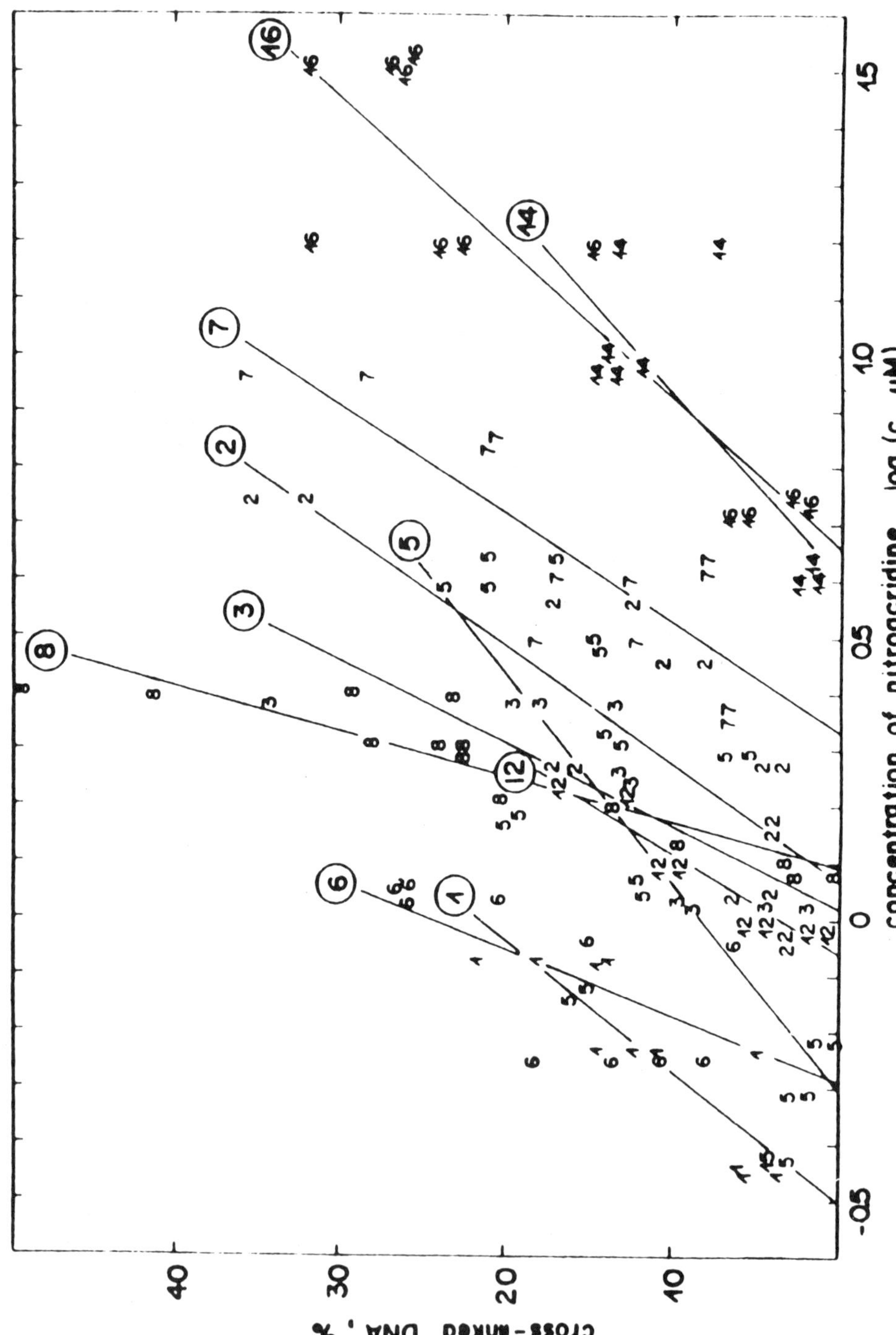

FIG. 7-5. Fraction of cross-linked DNA from HeLa S_3 cells treated with different concentrations of 1-nitro-9-aminoacridines listed in Table 7-1. The numbers in circles correspond to the code numbers of 1-nitroacridines listed in Table 7-1. The data points relate to the assigned 1-nitroacridine code numbers (Table 7-1) to the experimentally determined values. (From Konopa et al. (1984).)

TABLE 7-1. *Cytotoxic Activity of 1-Nitro-9-aminoacridines Against HeLa S_3 Cells in Culture*

1-Nitro-acridine code no.	Synthetic designation	—R	EC_{50} (μM)*
2	C-857	$-NH-(CH_2)_2-OH$	0.0005
1	C-609	$-NH-(CH_2)_5-N(CH_3)_2$	0.0016
3	C-849	$-NH-(CH_2)_3-NH(CH_3)$	0.0028
6	C-835	$-NH-(CH_2)_2-N(CH_2CH_2OH)_2$	0.0031
8	C-283	$-NH-(CH_2)_3-N(CH_3)_2$	0.0037
5	C-846	$-NH-(CH_2)_3-NH-CH(CH_3)_2$	0.0041
12	C-516	$-NH-(CH_2)_2-N(C_2H_5)_2$	0.0077
7	C-1006	$-NH-(CH_2)_3-NH-(CH_2)_5-CH_3$	0.013
14	C-878	$-NH-CH(CH_3)COOC_2H_5$	0.028
16	C-684	$-NH-(CH_2)_3-N(CH_3)_2$-oxide	0.074

*EC_{50} values are drug concentrations inhibiting cell growth by 50% after 72 hr treatment as described elsewhere.

From K. Pawlak et al. (1984).

dines and their cytotoxic activity against HeLa S_3 cells and antitumor activity against sarcoma 180 in mice (Pawlak, K., et al., 1984). These correlation studies strongly suggest that interstrand DNA cross-linking potency is very likely a basis for potent cytotoxic and antitumor activity of 1-nitro-9-aminoacridines.

Following the finding that 1-nitro-9-aminoacridines, which were believed to belong to a group of classical DNA intercalating agents, exert their cytotoxic and antitumor activity by virtue of interstrand cross-linking of DNA in tumor cells, it was logical to consider that other very active antitumor compounds, which intercalate to DNA, might also form interstrand DNA cross-links.

3.2. ANTHRACYCLINES

To check this hypothesis, a group of antitumor anthracyclines, from which currently about 20 are under clinical trials, with adriamycin one of the most potent and widely used antitumor drugs, have been selected. Several mechanisms of action of this important group of compounds have been proposed: (1) high-affinity binding to DNA through intercalation, (2) generation of reactive radicals, (3) cell membrane effects leading to altered membrane fluidity, and (4) inhibition of topoisomerase II (for extensive review, see Gianni et al., 1983). None of these mechanisms has been convincingly proved, and binding to DNA by intercalation is widely accepted as a basis of antitumor activity of anthracyclines.

In all methods used for the detection of interstrand DNA cross-links, DNA must be denatured, usually by heating or alkalization. The additional assumption was also made that DNA cross-links formed by anthracyclines, as well as by other intercalating agents, might be alkali and/or thermolabile, so that they could escape detection by most of the well-established methods. To circumvent this, two mild and sensitive procedures for detection of interstrand DNA cross-links, shown in Fig. 7-6, in which DNA is denatured without using either high temperature or alkalization, were developed. In the first method (A), DNA without isolation, only after partial purification, delipidation, and deproteinization, is denatured by formamide at 40°C (Konopa, 1983). In the second (B), DNA in cell lysates, without isolation and purification, is denatured in concentrated sodium perchlorate solution, in the presence of methanol and elevated temperature up to 50°C (Konopa & Składanowski, 1988). The fraction of cross-linked DNA in both procedures is determined by nuclease S_1 assay.

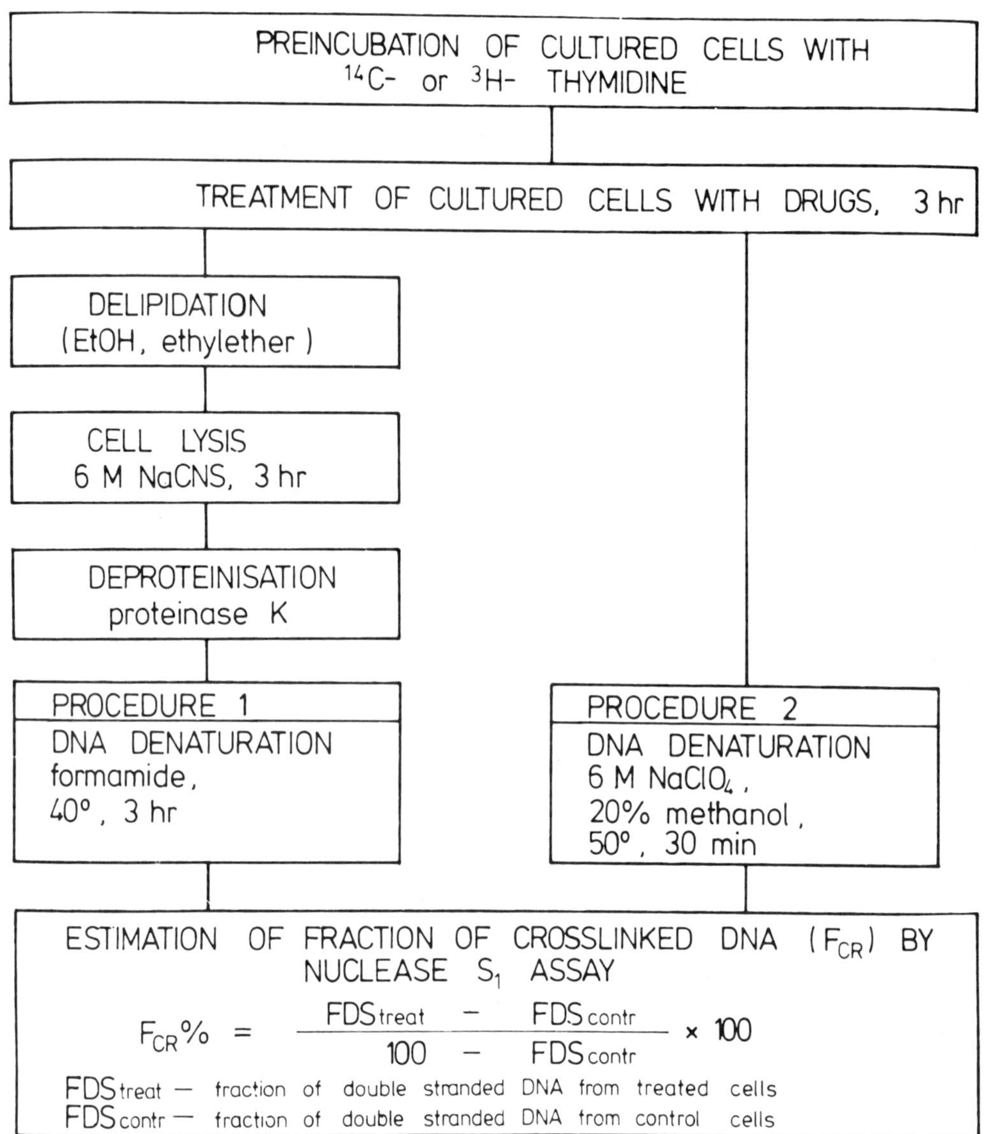

Fig. 7-6. Procedures for detection of interstrand cross-links in DNA of tumor cells.

Using procedure A, it was found that adriamycin and daunomycin form interstrand DNA cross-links in HeLa S_3 cells in a dose-dependent manner (Table 7-2) (Konopa, 1983). Similarly, by using procedure B, it was determined that anthracyclines of the so-called second class, aclacinomycin A, marcellomycin, and cinerubin A, induce interstrand cross-links in DNA of HeLa S_3 cells in a dose-dependent manner (Table 7-3) (Konopa & Składanowski, 1988).

The increased capability of renaturation of DNA from HeLa S_3 cells treated with anthracyclines, which is the basis for detection of interstrand DNA cross-links, cannot be attributed to strong binding of anthracyclines to DNA by intercalation. Fractions of cross-linked DNA, detected in cell lysates obtained from nontreated cells and then mixed with anthracyclines, are very low when compared with fractions of cross-linked DNA in lysates from cells treated with anthracyclines at the same 50 μM concentration (Tables 7-2, 7-3). From these studies in cell-free systems, a second important conclusion emerges. Inability of anthracyclines to induce DNA cross-links in cell-free systems means that metabolic activation is a prerequisite for interstrand DNA cross-linking by anthracyclines. Interstrand

TABLE 7-2. *Interstrand DNA Cross-linking in HeLa S_3 Cells after Treatment with Anthracyclines*

Concentration (μM)	Fraction of cross-linked DNA, F_{CR} (%)	
	Adriamycin	Daunomycin
10	11.0 = 2	15.3 = 1
20	–	16.2 = 1
50	24.8 = 2	20.8 = 3
150	41.7 = 5	–
50 μM Cell-free system	−0.5 = 2	−3.7 = 2

From Konopa (1983).

TABLE 7-3. *Interstrand DNA Cross-linking in HeLa S_3 Cells after Treatment with Second-class Anthracyclines*

Concentration (μM)	Fraction of cross-linked DNA, F_{CR} (%)		
	Aclacinomycin A	Marcellomycin	Cinerubin A
5	10.6 = 4	12.7 = 2	–
10	14.8 = 1	28.9 = 10	6.9 = 5
20	32.6 = 14	56.0 = 3	23.7 = 2
50	53.0 = 13	70.1 = 6	66.2 = 11
150	–	–	69.1 = 27
50-μM Cell-free system	−1.79	−3.06	−7.52

From Konopa and Składanowski (1988).

DNA cross-links formed by anthracyclines are thermal and alkali labile because almost no cross-linking of DNA was observed when DNA from cells treated with anthracyclines was denatured by high temperature or alkalization (Table 7-4). These findings explain also why formation of DNA cross-links by anthracyclines could not be detected by other currently used methods, especially by the widely used alkaline elution method (Konopa, 1983; Konopa & Składanowski, 1988).

3.2.1. *Relevance to Biological Activity*

Two approaches were adopted for studies on establishing the relevance of interstrand DNA cross-linking by anthracyclines to cytotoxic activity of these antibiotics. First, the ability of anthracyclines to interstrand cross-link DNA in cells sensitive and resistant to

TABLE 7-4. *Alkali and Thermal Lability of DNA Cross-links Formed by Anthracyclines after Treatment with 50 μM for 3 hr*

Compound	Fraction of cross-linked DNA, F_{CR} (%)	
	After alkaline* denaturation	After thermal† denaturation
Adriamycin	−1.1 = 0.6	−1.0 = 0.1
Daunomycin	0.7 = 1	−0.9 = 0.5
Aclacinomycin	−4.2 = 0.5	−0.1 = 0.4

*Alkaline denaturation, pH 12, 1 hr.
†Thermal denaturation, 100°, 15 min.

From Konopa and Składanowski (1988).

these antibiotics was studied. As shown in Fig. 7-7, interstrand DNA cross-linking by adriamycin in sensitive LoVo cells is considerably higher than in an adriamycin-resistant LoVo cell line. It is also very interesting that iododoxorubicin, which exhibits similar cytotoxic activity against both sensitive and resistant cells, is able to interstrand cross-link DNA of both lines to the same extent (A. Składanowski and J. Konopa, unpublished data). In the second approach, correlation between cytotoxic activity of anthracyclines and their ability to interstrand cross-link DNA were studied. As the results presented in Fig. 7-8 show, there is positive correlation between cytotoxic activity and ability to form interstrand DNA cross-links by anthracyclines studied. N-acetyl-daunomycin and 3′-N-(λ-/L/-alanyl)-daunomycin, DR-31, which exhibit low cytotoxic activity, exhibit also lower interstrand DNA cross-linking ability, in comparison to daunomycin. Biologically inactive 3′-N-(N,N-dibenzyl-λ-/L/-alanyl)-daunomycin, DR-28, does not form interstrand cross-links in DNA of HeLa S_3 cells, even at very high concentrations (A. Składanowski and J. Konopa, unpublished results). Results from these preliminary studies strongly suggest that ability to form interstrand DNA cross-links may be considered as a basis for cytotoxic and antitumor activity of anthracyclines.

3.3. Aminoanthraquinones

Another group of antitumor DNA intercalating agents which were studied for their ability to induce interstrand DNA cross-links are aminoanthraquinones. Like the anthracyclines, mitoxantrone and ametantrone were shown to induce interstrand cross-links in DNA of HeLa S_3 cells in a dose-dependent manner (Table 7-5). These cross-links, as in the case of anthracyclines, are thermal and alkali labile. When added directly to lysates of non-treated cells, neither drug forms interstrand DNA cross-links (Table 7-5); hence, their metabolic activation is necessary for interstrand DNA cross-linking to take place (Konopa & Składanowski, 1985, 1988). From a comparison of mitoxantrone and its close analog NSC 321458, which does not possess a distal amino group in the side chains, it does not exhibit cytotoxic and antitumor activity and also does not form interstrand DNA cross-links (Table 7-5). Two important conclusions emerge: First, the ability to induce DNA cross-links is important for biological activity of aminoanthraquinones, and second, ethylenediamino groups in the side chains are important not only for biological activity of aminoanthraquinones, which is well known from structure–activity relationship studies (Cheng et al.,

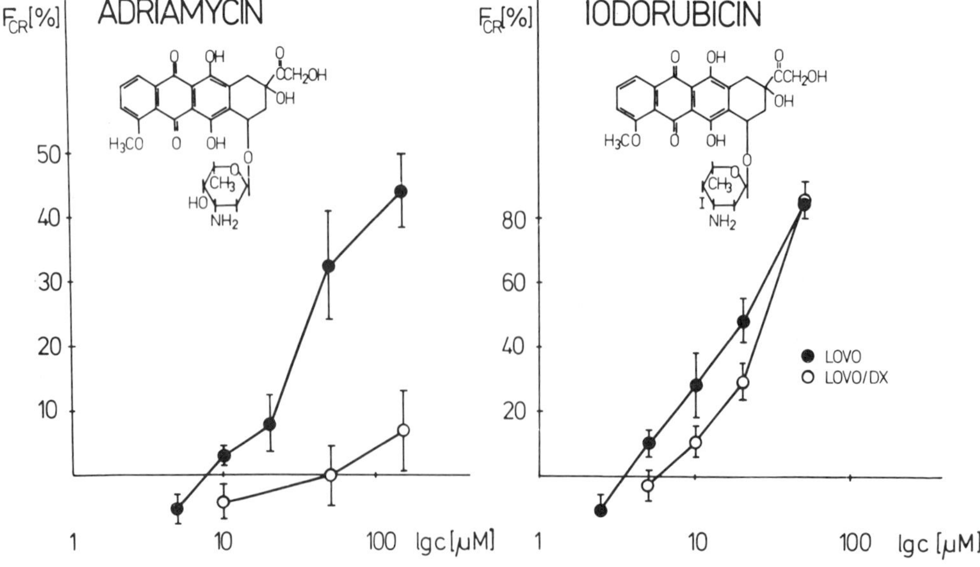

Fig. 7-7. Interstrand DNA cross-linking formed by anthracyclines in LoVo-sensitive and LoVo/DX adriamycin-resistant cells.

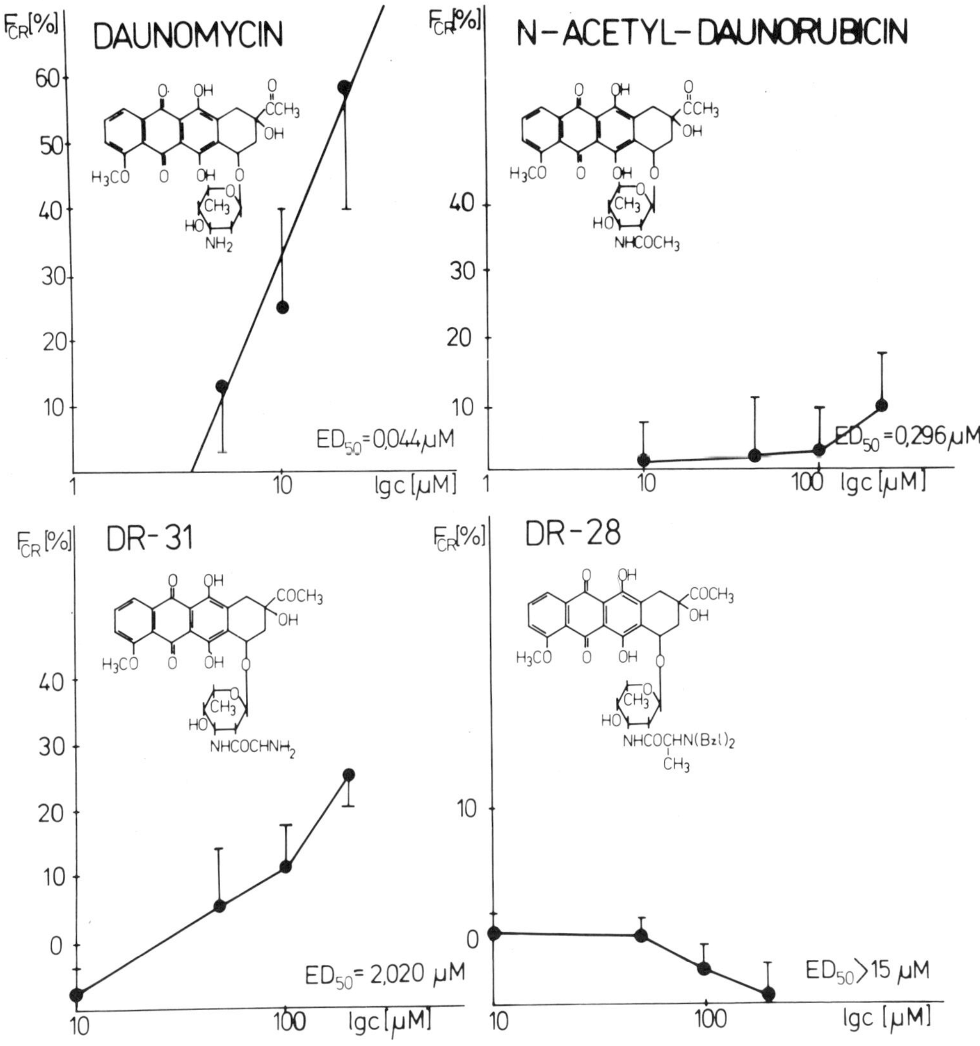

FIG. 7-8. Interstrand cross-linking of DNA of HeLa S_3 cells by daunomycin and its derivatives of lower cytotoxic activity.

TABLE 7.5. *Interstrand DNA Cross-linking in HeLa S_3 Cells after Treatment with Aminoanthraquinones*

MITOXANTRONE: $NHCH_2CH_2NHCH_2CH_2OH$ (×2), HO, O

NSC 321458: $NHCH_2CH_2CH_2CH_2CH_2OH$ (×2), HO, O

Concentration (μM)	Fraction of cross-linked DNA, F_{CR} (%) Ametantrone	Mitoxantrone	NSC 321458
20	12.8 = 8	10.6 = 2	–
50	25.4 = 15	36.2 = 7	–
100	37.5 = 12	–	−2.3 = 1
150	48.2 = 9	53.9 = 15	–
200	–	–	−2.6 = 2
50-μM Cell-free system	0.92	6.36	−2.46

From Konopa and Składanowski (1988).

1983) but are also important for interstrand DNA cross-linking (Konopa & Składanowski, 1988). One could speculate that these groups are involved in the formation of interstrand DNA cross-links, and also that these ethylenediamino groups undergo metabolic activation within the cell. Verification of this hypothesis calls for further studies.

REFERENCES

Bartoszek, A., and Konopa, J. (1989) ^{32}P-post-labeling analysis of DNA adduct formation by antitumor drug Nitracrine and other nitroacridines in different biological systems. *Biochem. Pharmacol.*, **38**:1301–1312.

Bartoszek, A., and Konopa, J. (1987) ^{32}P-post-labeling analysis of DNA adducts formed by antitumor 1-nitro-9-aminoacridines with DNA of HeLa S_3 cells. *Biochem. Pharmacol.* **36**:4169–4171.

Cheng, C. C., Robert, K. Y., and Zee-Cheng, B. S. (1983) The design, synthesis, and development of a new class of potent antineoplastic anthraquinones. In *Progress med. chem.*, G. P. Ellis and G. B. West, eds., Vol. 20, pp. 83–118. New York: Elsevier.

Dauter, Z., Bogucka-Ledóchowska, M., Hempel, A., Ledóchowski, A., and Kosturkiewicz, Z. (1976) X-ray investigation on acridine derivatives. I. Crystal and molecular structure of 1-nitro-9-(3-dimethylaminopropylamino)-acridine hydroiodide. *Ann. Soc. Chim. Polonorum/Roczniki Chemii* **50**:1573–1585.

Dauter, Z., Bogucka-Ledóchowska, M., Hempel, A., Ledóchowski, A., and Kosturkiewicz, Z. (1975) Crystal and molecular structure of 1-nitro-9-(3-dimethylaminopropylamino)-acridine (C-283) monoiodide. *Ann. Soc. Chim. Polonorum/Roczniki Chemii* **49**: 859–861.

Filipski, J., Marczyński, B., Sadzińska, L., Chałupka, G., and Chorąży, M. (1977) Interactions of some nitroderivatives of substituted 9-aminoacridine with DNA. *Biochim. Biophys. Acta* **478**: 33–43.

Gianni, L., Corden, B. J., and Myers, C. E. (1983) The biochemical basis of anthracyclines toxicity and antitumor activity. In *Reviews in biochemical toxicology*, E. Hodgson, J. R. Bend and R. M. Philpot, eds., Vol. 5, pp. 1–82. New York, Amsterdam, Oxford: Elsevier Biomed.

Gniazdowski, M., Ciesielska, E., and Szmigiero, L. (1981) Some properties of the irreversible complexes of Nitracrine (Ledakrin, C-283) with polynucleotides. *Chem.-Biol. Interact.* **34**: 355–366.

Hrabowska, M., Mazerska, Z., Pawadziej-Lukowicz, J., Onoszko, K., and Ledóchowski, A. (1982) Antitumor activity of 1-nitro-9-aminoacridine derivatives. *Arzneim.-Forsch./Drug Res.* **32**: 1013–1016.

Konopa, J. (1983) Adriamycin and daunomycin induce interstrand DNA cross-links in HeLa S_3 cells. *Biochem. Biophys. Res. Comm.* **110**: 819–826.

Konopa, J., and Składanowski, A. (1988) Anthracyclines and anthracenediones induce covalent interstrand DNA cross-links in tumor cells. In *Proc. 15th Int. Congress Chemother.*, Istanbul, 1987, Ecomed, ed., Landsberg/Lech, in press.

Konopa, J., and Składanowski, A. (1985) Mitoxantrone induces covalent interstrand DNA cross-linking in tumor cells. In *Proc. 14th Int. Congress Chemother.*, Kyoto, 1985, J. Ishigami, ed., University of Tokyo Press, pp. 633–634.

Konopa, J., Pawlak, J. W., and Pawlak, K. (1983) The mode of action of cytotoxic and antitumor 1-nitroacridines. III. *In vivo* interstrand cross-linking of DNA of mammalian or bacterial cells by 1-nitroacridines. *Chem.-Biol. Interact.* **43**: 175–197.

Konopa, J., Kołdej, K., and Pawlak, J. W. (1976) Covalent binding of 1-nitro-9-(3′-dimethyl-amino-N-propylamino)acridine, a new antitumor drug, to DNA of Ehrlich ascites tumor cells *in vivo*. *Chem.-Biol. Interact.* **13**: 99–103.

Konopa, J., Ledóchowski, A., Matuszkiewicz, A., and Jereczek-Morawska, E. (1969) *In vitro* studies on the cytotoxic properties of 9-amino-nitroacridine derivatives. *Neoplasma* **16**: 171–179.

Pawlak, J. W., Pawlak, K., and Konopa, J. (1983) The mode of action of cytotoxic and antitumor 1-nitroacridines. II. *In vivo* enzyme-mediated covalent binding of a 1-nitroacridine derivative, Ledakrin or Nitracrine, with DNA and other macromolecules of mammalian or bacterial cells. *Chem.-Biol. Interact.* **43**: 151–173.

Pawlak, J. W., and Konopa, J. (1979) *In vitro* binding of metabolically activated (^{14}C)-Ledakrin, or 1-nitro-9-^{14}C-(3′-dimethylamino-N-propylamino)acridine, a new antitumor and DNA cross-linking agent, to macromolecules of subcellular fractions isolated from rat liver and HeLa cells. *Biochem. Pharmacol.* **28**: 3391–3402.

Pawlak, K., Pawlak, J. W., and Konopa, J. (1984) Cytotoxic and antitumor activity of 1-nitroacridines as an aftereffect of their interstrand DNA cross-linking. *Cancer Res.* **44**: 4289–4296.

Pawlak, K., Matuszkiewicz, A., Pawlak, J. W., and Konopa, J. (1983) The mode of action of cytotoxic and antitumor 1-nitroacridines. I. The 1-nitroacridines do not exert their cytotoxic effects by physicochemical binding with DNA. *Chem.-Biol. Interact.* **43**: 131–149.

Szmigiero, L., and Gniazdowski, M. (1981) Complexes of Nitracrine with DNA. *Arzneim.-Forsch./Drug Res.* **31**: 1875–1877.

CHAPTER 8

TARGETING OF ANTICANCER AGENTS TO CELLULAR MEMBRANES OF CANCER CELLS

George Deliconstantinos

Department of Experimental Physiology,
University of Athens Medical School, Athens, Greece

Abstract—Alterations in plasma membrane fluidity in cancer cells with concomitant modifications in cell surface syndromic and/or antidromic proteins give rise to (1) ligand-induced redistribution of cell surface antigens and receptors, leading to "patching" or "capping"; (2) expression or exposition of cryptic antidromic antigens and/or receptors; (3) enzymatic activity; (4) microaggregation of receptors, essential for signal transduction of various hormones; and (5) transduction mechanism translating the external signal into internal signal carried by second messengers.

Advances in cancer therapy may be derived from the elucidation of the regulation of cell proliferation and differentiation by transforming growth factors (TGFs) (low-molecular-weight proteins). Such factors may be induced and/or activated by oncogene(s) rather than as a consequence of cellular changes during the process of transformation. Current trends toward these directions include (1) manipulation of the membrane fluidity using specific membrane modifiers and (2) interference with the synthesis, processing, and secretion of the growth factors. It should be expected that compounds which disrupt the activity of tyrosine kinases, protein kinase C, ion channels, and other transduction mechanisms would provide a new approach for the treatment of neoplastic diseases. Attempts could also focus on alteration of the availability and/or the function of the membrane receptors by designing compounds that alter receptor internalization and recycling. The wide chemical variability of synthetic ether lipids and related compounds may open a new perspective in the therapy of leukemia and cancer in humans. The possibility that cancer cell plasma membranes expose various proteins (e.g., membrane-bound enzymes) by altering the membrane fluidity has triggered a potentially new approach in the treatment of neoplastic diseases.

1. INTRODUCTION

The fluid mosaic model for the structure of the cell membrane proposed by Singer and Nicolson (1972) has brought in its wake an increasing realization that many of the roles played by the plasma membrane may be mediated by the intrinsic fluidity of the membrane. The fluidity of the plasma membrane has considerable implications for cell behavior *in vitro* and *in vivo*. Membrane fluidity can affect cell shape and adhesion *in vitro*. Deformability of the cell can affect adhesion-dependent phenomena such as cellular aggregation and cellular motility. The mobility of membrane antigens and lectin receptors is attributable to fluidity, and compatible with this is the demonstration that changes in ambient temperature reduce lateral mobility of membrane components (Edidin, 1974; Inbar et al., 1974).

Membrane-associated proteins which are amphipathic in nature may be immersed to different degrees and also interact with submembranous peripheral and cytoskeletal proteins (Golan & Veatch, 1980), and both fluidity and anchorage may determine their lateral mobility. Furthermore, the protein content can raise the viscosity of the membrane (Jacobson et al., 1981). Membrane lipid fluidity affects receptor function at both static and dynamic levels. At the steady-state equilibrium of the membrane, the lipid fluidity operates as a determinant of the lipid-free volume, which determines the degree of submergence of freely diffusible receptor molecules in the membrane lipid bilayer. This, in turn, is reflected in the available portion of the total receptor capacity for ligand binding. On the dynamic level the lipid microviscosity acts as a retarding force in lateral and rotational diffusion processes. These processes presumably determine the rate of coupling between the occupied receptor with other receptors or second messenger to form the signaling unit. The dependence of the overt receptor activity on the membrane lipid fluidity is a combination of static and dynamic effects (Shinitzky & Henkart, 1979). The application of molecular genetic techniques to membrane biology began in the late 1970s and already has had a major impact. This is particularly true in growth regulation. Membrane growth factor receptors have been purified, sequenced, and cloned (Ullrich et al., 1984, 1985; Schlessinger, 1988).

In therapeutics, alterations of tumor cell membrane fluidity have been identified which could serve as a target for pharmacological intervention (Shinitzky, 1984; Deliconstantinos, 1987a). It is not unreasonable to speculate that over the coming years, the plasma membrane will emerge as a major focus for the diagnosis and therapy of malignant tumors. The ability to insert, modify, and delete genes coding for membrane molecules will provide valuable insight into the function of individual membrane (glyco)proteins and how they interact with other membrane components to confer particular biology of signal transduction. The mechanism by which extracellular signals are conveyed across the plasma membrane to the cytoplasm and the nucleus remains relatively obscure. Signal transduction is a crucial membrane property and advances in this area are likely to have substantial impact on our understanding of cell biology. The participation of arachidonic acid metabolites in regulating signal transduction, second messenger levels, and gene expression will likely emerge as a critical focus for understanding how membrane biochemistry can influence overall cell metabolism (Berridge, 1987). Advances in cancer therapy may also be expected from an increased understanding of the regulation of cell proliferation and differentiation by specific growth factors (acting through autocrine, paracrine, or endocrine mechanisms), whose aberrant expression can be implicated in neoplastic proliferation (Goustin et al., 1986). One approach is to interfere with the synthesis, processing, and secretion to the growth factor. An additional strategy is to usurp the availability and/or the function of their corresponding membrane-bound receptors. In this situation, the purpose is to design compounds that could alter the binding of growth factors to their receptors, and/or to alter receptor internalization and recycling. Compounds able to disrupt the activity of tyrosine kinases, protein kinase C, ion channels, and other transduction mechanisms will prove useful tools in examining growth regulation and some may hold the prospect of clinical utility.

2. EFFECT OF ANTINEOPLASTIC AGENTS ON MEMBRANE FLUIDITY OF CANCER CELLS

The possibility that membrane fluidity may be involved in the processes leading to changes in the biological behavior of cells following neoplastic transformation was recognized several years ago. A solid tumor that has been most extensively studied, in experimental animals, with respect to the fluidity of the plasma and mitochondria membranes is the hepatoma. The higher diphenylhexatriene (DPH) fluorescence polarization values in hepatoma plasma membranes indicate a lower lipid fluidity in these membranes as compared to normal. The mechanism of "homeoviscous adaptation," which operates mostly *via* alterations in the degree of unsaturation of the membrane phospholipids and in the level of cholesterol, may be responsible for the decreased fluidity of the hepatoma (Sinensky, 1974). An increased level of monounsaturated fatty acyl groups, mostly oleic acid (18:1), in the phospholipids of plasma membranes (Van Hoeven et al., 1975) and an increased ratio of oleic acid to polyunsaturated fatty acids in microsomes of Morris hepatoma 7777 (Waite et al., 1977) have been observed. Walker-256 tumor membranes are characterized by a low membrane fluidity, as compared to normal cell membranes (Deliconstantinos et al., 1988), resulting in an increased intracellular acidity relative to normal tissue, due to accumulation of lactic acid formed by glycolysis. The administration of aniline mustard glucuronide in combination with glucose produced an inhibition of tumor growth due to increased activity of β-glucuronidase at lower tumor intracellular pH, which converts the aniline mustard glucuronide to the more toxic p-hydroxyaniline mustard (Deliconstantinos & Ramantanis, 1983).

Differences in plasma membrane fluidity between normal and leukemic cells have been proposed. Using the fluorescence lipid probe, diphenylhexatriene (DPH), it was demonstrated that the fluidity of the mouse lymphoma cell membrane was greater (by as much as 65%) than that of normal lymphocytes (Shinitzky & Inbar, 1976). Human leukemic cell membranes were also found more fluid than those of lymphocytes from healthy donors, and the differences in fluidity were maintained in intact cells or isolated plasma membranes (Inbar et al., 1977; Deliconstantinos et al., 1987a; Daefler et al., 1987). The increase in membrane fluidity of the leukemic cells was directly related to the degree of cell proliferation (Collard et al., 1977). Estimation of the membrane fluidity of peripheral blood T lymphoyctes, obtained from untreated patients with Hodgkin's disease, using the fluorescence polarization of DPH, showed increased whole-cell P values as compared to normal T lymphocytes, suggesting that Hodgkin's disease lymphocyte membranes are more rigid. The increased rigidity of T-lymphocyte membrane was observed in all Hodgkin's disease patients tested without any relation to the clinical stage of the disease (Aleksijevic et al., 1986). The main physiological factors influencing the lipid fluidity in leukemia cell membranes are (1) the shedding of rigid membrane vesicles from the cell surface, (2) the site of growth of the tumor cells, and (3) the interaction with the plasma lipoproteins, in combination with cellular cholesterol biosynthesis (Van Blitterswijk et al., 1977; Petitou et al., 1978; Van Blitterswijk et al., 1982).

Fluidity of the membrane may be involved in the physiological regulation of the activity of membrane-bound enzymes. We have shown that increased cholesterol content reduced the activity of plasma membrane-bound ($Na^+ + K^+$) ATPase by decreasing the membrane fluidity (Deliconstantinos et al., 1986; Deliconstantinos, 1987c). One of the best-known effects of cholesterol on the properties of membrane lipid bilayer is the dramatic change in the enthalpy and cooperativity of the gel-to-liquid crystalline phase transition. Cholesterol causes the elimination of the sharp, highly cooperative phase transition in leukemia cell membranes and the size of the cooperativity unit for the sharp transition also increases as the cholesterol content of the normal lymphocyte cell membranes increases (Deliconstantinos et al., 1987a,b). Adenylate cyclase and ($Na^+ + K^+$)ATPase activities of plasma membranes of EL_4 tumor cells were inhibited by saturated fatty acids, while unsaturated fatty acids produced a moderate enhancement of enzyme activities (Poon et al., 1981). Malignant lymphoid diseases are accompanied by alterations of the activities of ectonucleotide phosphohydrolases (ecto-ATPase) associated with the outer surface of the cell membrane (Gutmann et al., 1983; Segel et al., 1985). The increase in the ecto-ATPase activity observed in CLL lymphocytes compared to normal lymphocytes is presumably due to the increased fluidity of their plasma membrane, resulting in an increase of the conformational flexibility of the enzyme achieved by a relief of the physical constraint imposed by the membrane annular lipids upon the protein molecule (Deliconstantinos et al., 1987a). It has been reported that membrane fluidity can modulate excision repair of DNA damage in prokaryotes (Todo et al., 1983). No information is available concerning the relationship between DNA repair synthesis and membrane fluidity in eukaryotic membranes.

Membrane fluidity, considered in all its bearing, has obvious implications for the process of metastatic dissemination. The property of cell deformability and modulation of shape afforded by membrane fluidity, the regulation of expression of membrane antigens, and the activities of enzymes associated with the plasma membrane can exert major influences on the biological behavior of the cell. Recently, considerable effort has gone into investigations of the possible role of membrane fluidity in cancer metastasis. Fluidizing compounds disturb the lipid–protein interactions. Some authors have discussed the appearance of cryptic binding sites. The missing link between binding at the accessory site and receptor inhibition could be the membrane fluidity, which could expose new binding sites. The direction of the induced changes in ligand binding depends on whether the lipid modulator fluidizes or rigidizes the membrane and also on the type of the membrane-bound proteins. "Syndromic proteins" is the name used to refer to the proteins which are "upregulated" by an increase in membrane fluidity and "downregulated" by a decrease in membrane fluidity. "Antidromic proteins" are those which are "downregulated" when the fluidity increases and "upregulated" when the fluidity decreases. There is also a group of membrane-bound proteins which appears to be unaltered by changing the membrane fluidity (Muller & Krueger, 1986). Modulation of the ability of the F1 variant of B16 melanoma cells to metastasize is associated with changes in the expression of membrane proteins. Thus, when F1 cells are grown as spheroids on a nonadhesive surface, they showed greater ability to metastasize. Concomitantly, there occurred a decrease in protein accessible to labeling by radioiodination (Raz & Ben-Ze'ev, 1983). L5178Y-ES lymphoma, which has considerable metastasizing ability, has a higher membrane fluidity than the L517Y-E variant, which is not malignant (Sherbet & Jackson, 1986), consistent with their phospholipid-to-cholesterol ratios reported by Barr and colleagues (1985). As compared to local tumor plasma membranes of LM fibroblasts, the lung metastasis plasma membranes had elevated $(Na^+ + K^+)$ATPase specific activity, phospholipid oleic and arachidonic acid content, and fluidity. In contrast, the 5′-nucleotidase specific activity, the content of cholesterol, phospholipid, and phosphatidylethanolamine were decreased in lung metastasis plasma membranes (Kier et al., 1988).

There is increasing experimental evidence that certain ether lipids and derivatives that are related to platelet-activating factor (PAF) [e.g., various 1-0-alkyl lysophospholipid derivatives (ALP), thioether lysophospholipid derivatives (TLP), ether-linked lipoidal amines, sn-2 analogs of PAF, and conjugates of ether lipids and cytosine arabinoside] represent a new group of antineoplastic agents. This notion is supported by the results of clinical pilot trials (Berdel et al., 1982). The activity of these compounds is partially due to their direct effects on neoplastic cell. These direct effects consist of cytostatic–cytotoxic properties and also consist of the induction of differentiation in neoplastic cells and an inhibition of the invasive properties of such cells (Storme et al., 1985). The molecular mechanism leading to these direct effects appears to be the destruction of cell membranes. Extensive incorporation of the antineoplastic agent 1-0-alkyl-2-0-methylglycero-3-phosphocholine (AMG-PC) in the plasma membrane of tumor cells LLC-H61 (a highly metastatic subclone of the Lewis lung carcinoma cell line) resulted in a decrease in plasma membrane fluidity and inhibition of tumor cell invasiveness in embryonic chick heart fragments (van Blitterswijk et al., 1987a; Eible, 1988). Various modifications of the basic structure of platelet-activating factor (PAF) lead to different ether lipids and analogs. Data from the evaluation of thioalkyl and amidoalkyl glycerophosphocholine and of glycerophosphoinositol ether lipids analogs against different experimental tumors *in vitro* (HL60 and K562 human leukemia cells, BG1 and BG3 ovarian adenocarcinomas) indirectly confirm that the plasma membrane of the tumor cells is a specific target for these compounds, causing alterations of the membrane fluidity. Combined use of ether lipid analogs, which are membrane interactive, with classical DNA-interactive chemotherapeutic drugs revealed that the combinations have additive antiproliferative effects (Noseda et al., 1987). Several kinds of alkyl-lysophospholipids enhanced the accumulation of vincristine (VCR) in both drug-sensitive and -resistant K562 cells. Verapamil specifically inhibits the efflux of VCR from the cells, especially in drug-resistant tumor cells, thereby enhancing the accumulation of antitumor agent in the cells. Thus the actions of alkyl-lysophospholipids and verapamil in tumor cells are obviously different. Furthermore, the combined effect of alkyl-lysophospholipids and verapamil were additive or synergistic, indicating that their sites of action may be different. Alkyl-lysophospholipids alter the membrane fluidity and modify the membrane functions of cells (Tsuruo & Saito, 1987). Cholesterol, which decreases the membrane fluidity, modulated the cytotoxicity and antiproliferative effects of lysophosphatidylcholine and alkyl-lysophospholipids in Novikoff rat hepatoma cells. The resistance of the cells to cytotoxic attack by these compounds, increased with increasing cell cholesterol level (Malewicz, 1988). The anthracycline antibiotic adriamycin has been shown to influence many properties of cellular membranes and model membrane systems. These include drug modulation of lectin-induced cell agglutination, transport of ions, membrane fluidity, organization of lipids, and membrane morphology. Modulation of membrane fluidity, with consequent effects on the expression of membrane-bound enzymes as well as on other cell surface functional properties, may initiate the series of events leading to cytotoxicity (Goormaghtich & Ruysschaert, 1984). Adriamycin achieves these effects through asymmetric perturbations of the membrane lipid structure and changes in membrane fluidity may be an early key event in adriamycin-induced cytotoxicity (Deliconstantinos et al., 1987b).

3. INTERACTIONS OF ANTINEOPLASTIC AGENTS WITH PROTEIN KINASE C

There is considerable experimental evidence that some ether lipids and derivatives represent a new class of anticancer and antimetastatic agents acting on cell membranes as shown by electron microscopy and this may account for direct cytotoxicity. However, interference of the ether lipids or their metabolites with other vital metabolic events within the target cells, for example, the inhibition of protein kinase systems or other enzymes, could lead to cell death. The wide chemical variability of synthetic ether lipids and related compounds might open a new perspective in the therapy of leukemia and cancer in humans. In addition, these compounds might be combined with conventional cytotoxics and thus potentiated in their cytotoxic action as synergistic effects. On the other hand, it might be worthwhile to seek more experimental information on the putative toxification–detoxification steps within the metabolism of these ether lipids. This might lead to the design of more specific compounds, which as enzymatic substrate analogs could accumulate in certain target cells that exhibit metabolic insufficiencies.

The autocrine mechanism of control of growth occurring in neoplasms naturally leads one to examine whether these might be a common mechanism by which the effects of growth factors, tumor promoters, and oncogene function are achieved. Protein kinase C, a serine- and threonine-specific kinase, has been firmly implicated in recent years in the activation of cellular function and proliferation as a transducer of extracellular signals. The initiation of a number of biological responses by hormones, neurotransmitters, and growth factors is dependent upon second messengers such as cAMP, Ca^{2+}, and diacylglycerol and inositol triphosphate. The formation of the latter two compounds is mediated by an inositide-specific phospholipase which is stimulated when the agents which have the capability to modify biological responses interact with specific membrane receptors (Lapetina et al., 1985). One of the most interesting aspects of the biology of protein kinase C is its mechanism of activation. Under quiescent conditions, the enzyme is cytoplasmic and inactive; when stimulated, the kinase is translocated to the membrane where it can actively phosphorylate its substrates at selected threonine or serine residues (Nishizuka, 1986). The demonstration that protein kinase C is the cellular phorbol diester receptor also implies that protein kinase C is involved in the mechanism of tumor promotion. Phorbol diester, on the other hand, was shown to stimulate protein kinase C by altering the membrane fluidity (Sugimoto et al., 1986). Recent studies have shown that protein kinase C activation requires phosphatidylserine, Ca^{2+}, and diacylglycerol binding to the kinase with a stoichiometry of 4:1, 1:1, and 1:1, respectively (Rando, 1988). When cells are stimulated by growth factors the inositide-specific phospholipase hydrolyzes phosphoinositides to yield diacylglycerol and inositol (1,4,5)-triphosphate (IP_3). Both these molecules are intracellular second messengers; diacylglycerol stimulates protein kinase C and IP_3 causes an increase in the concentration of intracellular Ca^{2+} (Berridge, 1987).

Several oncogenes have been shown to encode altered forms of normal components of the signal transduction pathways. These include altered forms of growth factors (sis) (Doolittle et al., 1983), growth factor receptors (erbB) (Downward et al., 1984), and GTP-binding proteins (ras) (Shih et al., 1980), which may lead to altered expression of protein kinase C. All these studies indicate the importance of protein kinase C in growth control and signal transduction and indicate that inhibitors of protein kinase C would be useful in defining the role of protein kinase C in cellular function. In addition, these inhibitors are of potential importance as chemotherapeutic agents. Several classes of protein kinase C inhibitors include calmodulin antagonists (Schatzman et al., 1983), vinblastine, daunomycin (Palayoor et al., 1987), and palmitoylcarnitine (Nakadate & Blumberg, 1987).

Analogs of 2-lysophosphatidylcholine (2-LPL) (e.g., the alkyl-lysophospholipid derivative (ALP)) have previously been shown to possess antitumor activity. They destroy leukemic and tumor cells *in vitro*, inhibit the growth and metastasis of syngeneic murine tumors, and have been used successfully in treating experimental rat tumors. This activity is suggested to be partially mediated by the inhibition of protein kinase C (Fromm et al., 1987; Schick et al., 1987). Inhibition of transmembrane signaling via protein kinase

C was observed by 1-0-hexadecyl-2-0-methylglycerol in mouse fibrosarcoma cells, by rac-1-0-octadecyl-2-0-methylglycerol-3-β-D-glucopyranoside (Weber & Benning, 1988) in Ehrlich ascites tumor cells and by a series of halogen-containing alkylglycerolipid analogs in Ehrlich ascites tumor cell and also in Lewis lung carcinoma in mice (Brachwitz et al., 1987). Investigation of the mechanisms by which the drug 1-0-alkyl-2-0-methylglycero-3-phosphocholine (AMG-PC) inhibits tumor growth and metastasis led to detection of a metabolite, 1-0-alkyl-2-0-methylglycerol (AMG), in membranes of MO_4 mouse fibrosarcoma cells grown in the presence of the drug. Synthetic AMG inhibited the activation of highly purified human protein kinase C by diacylglycerol in the presence of phosphatidylserine. Furthermore, AMG also inhibited the receptor-specific binding of ^{3}H-phorbol-12, 13-dibutyrate to human HL-60 promyeloid leukemia cells in a dose-dependent fashion. It was suggested that interaction of the metabolite AMG with protein kinase C may inhibit stimulus–response coupling in tumor cells and may thus potentially contribute to the mechanism by which AMG-PC exerts its anticancer activities (Van Blitterswijk et al., 1987b).

While EGF stimulation of normal cells produces tyrosine phosphorylation, EGF receptors from phosphorylated membranes of *ki-ras* transformed cells show an increase in serine and threonine phosphorylation. This appears to be due to an enhanced constitutive level of protein kinase C in the transformed cells (Chua & Ladda, 1986). Breast cancer lines which have high estrogen receptor content have been found to have low levels of protein kinase C activity and a small number of high-affinity EGF receptors. In contrast, cell lines which are independent of estrogen show high protein kinase C activity and, most interestingly, a high number of low-affinity EGF receptors (Iwashita & Fox, 1984). There is thus a strong possibility that the phosphorylation of the EGF receptor by the kinase might be modulating the binding of the ligand (Chua & Ladda, 1986). It seems, therefore, that the physiological effects of EGF and other growth factors may involve the protein kinase C. With the demonstrable relationship between EGF receptor and the *erbB* oncogene, this would now suggest an involvement of protein kinase C in oncogene activity as well.

The anticancer drug vinblastine has been reported to act on cell membranes and to inhibit polypeptide hormone receptor binding. Binding of ^{125}I-insulin to its receptor on rat heart cells is inhibited by the drug due to a decrease in receptor concentration. This was interpreted to indicate a role for microtubules in the interaction of the hormone with its receptor (Eckel & Reinauer, 1980). A decrease in EGF binding to MCF-7 cells after incubation with vinblastine was also observed (Hanauske et al., 1987). *Cis*platin has been reported to affect cell membranes of normal and malignant cells, leading to a disappearance of cell surface nucleic acids in mouse tumor cells (Juckett & Rosenberg, 1982). *Cis*platin also interacts with the cell membrane of MCF-7 cells and alters the binding of EGF. Thus, disturbance of the EGF receptor might result in reduced tumor growth. The mechanisms leading to the observed affinity changes may comprise three possible events: direct competition with the natural ligand for binding to the receptor, binding to cell membrane compounds with secondary changes of receptor conformation, and secondary receptor alterations resulting from intracytoplasmatic drug action (Hanauske et al., 1987). In summary vinblastine and *cis*plastin affect the plasma membrane of MCF-7 human breast cancer cells and reduce EGF binding. Reduction in growth factor binding is a potential mechanism for the antineoplastic activity of these drugs.

The activity of EGF receptor may be affected by alterations in membrane fluidity, since clustering of occupied EGF receptors can occur in the absence of metabolic energy and external interactions, for example, with components of the cytoskeleton, and thus reflects inherent properties of the receptor protein in its natural environment (Carpenter & Zendegui, 1986). It is suggested that the EGF-receptor-mediated increase in membrane fluidity is an early key event where transduction mechanisms translate the EGF external signal into internal signal carried by second messengers.

REFERENCES

Aleksijevic, A., Cremel, G., Muter, Ch., Giron, C., Hubert, P., Waksman, A., Falkenrodt, A., Oberling, F., Mayer, S., and Lang, J. M. (1986) Decreased membrane fluidity of T lymphocytes from untreated patients with Hodgkin's disease. *Leukemia Res.* **10**: 1477–1484.

Barr, D., Goppelt, M., Schirrmacher, V., and Resch, K. (1985) Characterization of cellular and extracellular plasma membrane vesicles from a non-metastasizing lymphoma (EB) and its metastasizing variant (ESB). *Biochim. Biophys. Acta* **814**: 77–84.

Berdel, W. E., Schlehe, H., Fink, V., Emmerich, B., Maubach, P. A., Emslander, H. P., Daum, S., and Rastetter, J. (1982) Early tumor and leukemia response to alkyl-lysophospholipids in a phase-1 study. *Cancer* **50**: 2011–2015.

Berridge, M. J. (1987) Inositol lipids and cell proliferation. *Biochim. Biophys. Acta* **907**: 33–45.

Brachwitz, H., Langen, P., Arudt, D., and Fishtner, I. (1987) Cytostatic activity of synthetic O-alkylglycerolipids. *Lipids* **22**: 897–903.

Carpenter, G., and Zendegui, Z. G. (1986) Epidermal growth factor, its receptor and related proteins. *Exper. Cell Res.* **164**: 1–10.

Chua, C. C., and Ladda, R. L. (1986) Protein kinase C and nonfunctional EGF receptor in K-rats transformed cells. *Biochem. Biophys. Res. Commun.* **135**: 435–444.

Collard, J. G., DeWildt, A., Oomen-Menlemans, E. P. M., Smeekens, J., Emmelot, P., and Inbar, M. (1977) Increase in fluidity of membrane lipids in lymphocytes, fibroblasts, and liver cells stimulated for growth. *FEBS Lett.* **77**: 173–178.

Daefler, S., Krueger, G. R. F., Mödder, B., and Deliconstantinos, G. (1987) Cell membrane fluidity in chronic lymphocytic leukemia (CLL). Lymphocytes and its relation to membrane receptor expression. *J. Exper. Pathol.* **3**: 147–154.

Deliconstantinos, G., Kopeikina, L., and Ramantantis, G. (1988) Evoked effects of PGE_2 and PGA_2 on lipid fluidity and Ca^{2+}-stimulated ATPase of Walker-256 tumor microsomal membranes. *Ann. N.Y. Acad. Sci.* (in press).

Deliconstantinos, G. (1987a) Physiological aspects of membrane lipid fluidity in malignancy. *Anticancer Res.* **7**: 1011–1022.

Deliconstantinos, G. (1987b) Interaction of liposomes containing cholesterol with mouse spleen cells. Studies on the mode and on the consequences of interaction. *Cell Mol. Biol.* **33**: 413–422.

Deliconstantinos, G. (1987c) Effect of rat serum albumin-cholesterol on the physical properties of biomembranes. *Biochemistry International* **15**: 464–474.

Deliconstantinos, G., Daefler, S., and Krueger, G. R. F. (1987a) Cholesterol modulation of membrane fluidity and ecto-nucleotide triphosphatase activity in human normal and CLL lymphocytes. *Anticancer Res.* **7**: 347–352.

Deliconstantinos, G., Kopeikina-Tsiboukidou, L., and Villioutou, V. (1987b) Evaluation of membrane fluidity effects and enzyme activities alterations in adriamycin neurotoxicity. *Biochem. Pharmacol.* **36**: 1153–1161.

Deliconstantinos, G., Tsopanakis, Ch., Karayiannakos, P., and Skalkeas, G. R. (1986) Evidence for the existence of nonesterified cholesterol carried by albumin in rat serum. *Atherosclerosis* **61**: 67–75.

Deliconstantinos, G., and Ramantanis, G. (1983) Cytotoxicity of aniline mustard glucuronide alone or in a combination with glucose in Walker cells in culture and sarcoma-180 tumor bearing animals. *Biomedicine and Pharmacotherapy* **37**: 339–343.

Doolittle, R. F., Hankapiller, M. W., Hood, L. E., Devare, S. G., Robbins, K. C., Aaronson, H. N., Antoniades, H. N. (1983) Simian sarcoma virus oncogene, v-sis, is derived from the gene (or genes) encoding a platelet-derived growth factor. *Science* **221**: 275–279.

Downward, J., Yarden, Y., Mayes, E., Scrace, G., Totty, N., Stockwell, P., Ullrich, A., Schlessinger, J., and Waterfield, M. D. (1984) Close similarity of epidermal growth factor receptor and v-erb-B oncogene protein sequences. *Nature* **307**: 521–524.

Eckel, J., and Reinauer, H. (1980) Effect of vinblastine on insulin-receptor interaction in mammalian heart muscle. *Biochem. Biophys. Res. Commun.* **92**: 1403–1408.

Edidin, M. (1974) Rotational and translational diffusion in membranes. *Ann. Rev. Biophys. Bioeng.* **3**: 179–203.

Eible, H. (1988). Alkylphosphocholines: A new class of antitumor drugs. *J. AOCS* **65**: 517.

Fromm, M., Berdel, W. E., Schick, H. D., Fink, V., Pahlke, W., Bicker, V., Reichejt, A., and Rastetter, J. (1987) Antineoplastic activity of the thioether lysophospholipid derivative BM 41.440 *in vitro*. *Lipids* **22**: 916–918.

Golan, D. E., and Veatch, W. (1980) Lateral mobility of band-3 in the human erythrocyte membrane studied by fluorescence photobleaching recovery. Evidence for control by cytoskeletal interactions. *Proc. Natl. Acad. Sci. USA* **77**: 2537–2541.

Goormaghtigh, E., and Ruysschaert, J. M. (1984). Anthracycline glycoside–membrane interactions. *Biochim. Biophys. Acta* **79**: 271–288.

Goustin, A. J., Neof, E. B., Shipley, G. D., and Moses, H. L. (1986) Growth factors and cancers. *Cancer Res.* **46**: 1015–1029.

Gutmann, H. R., Chow, M. Y., Vessella, R. L., Schuetzle, B., and Kaplan, M. E. (1983) The kinetic properties of the ecto-ATPase of human peripheral blood lymphocytes and of chronic lymphatic leukemia cells. *Blood* **62**: 1041–1046.

Hanauske, A. R., Osborne, C. K., Chamness, G. C., Clark, G. M., Forseth, J., Buchok, J. B., Artaega, C. L., and Von Hoff, D. D. (1987) Alteration of EGF-receptor binding in human breast cancer cells by antineoplastic agents. *Eur. J. Cancer Clin. Oncol.* **23**: 545–551.

Inbar, M., Goldman, R., Inbar, L., Barsaker, B., Goldman, B., Akstein, E., Segal, P., Ipp, E., and Ben-Busset, I. (1977) Fluidity differences of membrane lipids in human normal and leukemic lymphocytes as controlled by serum components. *Cancer Res.* **37**: 3037–3041.

Inbar, M., Shinitzky, M., and Sachs, L. (1974). Microviscosity in surface membrane lipid layer of intact normal lymphocytes and leukemic cells. *FEBS Lett.* **38**: 268–273.

Iwashita, S., and Fox, C. F. (1984) Epidermal growth factor and potent phorbol tumor promoters induce epidermal growth factor receptor phosphorylation in a similar but distinctively different manner in human epidermoid carcinoma-A431 cells. *J. Biol. Chem.* **259**: 2559–2567.

Jacobson, K., Hou, Y., Derrko, Z., Wojcieszyn, J., and Organisciak, D. (1981) Lipid lateral diffusion in the surface membrane of cells and in multibilayers formed from plasma membrane lipids. *Biochemistry* **20**: 5268–5275.

Juckett, D. A., and Rosenberg, B. (1982) Actions of cis-diamine-dichloroplatinum on cell surface nucleic acids in cancer cells as determined by cell electrophoresis techniques. *Cancer Res.* **42**: 3565–3573.

Kier, A. B., Parker, M. T., Schroeder, F. (1988) Local and metastatic tumor growth and membrane properties of LM fibroblasts in athymic (nude) mice. *Biochim. Biophys. Acta* **938**: 434–446.

Lapetina, E. G., Reep, B., Ganong, B. R., Bell, R. M. (1985) Exogenous Sn-1,2-diacylglycerols containing saturated fatty acids function as bioregulators of protein kinase C in human platelets. *J. Biol. Chem.* **260**: 1358–1361.

Malewicz, B. (1988) The cytotoxicity and antiproliferative effects of lysophosphatidylcholine and alkyl-lysophospholipids are modulated by cholesterol. *J. AOCS* **65**: 532.

Muller, C. P., and Krueger, G. R. F. (1986) Modulation of membrane proteins by vertical phase separation and membrane lipid fluidity. Basis for a new approach to tumor immunotherapy. *Anticancer Res.* **6**: 1181–1194.

Nakadate, T., and Blumberg, P. M. (1987) Modulation by palmitoylcarnitine of protein kinase C activation. *Cancer Res.* **47**: 6537–6546.

Nishizuka, Y. (1986) Studies and perspectives of protein kinase C. *Science* **233**: 305–312.

Noseda, A., Berens, M. E., Piantadosi, C., and Modest, E. J. (1987) Neoplastic cell inhibition with new ether lipid analogs. *Lipids* **22**: 878–883.

Palayoor, S. T., Stein, J. M., and Hait, W. N. (1987) Inhibition of protein kinase C by antineoplastic agents: Implications for drug resistance. *Biochem. Biophys. Res. Commun.* **148**: 718–729.

Petitou, M., Tuy, R., Rosenfeld, C., Mishal, Z., Paintrand, M., Jasmin, C., Mathé, G., and Inbar, M. (1978) Decreased microviscosity of membrane lipids in leukemic cells: Two possible mechanisms. *Proc. Natl. Acad. Sci. USA* **75**: 2306–2310.

Poon, R., Richards, J. M., and Clark, W. R. (1981) The relationship between plasma membrane lipid composition and physical chemical properties. Effect of phospholipid fatty acid modulation on plasma membrane physical properties and enzymatic activities. *Biochim. Biophys. Acta* **649**: 58–66.

Rando, R. R. (1988) Regulation of protein kinase C activity by lipids. *FASEB J.* **2**: 2348–2355.

Raz, A., and Ben-Ze'ev, A. (1983) Modulation of the metastatic capability in B-16 melanoma by cell shape. *Science* **221**: 1307–1310.

Schatzman, R. C., Raynor, R. L., and Kuo, J. F. (1983) N-(6-Amino-hexyl)-5-chloro-1-naphthalenesulfonimide (W-7), a calmodulin antagonist, also inhibits phospholipid-sensitive calcium-dependent protein kinase. *Biochim. Biophys. Acta* **755**: 144–151.

Schick, H. D., Berdel, W. E., Fromm, M., Fink, V., Jehn, V., Ulm, K., Reichert, A., Eible, H., Unger, C., and Rastetter, J. (1987) Cytotoxic effects of ether lipids and derivatives in human nonneoplastic bone marrow cells and leukemic cells *in vitro*. *Lipids* **22**: 904–910.

Schlessinger, J. (1988) The epidermal growth factor receptor as a multifunctional allosteric protein. *Biochemistry* **27**: 3119–3123.

Segel, G. B., Ryan, D. H., and Lichtman, M. A. (1985) Ecto-nucleotide triphosphatase activity of human lymphocytes. Studies of normal and lymphocytes CLL. *J. Cell Physiol.* **124**: 424–432.

Sherbet, G. V., and Jackson, S. (1986) Temperature-dependent surface charge modulation, membrane fluidity, and metastatic ability of L51178 Y lymphoma. *Anticancer Res.* **6**: 129–134.

Shih, T. Y., Papageorge, A. G., Stokes, P. E., Weeks, M. O., and Scolnick, E. M. (1980). Guanine nucleotide-binding and autophosphorylating activities associated with the $p21^{scr}$ protein of Harvey murine sarcoma virus. *Nature* **287**: 686–688.

Shinitzky, M. (1984) Membrane fluidity in malignancy. *Biochim. Biophys. Acta* **738**: 251–261.

Shinitzky, M., and Henkark, P. (1979) Fluidity of cell membranes. Current concepts and trends. *Int. Rev. Cytol.* **60**: 121–147.

Shinitzky, M., and Inbar, M. (1976) Microviscosity parameters and protein mobility in biological membranes. *Biochim. Biophys. Acta* **433**: 133–149.

Sinensky, M. (1974) Homeoviscous adaptation—a homeostatic process that regulates the viscosity of membrane lipids in *Escherichia coli* (spin labeling/phase transition). *Proc. Natl. Acad. Sci. USA*. **71**: 522–525.

Singer, S. J., and Nicolson, G. L. (1972) The fluid mosaic model of the structure of cell membranes. *Science* **175**: 720–731.

Storme, G. A., Berdel, W. E., Van Blitterswijk, W. J., Bruyneel, E. A., De Bruyne, G. K., and Mareel, M. M. (1985) Antiinvasive effect of racemic 1-0-octadecyl-2-0-methylglycero-3-phosphocholine on MO_4 mouse fibro-sarcoma cells *in vitro*. *Cancer Res.* **45**: 351–357.

Sugimoto, Y., Saito, H., Tabeta, R., and Kodama, M. (1986) An NMR study on alterations of the membrane organization of mouse B16 melanoma cells treated with 12-0-tetradecanoylphorbol-13-acetate,6. *J. Biochem. (Tokyo)* **100**: 867–874.

Todo, T., Yonei, S., and Kato, M. (1983) The modulating influence of the fluidity of cell membrane on excision repair of DNA in UV-irradiated *Escherichia coli*. *Biochem. Biophys. Res. Comm.* **110**: 609–615.

Tsuruo, T., and Saito, H. (1987) Difference in effects of alkyl-lysophospholipids and verapamil on vincristine transport in vincristine-sensitive and -resistant human myelopenous leukemia K562. *Anticancer Res.* **7**: 39–44.

Ullrich, A., Bell, J. R., Chen, E. Y., Herrera, R., Petruzzelli, L. M., Dull, T. J., Gray, A., Coussens, L., Liao, Y. C., Tsubokawa, M., Mason, A., Seeburg, P. H., Grunfeld, C., Rosen, O. M., and Ramachandran, J. (1985) Human insulin receptor and its relationship to the tyrosine kinase family of oncogenes. *Nature* **313**: 756–761.

Ullrich, A., Coussens, L., Hayflick, J. S., Dull, T., Gray, A., Tam, A. W., Lee, J., Yarden, Y., Liberman, T. A., Schlessinger, J., Downward, J., Mayes, E. L. F., Whittle, N., Waterfield, M. D., and Seeburg, P. H. (1984) Human epidermal growth factor receptor cDNA sequence and aberrant expression of the amplified gene in A431 epidermoid carcinoma cells. *Nature* **309**: 418–425.

Van Blitterswijk, W. J., Hilkmann, H., and Storme, G. A. (1987a) Accumulation of an alkyl-lysophospholipid in tumor cell membranes affects membrane fluidity and tumor cell invasion. *Lipids* **22**: 820–823.

Van Blitterswijk, W. J., van der Bend, R. L., Kramer, I. M., Verhoeven, A. J., Hilkmann, H., and de Widt,

J. (1987b) A metabolite of an antineoplastic ether phospholipid may inhibit transmembrane signaling via protein kinase C. *Lipids* **22**: 842–846.

Van Blitterswijk, W. J., DeVeer, G., Krol, J. J., and Emmelot, P. (1982) Comparative lipid analysis of purified plasma membranes and shedded extracellular membrane vesicles from normal murine thymocytes and leukemic GRSL cells. *Biochim. Biophys. Acta* **688**: 495–504.

Van Blitterswijk, W. J., Emmelot, P., Hilkmann, H. A. M., Oomen-Menlemans, E. P. M., and Inbar, M. (1977) Differences in lipid fluidity among isolated plasma membranes of normal and leukemic lymphocytes and membranes exfoliated from their cell surface. *Biochim. Biophys. Acta* **467**: 309–318.

Van Hoeven, R. P., Emmelot, P., Krol, J. H., and Oomen-Meulemans, E. P. (1975) Studies on plasma membranes. XXII. Fatty acid profiles of lipid classes in plasma membranes of rat and mouse livers and hepatomas. *Biochim. Biophys. Acta* **380**: 1–12.

Waite, M., Parce, B., Morton, R., Cunningham, C., and Morris, H. P. (1977). The deacylation and reacylation of phosphoglyceride in microsomes of Morris hepatoma 7777 and host rat liver. *Cancer Res.* **37**: 2092–2098.

Weber, N., and Benning, H. (1988). Metabolism of ether glycolipids with potentially antineoplastic activity by Ehrlich ascites tumor cells. *Biochim. Biophys. Acta* **959**: 91–94.

CHAPTER 9

DNA POLYMERASE DELTA: A TARGET FOR SELECTIVE INHIBITOR DESIGN

ROBERT TALANIAN,* FEDERICO FOCHER,† NEAL BROWN,* ULRICH HÜBSCHER,† NASEEMA KHAN,* AND GEORGE WRIGHT*

**Department of Pharmacology, University of Massachusetts Medical School, Worcester, Massachusetts, United States,*
†Department of Pharmacology and Biochemistry, University of Zürich-Irchel, Zürich, Switzerland

Abstract—DNA polymerase δ has been identified recently in several mammalian tissues and cultured cell lines together with the classical "replicative" DNA polymerase α. Although separable by hydroxylapatite chromatography, the enzymes share several properties such as sensitivity to aphidicolin. DNA polymerase δ, however, possesses a 3′ to 5′ exonuclease and prefers homopolymer primer: templates. Much circumstantial evidence has suggested that DNA polymerases α and δ participate in DNA replication and repair *in vivo*.

Reagents that can distinguish between the two enzymes include DNA polymerase α-neutralizing monoclonal antibodies and the DNA polymerase α inhibitors BuPdGTP and BuAdATP. We have sought to develop selective inhibitors of DNA polymerase δ to aid in determining its role in *in vivo* DNA metabolism. To this end we have screened many nucleotides, aphidicolin derivatives, and pyrophosphate analogs against DNA polymerases α and δ isolated from calf thymus. One compound, difluoromethylenebisphosphonate, emerged as an inhibitor of DNA polymerase δ without apparent effect on DNA polymerase α.

1. INTRODUCTION

1.1. ANIMAL CELL DNA POLYMERASES

Until 1976 three DNA polymerases had been identified in animal cells: DNA polymerases α, β, and γ (for review, see Fry & Loeb, 1986). The high-molecular-weight DNA polymerase α (pol α), the most abundant of the three, was long thought to be the enzyme responsible for semiconservative DNA replication. The lower-molecular-weight DNA polymerase β is at least partially responsible for repair synthesis, and DNA polymerase γ (mitochondrial DNA polymerase) mediates mitochondrial DNA synthesis.

Evidence for the role of DNA polymerase α in cellular DNA replication is based on several experimental observations: Inhibitors of DNA polymerase α such as aphidicolin also inhibit DNA replication (see, e.g., Huberman, 1981); pol α activity rises in cells synthesizing DNA (Chiu & Baril, 1975); microinjection of pol α-neutralizing monoclonal antibodies into cells inhibits DNA replication (Kaczmarek et al., 1986); cell mutants that are temperature sensitive (ts) in DNA replication have yielded ts pol α (Murakami et al., 1985). Isolated forms of DNA polymerase α, however, are too error-prone to account for the high fidelity of DNA replication *in vivo*. DNA polymerase α does not possess a proofreading 3′ to 5′ exonuclease, an activity present in prokaryotic DNA polymerases, for example, *E. coli* DNA polymerase III, which acts to increase their fidelity (Fersht & Knill-Jones, 1983). [However, a cryptic 3′ to 5′ exonuclease has recently been detected in the polymerase subunit of *Drosophila* DNA polymerase α-primase complex (Cotterill et al., 1987).]

1.2. DISCOVERY OF DNA POLYMERASE δ

In 1976 Byrnes and colleagues (1976) isolated a novel DNA polymerase from rabbit hyperplastic bone marrow which appeared to possess an intrinsic 3′ to 5′ exonuclease. It had optimal activity on the alternating copolymer poly d(A-T) as primer:template in contrast to the preference of DNA polymerase α for activated DNA. This new enzyme, designated DNA polymerase δ, shared certain physical properties in common with DNA polymerase α, but could be separated from the latter by hydroxylapatite chromatography. Subsequently, DNA polymerase δ species have been isolated from other mammalian tissues such as calf thymus (Lee et al., 1980; Focher et al., 1988b) and human placenta (Lee et al., 1987). More recently DNA polymerase δ has been isolated from cultured cell lines, including monkey CV-1 (Hammond et al., 1987) and the human HeLa line (Nishida et al., 1988).

The most common source of DNA polymerase δ is calf thymus, and the groups of So (Lee et al., 1980), Bambara (Crute et al., 1986), and Hübscher (Focher et al., 1988b) have reported extensively on the properties of the enzyme from this tissue. Calf thymus DNA polymerase δ is generally separated from DNA polymerase α on hydroxylapatite, but these groups have used different methods for further purification of each enzyme. The δ enzymes are of high molecular weight, have 3′ to 5′ exonuclease activity, and have greater activity on homopolymer primer:templates such as oligo dT:poly dA or alternating copolymers such as poly d(A-T) than on activated DNA.

1.3. Relationship to DNA Polymerase α

In addition to sharing several physical properties, DNA polymerases δ and α respond similarly to certain inhibitors. Both enzymes are inhibited by N-ethylmaleimide (NEM), araATP, and aphidicolin, but are relatively resistant to ddTTP (Lee et al., 1981; Goscin & Byrnes, 1982; Lee et al., 1984). These similarities have supported speculation that DNA polymerase δ may be a form of DNA polymerase α isolated at an early stage of purification. Although evidence concerning the structural relationship between them is lacking, several reagents have been found which distinguish between DNA polymerase δ and α. Byrnes (1985) first found that a DNA polymerase α-neutralizing monoclonal antibody did not inhibit DNA polymerase δ from rabbit bone marrow, a finding that has been consistently demonstrated for DNA polymerase δ from other sources. Furthermore, a polyclonal antibody to human placenta pol δ did not cross-react with DNA polymerase α (Lee & Toomey, 1987). DNA polymerase δ showed significant resistance to the potent DNA polymerase α inhibitors BuPdGTP and BuAdATP (Byrnes, 1985; Lee et al., 1985). These nucleotides inhibit DNA polymerase α from all sources examined, with K_i values in the nanomolar range (Khan et al., 1984, 1985), but inhibit DNA polymerase δ species only in the 10–100 μm range (Byrnes, 1985; Lee et al., 1985). Table 9-1 summarizes inhibitor sensitivities of DNA polymerases α and δ from calf thymus.

1.4. Function of DNA Polymerase δ

Various studies have suggested roles for DNA polymerase δ in DNA replication and in DNA repair. Dresler and Frattini (1986, 1988) have shown that, although aphidicolin inhibits replicative DNA synthesis in permeabilized human fibroblasts at concentrations that completely inhibit both DNA polymerases α and δ, pol α-neutralizing monoclonal antibodies and BuPdGTP inhibit this process only at high concentrations. Microinjection of the DNA polymerase α-neutralizing monoclonal antibody SJK-287 raised against a

TABLE 9-1. *Inhibitory Activity Against Calf Thymus DNA Polymerases α and δ Assayed on oligo dT:poly dA*

	% Inhibition of	
Compound (concn.)	pol α	pol δ
SJK 132-20 MOAB (2.8 μg/tube)	80	2
Aphidicolin (300 μM)	87	96
N-Ethylmaleimide (5 mM)	97	99
BuPdGTP (5 μM)	84	3
BuAdATP (5 μM)	72	0
ddTTP (400 μM)	10	66

From Focher et al. (1988b). $[^3H]$dTTP was present at 10 μM.

human enzyme into nuclei of growing cells resulted in partial inhibition of DNA replication (Kaczmarek et al., 1986). Treatment of permeabilized CV-1 cells with aphidicolin, pol α-neutralizing monoclonal antibodies, and BuPdGTP led to similar conclusions with regard to the contribution of DNA polymerase δ to DNA replication (Miller et al., 1985; Hammond et al., 1987). These results suggest either that DNA polymerase α is in a form during DNA replication that is relatively resistant to antibodies and BuPdGTP, but highly sensitive to aphidicolin, or that another enzyme, possible DNA polymerase δ, is at least partially responsible for DNA replication. Replication of simian virus 40 chromatin *in vitro*, a process that requires the host cell DNA replication apparatus, has also been found to be resistant to BuPdGTP but sensitive to aphidicolin (Decker et al., 1987). Furthermore, simian virus 40 replication is also dependent on proliferating cell nuclear antigen (PCNA or cyclin) (Prelich et al., 1987a), an accessory protein of DNA polymerase δ (Bravo et al., 1987; Prelich et al., 1987b). Related inhibitor studies have also implicated DNA polymerase δ in UV-induced repair synthesis in permeabilized human fibroblasts (Dresler & Frattini, 1986, 1988). It should be noted that the *Drosophila* DNA polymerase α that contains a cryptic 3′ to 5′ exonuclease was also highly resistant to BuPdGTP and BuAdATP (Reyland et al., 1988).

Differential assays for detecting DNA polymerases α and δ and studies with selective inhibitors have strengthened the proposal that both enzymes are important in DNA replication. Levels of activity of both enzymes varied with the cell cycle of Chinese hamster ovary (CHO) cells, with an increase in the relative amount of δ observed at the G2/M portion and an increase of α at G_1 (Marraccino et al., 1987). Activity ratios of pol α and pol δ remained constant at each step of purification from human placenta (Lee & Toomey, 1987), and activity ratios of the two enzymes in calf thymus were found to be invariably 1:1, irrespective of the extraction procedure or subcellular localization (Focher et al., 1988a). Zhang and Lee (1987) have also shown that the pol α/pol δ ratio in neonatal rat heart did not change with time of development.

Consideration of the ubiquitous presence of DNA polymerases α and δ in equal amounts in mammalian cells has led Focher and colleagues (1988a) to hypothesize that both enzymes are crucial for semiconservative DNA replication. They have suggested that DNA polymerase δ catalyzes leading strand synthesis while DNA polymerase α catalyzes lagging strand synthesis. Consistent with this hypothesis, DNA polymerase α exists in a multiprotein form with a tightly associated primase and is only moderately processive, but DNA polymerase δ lacks a primase and is highly processive in the presence of PCNA.

1.5. Purpose of the Present Study

The genetic, structural, and functional relationships between DNA polymerase α and δ are unknown. Evidence is mounting, however, that DNA polymerase δ is an important contributor to animal cell DNA replication and repair. The search for and development of selective inhibitors of DNA polymerase δ is important for (1) providing tools with which to distinguish between the isolated enzymes, (2) studying the occurrence and function of this enzyme *in vivo*, (3) understanding of the mechanism of toxicity of drugs that may act on replicative or repair DNA synthesis, and (4) finding leads in the design of antitumor and other cytotoxic drugs that may act on DNA polymerase δ. The only reagents presently available to distinguish between DNA polymerases α and δ, that is, monoclonal antibodies, BuPdGTP, and BuAdATP, do so by inhibiting DNA polymerase α with high selectivity. One objective of our laboratories, the identification of a selective inhibitor whose target is DNA polymerase δ, is the purpose of the present study.

This study has relied on an abundant supply of holoenzyme forms of DNA polymerases α and δ from calf thymus, purified by a new efficient method (Focher et al., 1988b). Our strategy has been to test both enzymes with known and suspected DNA polymerase inhibitors available from commercial sources, from original synthesis in our laboratory, and from donation by colleagues. We have modified the enzyme assays in order that inhibitors could be tested under as similar conditions as possible for direct comparison of their relative potencies. These conditions involve incorporation of a labeled substrate into activated DNA assayed, where appropriate, in the absence of one of the substrates which might be competitive with the potential inhibitor ("truncated assay"), and whose presence might obscure weak inhibition.

2. MATERIALS AND METHODS

2.1. INHIBITORS

Certain nucleotide analogs were synthesized as described previously: BuPdGTP (N^2-(p-n-butylphenyl)deoxyguanosine 5′-triphosphate] (Wright & Dudycz, 1984); BuAdATP [2-(p-n-butylanilino)-deoxyadenosine 5′-triphosphate] (Khan et al., 1985); BuAA and BuAOMe (Wright et al., 1987). DCAdATP [2-(3,4-dichloroanilino)deoxyadenosine 5′-triphosphate] and its base DCAA were prepared according to Khan and colleagues (1985), and details will be published elsewhere. The tetraammonium salt of PCF_2P (difluoromethylenebisphosphonic acid) was prepared by the method of Blackburn and colleagues (1981).

AraATP, araCTP, ddTTP, tetrasodium pyrophosphate (PP_i), and trisodium phosphonoformate (PFA) were purchased from Sigma Chemical Co. Acycloguanosine triphosphate (ACGTP) and 3′-azidodeoxythymidine 5′-triphosphate (AZTTP) were gifts from Dr. Wayne Miller, Burroughs-Wellcome Co. Aphidicolin was a gift from the Natural Products Branch, National Cancer Institute; derivatives of aphidicolin were prepared as described (Dalziel et al., 1973).

2.2. ENZYMES

The calf thymus DNA polymerase α and δ preparations used in these studies were purified as described by Focher and colleagues (1988b). Briefly, crude extracts of quick-frozen tissue were passed through phosphocellulose, and DNA polymerases α and δ were separated by chromatography on a hydroxylapatite column. The polymerases were used without further purification and were free from cross-contamination based on assay of their primer:template preferences and inhibitor sensitivities.

2.3. DNA POLYMERASE ASSAYS

2.3.1. *Oligo dT:poly dA as Primer:template*

Assays of both DNA polymerases α and δ contained the following in 25 μL: 75 mM Hepes-K^+ (pH 7.5), 1.25 mM DTT, 20% (v/v) glycerol, 10 mM $MgCl_2$, 250 μg/mL BSA, 0.5 μg oligo dT:poly dA (base ratio 1:10), 10 μM [^{3}H]dTTP (1250 cpm/pmol), and about 0.005–0.02 units of the enzyme to be assayed. Incubations were done at 37°C for 30 min, and the trichloroacetic acid-precipitable material in these and the following assays was determined as described by Neville and Brown (1972). One unit is the amount of enzyme that catalyzes incorporation of 1 nmol of dTMP in 60 min at 37°C under standard assay conditions.

2.3.2. *Activated DNA as Primer:template*

For determination of DNA polymerase α, the assay contained the following in 25 μL: 20 mM potassium phosphate (pH 7.2); 0.1 mM EDTA; 4 mM DTT; 250 μg/mL BSA; 10 mM $MgCl_2$; 50 μM each of dATP, dGTP, and dCTP; 20 μM [^{3}H]dTTP (250–500 cpm/pmol); 10 μg DNAse-treated calf thymus DNA; and 0.1–0.5 units of enzyme. Incubations were done at 37°C for 30 min and were linear during this period. Optimal assay for DNA polymerase δ with this template included, in 25 μL; 75 mM Hepes-K^+ (pH 7.5); 1 mM DTT; 20% (v/v) glycerol; 250 μg/mL BSA; 10 mM $MgCl_2$; 100 mM KCl; 1 mM GMP [or AMP]; 25 μM each of dATP, dGTP, and dCTP; 10 μM [^{3}H]dTTP (1250 cpm/

pmol); 3 μg DNAse-treated calf thymus DNA; and 0.002–0.005 units of enzyme. Incubations were done at 37°C for 90 min; incorporation of [^{3}H]dTMP by activated DNA was linear throughout the incubation period.

2.3.3. *Truncated Assays*

DNA polymerase assays designed to magnify effects of potential competitive inhibitors (Wright & Brown, 1976) were identical to those described for activated DNA assays, except that one dNTP was omitted. When dTTP was the substrate to be omitted, [α-^{32}P]dGTP (1250 cpm/pmol) at 10 μM was used as the labeled substrate. Incorporation in the absence of one substrate, which was linear throughout the incubation period, corresponded to 5–25 pmol of labeled substrate per assay tube for DNA polymerase α and 1–5 pmol for DNA polymerase δ.

2.4. Inhibitor Assays

Stock solutions of nucleotides and pyrophosphate analogs were prepared in 10 mM Tris-Cl buffer (pH 7.5) and stored at −20°C. Stock solutions of water-insoluble bases and natural products were prepared in dimethylsulfoxide (DMSO). Suitable dilutions of the stock solutions were done in the appropriate enzyme assay buffer and added to assay solutions to achieve desired concentrations. Control assays contained, where appropriate, identical amounts of DMSO.

3. RESULTS AND DISCUSSION

3.1. Screening of Compounds for Inhibition of DNA Polymerases α and δ

Measurement of DNA polymerase δ activity by incorporation of labeled substrates into activated DNA is inefficient under conditions optimal for DNA polymerase α. We modified the standard assay, therefore, to obtain significant and reproducible counts of labeled DNA in DNA polymerase δ assays. These changes involved addition of 100 μM KCl and 1 mM GMP or AMP, the latter to inhibit the 3′ to 5′ exonuclease, and increase of the incubation time from 30 to 90 min. Under these conditions, >5000 cpm/assay tube were obtained for control reactions. These conditions also allowed us to perform truncated assays, those done in the absence of one of the four dNTP substrates, to enhance the ability to detect weak, competitive inhibitors (Wright & Brown, 1976). These assays required about twice the amount of enzyme as full assays and gave incorporation of >2000 cpm/assay tube. An additional advantage of truncated assays is that K_i values for competitive inhibitors can be obtained directly from dose–response curves; for true competitive inhibitors, such K_i values have been shown to be identical with those from conventional kinetic analysis (Wright & Brown, 1976). Using the truncated assay we screened various modified nucleotides and aphidicolin derivatives and, using the full assay, pyrophosphate analogs at 100 μM, and the results, which are summarized in Table 9-2, are discussed in the paragraphs that follow.

3.2. dATP Analogs

All the dATP analogs tested in the truncated assay gave significant inhibition of pol α, but several were weak or inactive against pol δ (Table 9-2). The arabinofuranosyl derivative araATP inhibited both enzymes with similar potency, a result in accord with reported sensitivities of the calf thymus enzymes purified by earlier methods (Lee et al., 1981). The potent and selective DNA polymerase α inhibitor BuAdATP completely inhibited pol α but was only partially effective on pol δ. Indeed, at lower concentrations (e.g., see Table 9-1) BuAdATP inhibited pol α without effect on pol δ. The high selectivity of this nucleotide is most clearly shown in Table 9-3 where K_i values for inhibition of pol α versus pol δ dif-

TABLE 9-2. *Inhibitory Activity Against Calf Thymus DNA Polymerases α and δ Assayed on Activated DNA**

Compound (100 μM)	% Inhibition of	
	pol α	pol δ
-dATP		
araATP	72	54
BuAdATP	90	40
BuAA	71	0
BuAOMe	78	16
DCAA	67	40
DCAdATP	90	79
-dGTP		
BuPdGTP	92	74
EMPdGTP	81	16
PhdGTP	73	15
HexdGTP	80	0
ACGTP	83	66
-dCTP		
araCTP	5	60
Aphidicolin†	90	96
17-Acetylaphidicolin	48	43
"16-Ketoaphidicolin"	74	64
-dTTP		
AZTTP	24	28
ddTTP	57	62
Full assay (4 dNTPs)		
PP_i	20	40
PFA	20	15
PCF_2P	8	36

*Enzymes were assayed as described in Section 2 under the normal assay conditions or in the absence of the expected competitive substrate.
†Assayed at 10 μM.

dATP ANALOGS

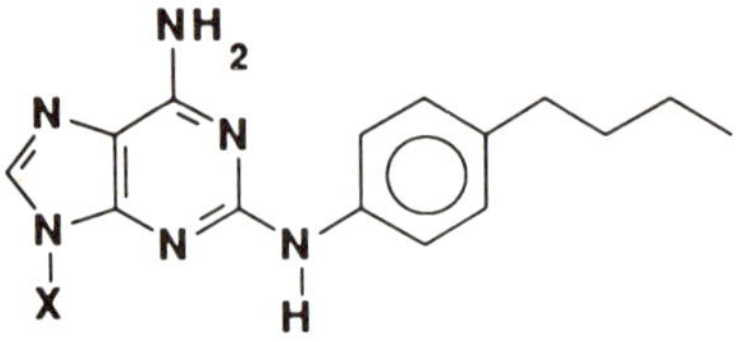

BuAA (X=H)

BuAdATP (X= $^{-4}O_9P_3O$–[2'-deoxyribose, OH])

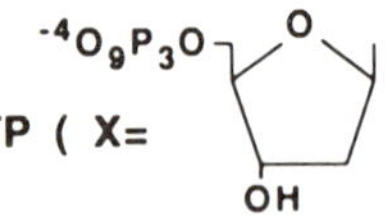

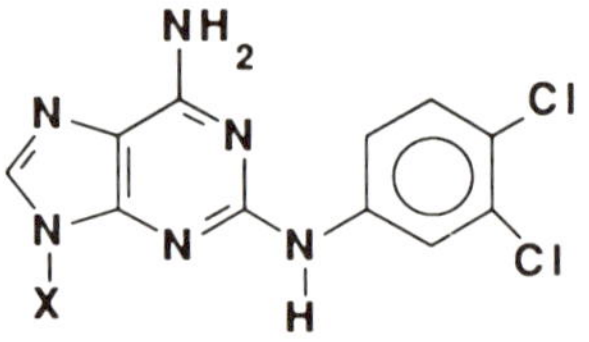

DCAA (X=H)

DCAdATP (X= $^{-4}O_9P_3O$–[2'-deoxyribose, OH])

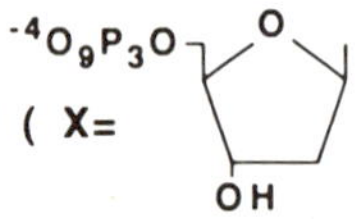

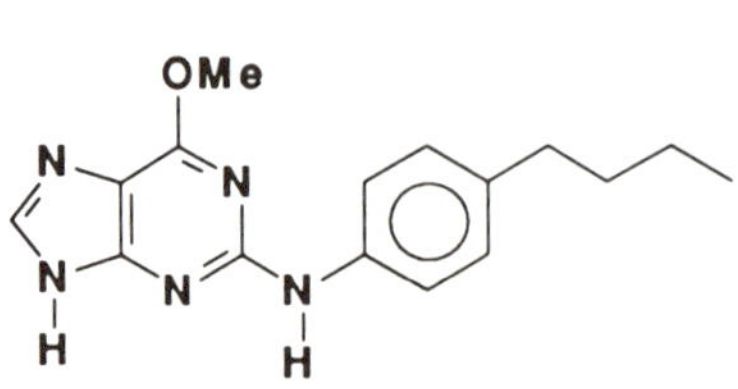

BuAOMe

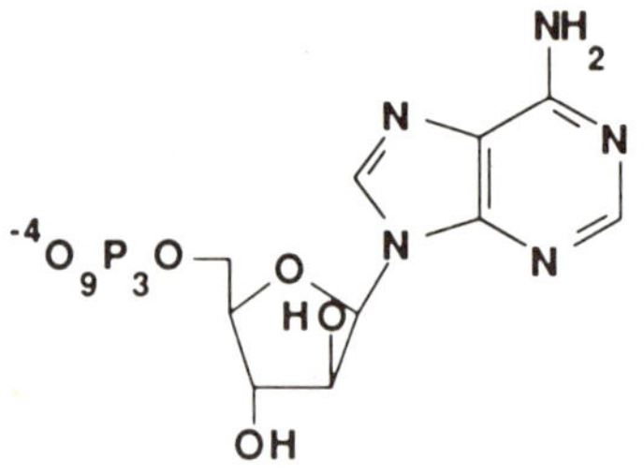

araATP

TABLE 9-3. *Potency of N^2-substituted Purine Deoxyribonucleotides as Inhibitors of Calf Thymus DNA Polymerases α and δ Assayed on Activated DNA*

	K_i (μM)*	
Compound	pol α	pol δ
BuPdGTP	0.005	25
BuAdATP	0.005	150
DCAdATP	3	66

*K_i values were determined from Dixon plots of each compound assayed with variable amounts of competitive substrates.

fer by a factor of 10^4. A similar result was reported previously for the placental DNA polymerases (Lee et al., 1985).

Although weaker than BuAdATP, the base analogs 2-(p-n-butylanilino)adenine (BuAA) and 2-(p-n-butylanilino)-6-methoxypurine (BuAOMe) strongly inhibited calf thymus pol α but were nearly ineffective at 100 μM against pol δ (Table 9-2). Although BuAA and BuAOMe were less potent pol α inhibitors than the nucleotide [K_i values of 14 and 1 μM, respectively, against CHO pol α (Wright et al., 1987)], they retain the selectivity that is a consequence of the p-n-butylphenyl group at position 2 of the 2-aminopurine nucleus (see structures). We have demonstrated that this 2-substituent represents the specificity site for inhibition of DNA polymerase α in a series of related N^2-substituted guanines (Wright et al., 1987). We therefore tested numerous guanine and adenine derivatives for their activity against DNA polymerase δ. Among a series of substituted adenines, 2-(3,4-dichloroanilino)adenine (DCAA) emerged as one of the few bases that showed observable inhibition of pol δ (Table 9-2). Based on this modest signal, and on observations that DCAA is a potent inhibitor of DNA synthesis in HeLa and CHO cells in culture (Talanian & Wright, in preparation), we synthesized the nucleotide derivative DCAdATP (see structures). A detailed analysis of this compound in the truncated assay gave a K_i of 66 μM against pol δ (see Fig. 9-1 and Table 9-3). DCAdATP was clearly not selective for pol δ, because in

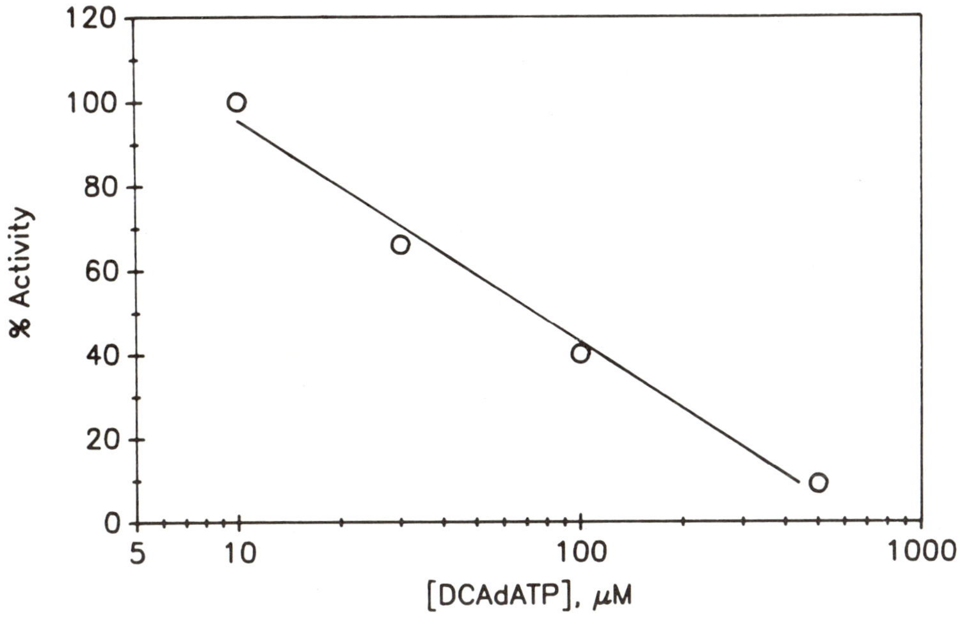

FIG. 9-1. Dose–activity curve for the effect of DCAdATP on calf thymus DNA polymerase δ. The enzyme was assayed on activated DNA in the absence of dATP (see Section 2).

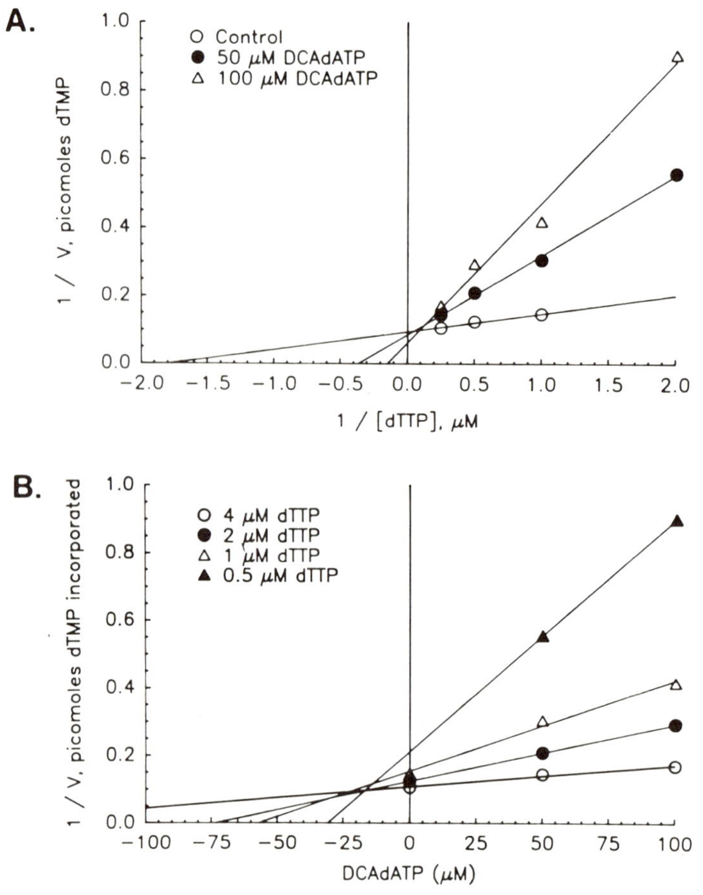

FIG. 9-2. Effect of DCAdATP on calf thymus DNA polymerase δ as a function of substrate concentration. The enzyme was assayed on oligo dT:poly dA with [^{3}H]dTTP as variable substrate as described in Section 2. (A) Lineweaver-Burk plot of the reciprocal of velocity against reciprocal of substrate concentration indicating that the drug is competitive with substrate. (B) Dixon plot of the same data indicating a K_i of approximately 20 μM.

the same conditions it inhibited pol α with K_i 3 μM (Table 9-3). Nevertheless, the replacement of the p-butylphenyl group by the dichlorophenyl group reduced pol α selectivity ($K_i,\alpha/K_i,\delta$) from 10^4 to 20. This drastic reduction in pol α selectivity suggests that further manipulation of substituents at the 2 position may generate an analog whose activity on the enzymes will cross over to give a selective inhibitor of pol δ.

A study of the mechanism of inhibition of DNA polymerases by DCAdATP is in progress. The results of Fig. 9-2, for example, show that this compound inhibited pol δ when the enzyme used oligo dT:poly dA as primer:template with kinetics that were competitive with dTTP (Fig. 9-2A), but not with dATP (data not shown), and with an apparent K_i of 20 μM (Fig. 9-2B). This behavior contrasts with that observed with BuAdATP in similar assays with CHO pol α, where the drug was competitive only with dATP (Khan et al., 1985). We must now determine the effect of DCAdATP and BuAdATP on calf thymus pol α with this "noncomplementary" primer:template to discover if the mechanism of inhibition by DCAdATP differs from that of BuAdATP.

3.3. dGTP ANALOGS

N^2-(p-n-Butylphenyl)deoxyguanosine 5′-triphosphate (BuPdGTP) is the guanine counterpart of BuAdATP (see structures). It inhibited calf thymus pol α nearly completely and 74% of pol δ activity at 100 μM in the truncated assay (Table 9-2). This similarity in inhi-

dGTP ANALOGS

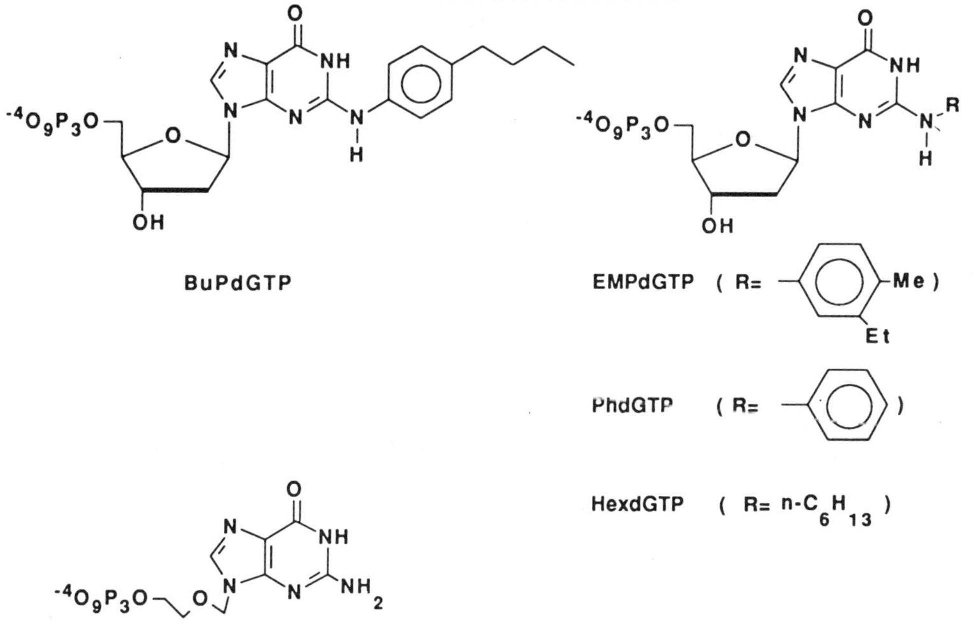

BuPdGTP

EMPdGTP (R= 3-ethyl-4-methylphenyl)

PhdGTP (R= phenyl)

HexdGTP (R= n-C_6H_{13})

ACG-TP

bition is more apparent than real, however. At concentrations at which pol δ is unaffected, pol α is completely inhibited by BuPdGTP (see, for example, Table 9-1). This selectivity is emphasized by the difference between K_i values of BuPdGTP for pol α and pol δ obtained in the truncated assay (Table 9-3).

Several N^2-substituted dGTP derivatives, EMPdGTP, PhdGTP, and HexdGTP (see structures), were also selective inhibitors of pol α, although they were considerably less potent against pol α (Table 2) than the prototype BuPdGTP. K_i values of these compounds against CHO pol α are, in fact, in the micromolar range (Freese & Wright, in preparation), in contrast to the nanomolar values for BuPdGTP (Khan et al., 1984).

The triphosphate of acycloguanosine (ACGTP), thought to be the active form of the antiherpetic drug acyclovir (Elion et al., 1977), inhibited both calf thymus pol α and pol δ to similar extents at 100 μM (Table 9-2). ACGTP has been reported to inhibit pol α from various sources with K_i values ranging from 0.1 to 1 μM (see, e.g., Derse et al., 1981). It is conceivable that inhibition of pol δ *in vivo* may contribute to the mechanism of cytotoxicity of acyclovir.

3.4. dCTP Analogs

AraCTP (arabinofuranosylcytosine 5′-triphosphate) did not significantly inhibit DNA polymerase α in the absence of dCTP, but it inhibited pol δ by 60% (Table 9-2). In the full assay, with all dNTPs present, however, araCTP at 100 μM inhibited calf thymus pol α by 40% and pol δ by 71%. The lack of effect of araCTP on pol α in the absence of dCTP was surprising for three reasons: (1) araCTP has been reported to be a potent inhibitor of pol α (Momparler, 1982), (2) araATP strongly inhibited pol α in the absence of dATP (see earlier discussion), and (3) araCTP inhibited pol α from CHO cells by 64% under truncated (-dCTP) conditions (results not shown). The result is consistent, however, with that of Yoshida and colleagues (1977) who reported, for calf thymus pol α, that the truncated synthesis on activated DNA remaining after dCTP was omitted was completely resistant to araCTP up to 200 μM. In contrast, araATP strongly inhibited the calf thymus enzyme in the absence of dATP (Okura & Yoshida, 1978). Whether this observation for araCTP

dCTP ANALOGS

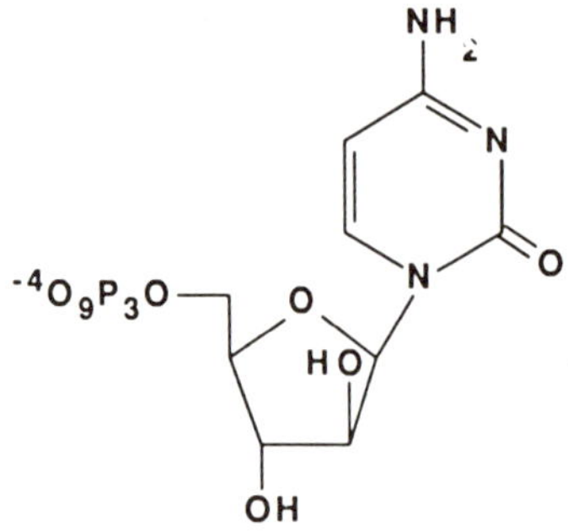

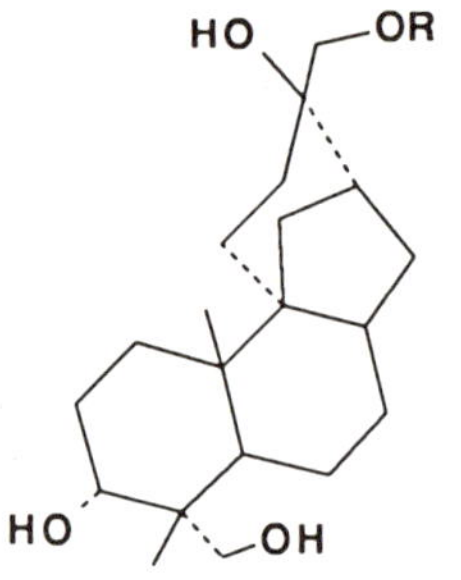

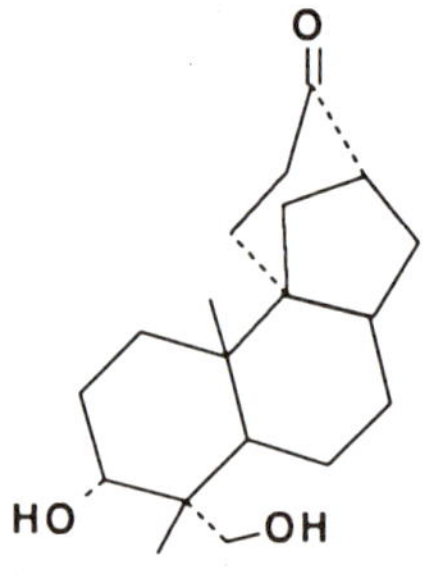

araCTP

Aphidicolin (R=H)

17-Acetylaphidicolin ($R=COCH_3$)

"16-ketoaphidicolin"

[3,18-dihydroxy-17-noraphidicolan-16-one]

is unique to the calf enzyme and whether it may suggest a different mechanism of araCTP inhibition compared with araATP are subjects for further study. Based on the results for araATP and araCTP, there does not appear to be any natural selectivity of arabinonucleotides for the α or δ polymerases, although the lack of inhibition of pol α by araCTP under truncated conditions could be used to differentiate between the two enzymes.

Aphidicolin and its derivatives were tested in the absence of dCTP because their inhibition of pol α's is commonly competitive with dCTP. Aphidicolin was a potent inhibitor of both DNA polymerases α and δ as expected (Table 9-2). Two derivatives, 17-acetylaphidicolin and "16-ketoaphidicolin," a product of periodic acid oxidation of aphidicolin (see structures), were weaker inhibitors of both enzymes but did not inhibit either selectively. Inhibition of pol δ by both compounds was completely reversed when assayed in the presence of dCTP at 25 μM.

We were surprised that "16-ketoaphidicolin" was the more potent derivative against pol α because 17-acetylaphidicolin is a more potent inhibitor of pol α from HeLa and CHO cells than is "16-ketoaphidicolin" (K_i's of about 5 and 40 μM, respectively) (Arabshahi et al., 1988). The resistance of calf thymus pol α to 17-acetylaphidicolin may be a consequence of the fact that the enzyme is partially purified, or it may reflect a fundamental difference between it and other more sensitive pol α's. For example, one group reported that 17-acetylaphidicolin inhibited sea urchin pol α with $K_i = 2.6$ μM (Haraguchi et al., 1983), but another group reported that it lacked activity against the KB cell enzyme (Hiranuma et al., 1987).

3.5. dTTP Analogs

2′,3′-Dideoxythymidine 5′-triphosphate (ddTTP) at 100 μM inhibited both DNA polymerases in the absence of dTTP to similar extents (Table 9-2). In the truncated assay the apparent K_i values for ddTTP were 60 and 25 μM for inhibition of pol α and pol δ, respectively. Thus, these enzymes have similar sensitivity to ddTTP, but it is only moderate when compared with the high sensitivity of DNA polymerases β and γ (Edenberg et al., 1978) and of reverse transcriptases (Smoler et al., 1971) to this and other 2′,3′-dideoxynucleotides.

3′-Azido-2′,3′-dideoxythymidine 5′-triphosphate (AZTTP), the putative active form of the human immunodeficiency virus inhibitor AZT (Mitsuya et al., 1985), showed little effect on either pol α or pol δ in the truncated assay (Table 9-2). The K_i values for both enzymes were >1 mM in the truncated assay, consistent with weak activity of AZTTP reported on DNA polymerase α from H9 cells (Furman et al., 1986).

dTTP ANALOGS

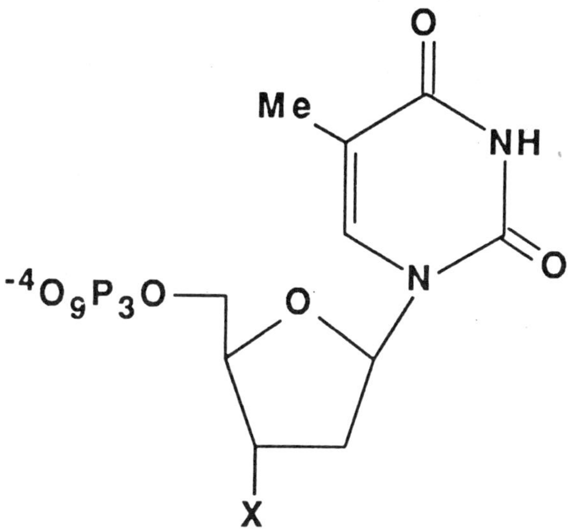

$^{-4}O_9P_3O$ — O — N — NH — Me — X

ddTTP (X=H)

AZTTP (X=N_3)

3.6. Pyrophosphate Analogs

We tested several pyrophosphate analogs (see structures) at 100 μM in the full assay. Phosphonoformate (PFA) weakly inhibited both pol α and pol δ similarly (Table 9-2). Pyrophosphate (PP_i) and a phosphonate isostere difluoromethylenebisphosphonate (PCF_2P) inhibited pol δ more than pol α in this screen and were studied further. The dose–response curves of Figure 9-3 show these results. Pyrophosphate was a moderately potent inhibitor of pol δ (IC_{50} = 0.15 mM), but was not very selective because its IC_{50} for pol α was 0.6 mM (Figure 9-3A). In contrast, although the difluoromethylene compound was a weaker inhibitor of pol δ (IC_{50} = 0.75 mM), it appeared to be highly selective. PCF_2P was without effect on pol α at concentrations up to 2 mM.

We next tested the influence of primer:template on the apparent selectivity of these compounds. Pyrophosphate inhibited both pol α and pol δ with similar potencies (IC_{50} ca. 0.6 mM) when oligo dT:poly dA was used as primer:template. In contrast, PCF_2P remained inhibitory to pol δ in the homopolymer assay (IC_{50} = 0.65 μM) and did not inhibit pol α at 2 mM.

The antiherpetic drug PFA and related compounds such as phosphonoacetate (PAA) inhibit DNA polymerases by a mechanism that likely involves interaction with the pyrophosphate binding region of sensitive enzymes. Although more effective against herpes virus DNA polymerases, PFA inhibits pol α (typical IC_{50} 40 μM) (Eriksson et al., 1980),

PYROPHOSPHATE ANALOGS

$^{-2}O_3POPO_3^{-2}$	$^{-2}O_3PCO_2^-$	$^{-2}O_3PCF_2PO_3^{-2}$
PP_i	PFA	PCF_2P

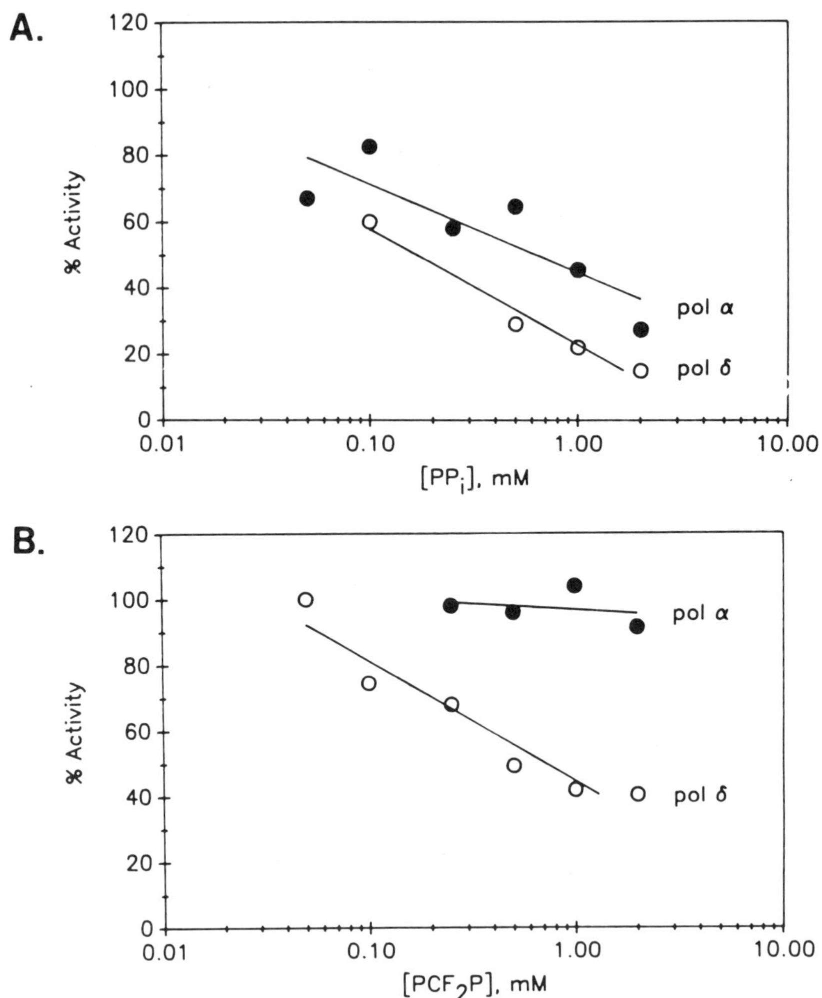

FIG. 9-3. Dose–activity curves for the effect of pyrophosphate analogs on calf thymus DNA polymerases α and δ. The enzymes were assayed on activated DNA in the presence of four dNTPs as described in Section 2. (A) Dose–activity curves for pyrophosphate (PP_i). (B) Dose–activity curves for difluoromethylenebisphosphonate (PCF_2P).

but most other pyrophosphate analogs were reported to be inactive against pol α (Eriksson et al., 1980). PCF_2P, the compound identified in this work as a selective inhibitor of calf thymus DNA polymerase δ, is one of a series of related methylenebisphosphonates that were recently reported to be without activity at 100 μM against human DNA polymerases α, β, and γ and several herpes virus DNA polymerases (McKenna et al., 1987).

Our current strategy is to examine the mechanism by which PCF_2P inhibits pol δ and to determine, in our and other laboratories, if the compound is a universal and selective inhibitor of DNA polymerase δ from other sources. We will also compare the activity of other phosphonocarboxylic acids and bisphosphonates as inhibitors of calf thymus DNA polymerases with the objective of discovering more potent and selective inhibitors of DNA polymerase δ.

4. CONCLUSIONS

Various modified nucleotides, aphidicolin derivatives, and pyrophosphate analogs were compared as inhibitors of calf thymus DNA polymerases α and δ. Most compounds inhibited the enzymes with approximately equal potency. Certain 2-substituted purines and their deoxyribonucleoside triphosphate derivatives were selectively inhibitory for pol α. Adenine and dATP derivatives with a p-n-butylanilino group at position 2 were highly selective for pol α, but analogs with a 3,4-dichloroanilino group at position 2 were much less selective. This result suggests that a search for a 2-substituted adenine or dATP derivative with selectivity for DNA polymerase δ might be fruitful.

One pyrophosphate analog, difluoromethylenebisphosphonate (PCF_2P), was selectively inhibitory for DNA polymerase δ. Using either activated DNA or oligo dT:poly dA as primer:template, PCF_2P inhibited pol δ with IC_{50} of about 0.7 mM, but the compound had no effect on pol α at 2 mM. Studies of the mechanism of PCF_2P and structure–activity relationships of analogs of this compound are in progress.

Acknowledgments—The authors thank Stephen Freese and Dr. Lili Arabshahi for the synthesis of dGTP and aphidicolin derivatives, respectively, and Dr. Wayne Miller for gifts of ddTTP and AZTTP. We are grateful to Matthew Wright for expert assistance in the preparation of the manuscript. This work was supported by National Institutes of Health grants GM21747 (to G.W.) and GM28775 (to N.B.) and by Swiss National Science Foundation grant 3.604-0.87 (to U.H.).

REFERENCES

Arabshahi, L., Brown, N., Khan, N., and Wright, G. (1988) Inhibition of DNA polymerase alpha by aphidicolin derivatives. *Nucleic Acids Res.* **16**: 5107–5113.

Blackburn, G. M., England, D. A., and Kolkmann, F. (1981) Monofluoro- and difluoromethylenebisphosphonic acids: Isopolar analogues of pyrophosphoric acid. *J. Chem. Soc. Chem. Comm.*, 930–932.

Bravo, R., Frank, R., Blundell, P. A., and MacDonald-Bravo, H. (1987) Cyclin/PCNA is the auxiliary protein of DNA polymerase δ. *Nature* **326**: 515–517.

Byrnes, J. J. (1985) Differential inhibitors of DNA polymerases alpha and delta. *Biochem. Biophys. Res. Commun.* **132**: 628–634.

Byrnes, J. J., Downey, K. M., Black, V. L., and So, A. G. (1976) A new mammalian DNA polymerase with 3′ to 5′ exonuclease activity: DNA polymerase δ. *Biochemistry* **15**: 2817–2823.

Chiu, R. W., and Baril, E. F. (1975) Nuclear DNA polymerases and the HeLa cell cycle. *J. Biol. Chem.* **250**: 7951–7957.

Cotterill, S. M., Reyland, M. E., Loeb, L. A., and Lehman, I. R. (1987) A cryptic proofreading 3′ to 5′ exonuclease associated with the polymerase subunit of the DNA polymerase-primase from *Drosophila melanogaster*. *Proc. Natl. Acad. Sci. USA* **84**: 5635–5639.

Crute, J. J., Wahl, A. F., and Bambara, R. A. (1986) Purification and characterization of two new high molecular weight forms of DNA polymerase δ. *Biochemistry* **25**: 26–36.

Dalziel, W., Hesp, B., Stevenson, K. M., and Jarvis, J. A. J. (1973) The structure and absolute configuration of the antibiotic aphidicolin: A tetracyclic diterpenoid containing a new ring system. *J. Chem. Soc. Perkin Trans.* I, 2841–2851.

Decker, R. S., Yamaguchi, M., Possenti, R., Bradley, M. K., and DePamphilis, M. L. (1987) *In vitro* initiation of DNA replication in simian virus 40 chromosomes. *J. Biol. Chem.* **262**: 10863–10872.

Derse, D., Cheng, Y.-C., Furman, P. A., St. Clair, M. H., and Elion, G. B. (1981) Inhibition of purified human and herpes simplex virus-induced DNA polymerases by 9-(2-hydroxyethoxymethyl)guanine triphosphate. Effects on primer-template function. *J. Biol. Chem.* **256**: 11447–11451.

Dresler, S. L., and Frattini, M. G. (1986) DNA replication and UV-induced DNA repair synthesis in human fibroblasts are much less sensitive than DNA polymerase α to inhibition by butylphenyl-deoxyguanosine triphosphate. *Nucleic Acids Res.* **14**: 7093–7102.

Dresler, S. L., and Frattini, M. G. (1988) Analysis of butylphenyl-guanine, butylphenyl-deoxyguanosine, and butylphenyl-deoxyguanosine triphosphate inhibition of DNA replication and ultraviolet-induced DNA repair synthesis using permeable human fibroblasts. *Biochem. Pharmacol.* **37**: 1033–1037.

Edenberg, H. J., Anderson, S., and DePamphilis, M. L. (1978) Involvement of DNA polymerase alpha in simian virus 40 DNA replication. *J. Biol. Chem.* **253**: 3273–3280.

Elion, G. B., Furman, P. A., Fyfe, J. A., de Miranda, P., Beauchamp, L., and Schaeffer, H. J. (1977) Selectivity of action of an antiherpetic agent, 9-(2-hydroxyethoxymethyl)guanine. *Proc. Natl. Acad. Sci. USA* **74**: 5716–5720.

Eriksson, B., Larsson, A., Helgstrand, E., Johansson, N.-G., and Öberg, B. (1980) Pyrophosphate analogs as inhibitors of herpes simplex virus type 1 DNA polymerase. *Biochim. Biophys. Acta* **607**: 53–64.

Fersht, A. R., and Knill-Jones, J. W. (1983) Contribution of 3′ to 5′ exonuclease activity of DNA polymerase III holoenzyme from *Escherichia coli* to specificity. *J. Mol. Biol.* **165**: 669–682.

Focher, F., Ferrari, E., Spadari, S., and Hübscher, U. (1988a) Do DNA polymerases δ and α act coordinately as leading and lagging strand replicases? *FEBS Lett.* **229**: 6–10.

Focher, F., Spadari, S., Ginelli, B., Hottiger, M., Gassmann, M., and Hübscher, U. (1988b) Calf thymus DNA polymerase δ: Purification, biochemical, and functional properties of the enzyme after its separation from DNA polymerase α, a DNA-dependent ATPase, and proliferating cell nuclear antigen. *Nucleic Acids Res.*, **6**:6279–6295.

Fry, M., and Loeb, L. A. (1986) *Animal cell DNA polymerases*. Boca Raton, FL: CRC Press.

Furman, P. A., Fyfe, J. A., St. Clair, M. H., Weinhold, K., Rideout, J. L., Freeman, G. A., Lehrman, S. N., Bolognesi, D. P., Broder, S., Mitsuya, H., and Barry, D. W. (1986) Phosphorylation of 3′-azido-3′-deoxythymidine and selective interaction of the 5′-triphosphate with human immunodeficiency virus reverse transcriptase. *Proc. Natl. Acad. Sci. USA* **83**: 8333–8337.

Goscin, L. P., and Byrnes, J. J. (1982) DNA polymerase δ: one polypeptide, two activities. *Biochemistry* **21**: 2513–2518.

Hammond, R. A., Byrnes, J. J., and Miller, M. R. (1987) Identification of DNA polymerase δ in CV-1 cells: Studies implicating both DNA polymerase δ and DNA polymerase α in DNA replication. *Biochemistry* **26**: 6817–6824.

Haraguchi, T., Oguro, M., Nagano, H., Ichihara, A., and Sakamura, S. (1983) Specific inhibitors of eukaryotic DNA synthesis and DNA polymerase α, 3-deoxyaphidicolin, and aphidicolin-17-monoacetate. *Nucleic Acids Res.* **11**: 1197–1209.

Hiranuma, S., Shimizu, T., Yoshioka, H., Ono, K., Nakane, H., and Takahashi, T. (1987) Chemical modification of aphidicolin and the inhibitory effects of its derivatives on DNA polymerase α *in vitro*. *Chem. Pharm. Bull.* **35**: 1641–1644.

Huberman, J. A. (1981) New views of the biochemistry of eucaryotic DNA replication revealed by aphidicolin, an unusual inhibitor of DNA polymerase α. *Cell* **23**: 647–648.

Kaczmarek, L., Miller, M. R., Hammond, R. A., and Mercer, W. E. (1986) A microinjected monoclonal antibody against human DNA polymerase α inhibits DNA replication in human, hamster, and mouse cell lines. *J. Biol. Chem.* **261**: 10802–10807.

Khan, N. N., Wright, G. E., Dudycz, L. W., and Brown, N. C. (1984) Butyl-phenyl dGTP: A selective and potent inhibitor of mammalian DNA polymerase alpha. *Nucleic Acids Res.* **12**: 3695–3706.

Khan, N. N., Wright, G. E., Dudycz, L. W., and Brown, N. C. (1985) Elucidation of the mechanism of selective inhibition of mammalian DNA polymerase alpha by 2-butylanilinopurines: Development and characterization of 2-(p-n-butylanilino)adenine and its deoxyribonucleotides. *Nucleic Acids Res.* **13**: 6331–6342.

Lee, M. Y. W. T., and Toomey, N. L. (1987) Human placental DNA polymerase δ: Identification of a 170-kilodalton polypeptide by activity staining and immunoblotting. *Biochemistry* **26**: 1076–1085.

Lee, M. Y. W. T., Toomey, N. L., and Wright, G. E. (1985) Differential inhibition of DNA polymerases δ and α by BuPdGTP and BuAdATP. *Nucleic Acids Res.* **13**: 8623–8630.

Lee, M. Y. W. T., Tan, C.-K., Downey, K. M., and So, A. G. (1984) Further studies on calf thymus DNA polymerase α purified to homogeneity by a new procedure. *Biochemistry* **23**: 1906–1913.

Lee, M. Y. W. T., Tan, C.-K., Downey, K. M., and So, A. G. (1981) Structural and functional properties of calf thymus DNA polymerase δ. *Prog. Nucl. Acid. Res. Mol. Biol.* **26**: 83–96.

Lee, M. Y. W. T., Tan, C.-K., So, A. G., and Downey, K. M. (1980) Purification of deoxyribonucleic acid polymerase α from calf thymus: Partial characterization of physical properties. *Biochemistry* **19**: 2096–2101.

Marraccino, R. L., Wahl, A. F., Keng, P. C., Lord, E. M., and Bambara, R. A. (1987) Cell cycle dependent activities of DNA polymerases α and δ in Chinese hamster ovary cells. *Biochemistry* **26**: 7864–7870.

McKenna, C. E., Khawli, L. A., Bapat, A., Harutunian, V., and Cheng, Y.-C. (1987) Inhibition of herpes virus and human DNA polymerases by α-halogenated phosphonoacetates. *Biochem. Pharmacol.* **36**: 3103–3106.

Miller, M. R., Ulrich, R. G., Wang, T. S.-F., and Korn, D. A. (1985) Monoclonal antibodies against human DNA polymerase α inhibit DNA replication in permeabilized human cells. *J. Biol. Chem.* **260**: 134–138.

Mitsuya, H., Weinhold, K. J., Furman, P. A., St. Clair, M. H., Lehrman, S. N., Gallo, R. C., Bolognesi, D., Barry, D. W., and Broder, S. (1985) 3′-Azido-3′-deoxythymidine (BW A509U): An antiviral agent that inhibits the infectivity and cytopathic effect of human T-lymphotropic virus type III/lymphadenopathy-associated virus *in vitro*. *Proc. Natl. Acad. Sci. USA* **82**: 7096–7100.

Momparler, R. L. (1982) Biochemical pharmacology of cytosine arabinoside. *Med. Ped. Oncol.* Suppl. 1, 45–48.

Murakami, Y., Yasuda, H., Miyazawa, H., Hanaoka, F., and Yamada, M. (1985) Characterization of a temperature-sensitive mutant of mouse FM3A cells defective in DNA replication. *Proc. Natl. Acad. Sci. USA* **82**: 1761–1765.

Neville, M. M., and Brown, N. C. (1972) Inhibition of a discrete bacterial DNA polymerase by 6-(p-hydroxyphenylazo)-uracil and 6-(p-hydroxyphenylazo)-isocytosine. *Nature New Biol.* **240**: 80–82.

Nishida, C., Reinhardt, P., and Linn, S. (1988) DNA repair synthesis in human fibroblasts requires DNA polymerase δ. *J. Biol. Chem.* **263**: 501–510.

Okura, A., and Yoshida, S. (1978) Differential inhibition of DNA polymerases of calf thymus by 9-β-D-arabinofuranosyladenine 5′-triphosphate. *J. Biochem.* **84**: 727–732.

Prelich, G., Kostura, M., Marshak, D. R., Mathews, M. B., and Stillman, B. (1987a) The cell-cycle regulated proliferating cell nuclear antigen is required for SV40 DNA replication *in vitro*. *Nature* **326**: 471–475.

Prelich, G., Tan, C.-K., Kostura, M., Mathews, M. B., So, A. G., Downey, K. M., and Stillman, B. (1987b) Functional identity of proliferating cell nuclear antigen and a DNA polymerase α auxiliary protein. *Nature* **326**: 517–520.

Reyland, M. E., Lehman, I. R., and Loeb, L. A. (1988) Specificity of proofreading by the 3′ to 5′ exonucleases of the DNA polymerase-primase of *Drosophila melanogaster*. *J. Biol. Chem.* **263**: 6518–6524.

Smoler, D., Molineux, I., and Baltimore, D. (1971) Direction of polymerization by the avian myeloblastosis virus deoxyribonucelic acid polymerase. *J. Biol. Chem.* **246**: 7697–7700.

Wright, G. E., Dudycz, L. W., Kazimierczuk, Z., Brown, N. C., and Khan, N. N. (1987) Synthesis, cell growth inhibition, and antitumor screening of 2-(p-n-butylanilino)purines and their nucleoside analogs. *J. Med. Chem.* **30**: 109–116.

Wright, G. E., anmd Dudycz, L. W. (1984) Synthesis and characterization of N^2-(p-n-butylphenyl)-2′-deoxyguanosine and its 5′-triphosphate and their inhibition of HeLa DNA polymerase α. *J. Med. Chem.* **27**: 175–181.

Wright, G. E., and Brown, N. C. (1976) Inhibition of *Bacillus subtilis* DNA polymerase III by arylhydrazinopyrimidines: Novel properties of 2-thiouracil derivatives. *Biochim. Biophys. Acta* **432**: 37–48.

Yoshida, S., Yamada, M., and Masaki, S. (1977) Inhibition of DNA polymerase α and β of calf thymus by 1-β-D-arabinofuranosyl-cytosine 5′-triphosphate. *Biochim. Biophys. Acta* **477**: 144–150.

Zhang, S. J., and Lee, M. Y. W. T. (1987) Biochemical characterization and development of DNA polymerases α and δ in the neonatal rat heart. *Arch. Biochem. Biophys.* **252**: 24–31.

CHAPTER 10

TOPOISOMERASE II AS A TARGET OF ANTITUMOR AGENTS

RONALD HANCOCK, MARTIN CHARRON, HERMAN LAMBERT, MARGOT LEMIEUX, ROUMEN PANKOV,* AND NORMAND PEPIN

Centre de Recherche en Cancérologie de l'Université Laval, Hôtel-Dieu, Québec, Canada

Abstract—We present a synthesis of current work on the important and successful antitumor agents adriamycin, daunomycin, and amsacrine (*m*AMSA) (intercalating agents), and the epipodophyllotoxins VM-26 and VP-16, which have as their intracellular target the enzyme topoisomerase II. The molecular processes underlying production of DNA strand breaks, selective G2 arrest of growing cells, inhibition of mitotic chromosome formation and segregation, chromosomal recombination, sister chromatid exchange, the cytostatic and cytocidal action, and the development of tumor resistance are reviewed. This work opens new perspectives for rational development of new antitumor agents and elucidating the cellular functions of topoisomerase II.

1. INTRODUCTION

Over the past ten years the concept has emerged and been experimentally established that two families of clinically important and successful antitumor agents have as their intracellular target the enzyme topoisomerase II. This development is an excellent example of the fertile convergence of two apparently unrelated areas of research: on the one hand, studies of the effects of these agents on the DNA of cells growing in culture and, on the other, enzymological studies of this enzyme and its reaction. The elucidation of the mechanism of action of these agents is both opening new perspectives for the rational development of new antitumor agents and stimulating advances in our understanding of the cellular functions of topoisomerase II by allowing the use of these agents as specific probes in cellular and molecular studies.

The first of these families of antitumor agents comprises adriamycin (doxorubicin), daunomycin (daunorubicin), and amsacrine (*m*AMSA) and their derivatives. The second family comprises the epipodophyllotoxins VM-26 (teniposide) and VP-16 (etoposide). These agents are of biological origin, with the exception of amsacrine, which was developed by systematic synthesis and screening of acridine derivatives (Denny et al., 1983).

We do not attempt here to review comprehensively all the available literature on these agents, but rather to present a synthesis of current understanding and concepts concerning their action, and to draw attention to areas of future importance and interest. Recent reviews consider in detail the intercalating agents (Neidle & Waring, 1983), amsacrine (Marshall & Ralph, 1984), the epipodophyllotoxin VP-16 (Issell et al., 1984), the molecular biology of topoisomerase II (Wang, 1985; Vosberg, 1985), and the general field of antitumor agents affecting topoisomerase II (Potmesil & Ross, 1987).

2. ANTITUMOR AGENTS AFFECTING TOPOISOMERASE II REACTIONS

2.1. INTERCALATING AGENTS

Adriamycin and daunomycin are derivatives of anthracycline (Fig. 10-1). They differ only in that a hydrogen atom in daunomycin is replaced by a hydroxyl group in adriamycin but have significantly different spectra of clinical effectiveness (Arcamone, 1981). In spite of extensive search for other natural anthracyclines and for semisynthetic and synthetic derivatives (Brown, 1983), other agents suitable for wide clinical use have not yet been discovered.

*Permanent address: Institute of Molecular Biology, Academy of Sciences, 1113 Sofia, Bulgaria.

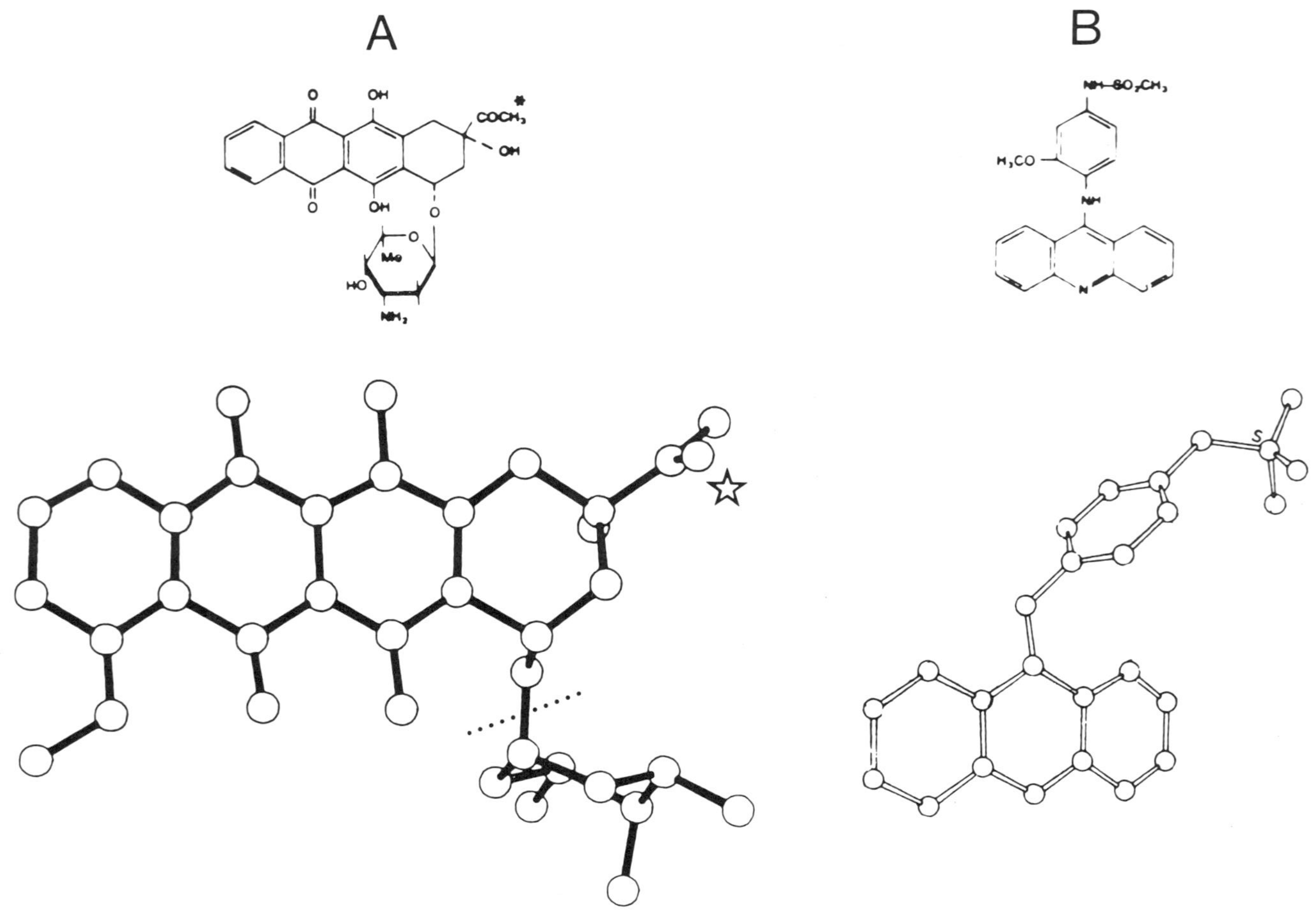

FIG. 10-1. The molecular structure (above) and three-dimensional conformation (below) of the intercalating antitumor agents daunomycin and *m*AMSA. (A) Daunomycin. In adriamycin an H atom at the position * is replaced by an —OH group. The dotted line separates the anthracycline chromophore and the amino sugar (Neidle & Sanderson, 1983). Reprinted with the kind permission of Dr. S. Neidle and the copyright holder, Elsevier Science Publishers, Amsterdam. (B) *m*AMSA (Hall et al., 1974). Figure kindly supplied by Dr. T. N. Waters.

Amsacrine (4′-[(9-acridinyl)amino] methansulfon-m-anisidide) is a synthetic derivative of acridine (Fig. 10-1). It is the only derivative successfully used in clinical chemotherapy out of many hundreds which have been synthesized and screened (Denny et al., 1983).

These agents bind to DNA by intercalation; the anthracycline and acridine ring systems fit snugly in the interior of the double helix between the base pairs, and the side chain lies in the minor groove on the exterior (e.g., Quigley et al., 1980) (Fig. 10-2).

2.2. Epipodophyllotoxins

The two epipodophyllotoxins in clinical use, VP-16 and VM-26, differ in structure only in an external substituent group (Fig. 10-3). Current evidence indicates that these agents do not bind to DNA (Chen et al., 1984).

3. USE IN TUMOR CHEMOTHERAPY

These agents are widely used in the chemotherapy of a range of human tumors, with significant long-term success (Table 10-1). In most situations they are employed in combination with other agents either simultaneously, or in alternating cycles designed to reduce the possibility of emergence of resistant tumor cells. Certain less common types of tumor respond to treatment by these agents alone (Table 10-1).

The optimism raised by the first observations of successful initial responses to these agents has been tempered by the finding that tumor cells resistant to them frequently emerge after a period of several months (Table 10-2). Present knowledge of the molecular basis for this resistance is discussed in Section 8.

4. EFFECTS ON CELLS IN CULTURE

4.1. Effects at the Cellular Level

All these agents show a characteristic spectrum of effects on mammalian cells growing in culture. These are seen most clearly in cells exposed to epipodophyllotoxins or to intercalating agents at minimal growth-inhibitory concentrations. At higher concentrations the latter agents show further effects, because when intercalative binding to DNA reaches a high enough level all functions of DNA which require strand separation are inhibited. Thus

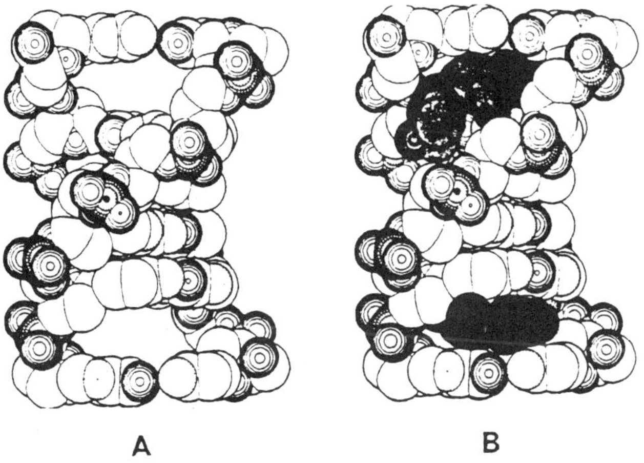

Fig. 10-2. The intercalation of daunomycin into a model DNA, the duplex hexanucleotide d(CpGpTpApCpGp), as shown in the structure determined by X-ray diffraction (Quigley et al., 1980). (A) The hexanucleotide duplex alone, (B) With two intercalated daunomycin molecules (atoms shaded). Reprinted with the kind permission of Dr. A. Rich, M.I.T.

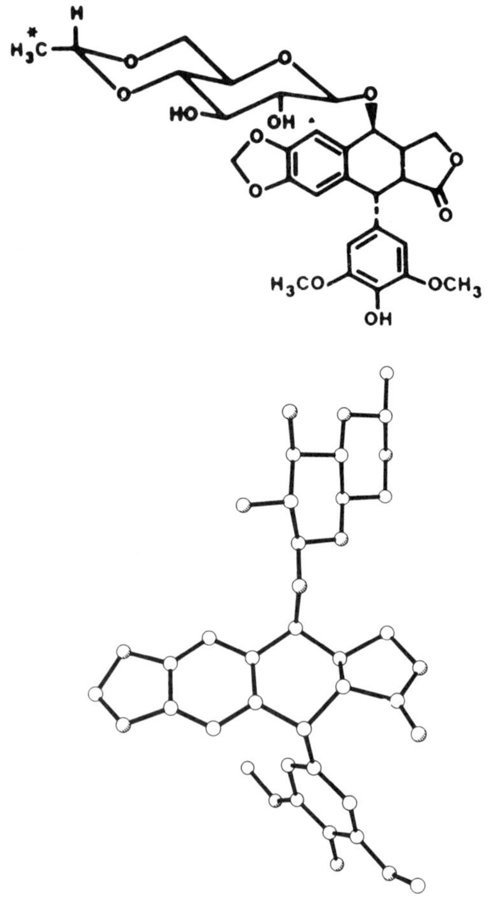

FIG. 10-3. The molecular structure (A) and three-dimensional conformation (B) of the epipodophyllotoxin VP-16 (Doyle, 1984). In VM-26 a thenylidine side chain replaces the methyl group at the position *. Figure kindly supplied by Dr. J. Clardy.

TABLE 10-1. *Examples of Long-Term Tumor Responses*

		Agents	% Remissions/Duration	Reference
Lymphomas				
Hodgkins	1984	VP-16 (+3 others)	84/1 year	McElwain & Selby (1984)
	1985	Adriamycin (+7)	80/7 years	Bonadonna (1985)
Non-Hodgkins	1985	VP-16, adriamycin (+6) (ProMace-MOPP)	65/3 years	Bonadonna (1985)
Leukemias				
Childhood AML	1987	VP-16 (+6)	33/3 years*	Amadori et al. (1987)
Adult AML	1981	Adriamycin (+3)	12/5 years	Keating et al. (1981)
Adult proML	1986	Adriamycin (+3)	43/5 years	Kantarjian et al. (1986)
Adult AL	1987	*m*AMSA (+3)	8/4 years	Keating et al. (1987)
Childhood sarcomas (various, relapsed)	1986	VP-16 (+ Ifosfamide)	35/1 year	Miser et al. (1987)
Trophoblastic tumors	1986	VP-16 alone	95/1–4 years	Wong et al. (1986)

*Extrapolated.

This table of representative results from published clinical trials is presented to illustrate the general efficacy of the agents discussed here, and not as a rigorous quantitative evaluation.

TABLE 10-2. *Examples of Development of Tumor Resistance*

	Agent	% Remissions/Duration	Reference
Non-Hodgkins, lymphoma (relapsed)			
1981	AMSA alone	7/1 year	Cabanillas et al. (1981)
1984	VP-16 alone	46/6 months	Young et al. (1984)
Small-cell lung cancer			
1987	VP-16 alone	30/9 weeks	Matsui et al. (1987)

RNA transcription and DNA synthesis are affected at higher concentrations of intercalating agents (e.g., Schwartz, 1983), and we do not consider these effects here although they may play a role in the inhibition of tumor cell growth by intercalating agents.

The characteristic effects seen in cells grown with these agents are

1. Accumulation of cells in the G2 phase of the cell cycle (Grieder et al., 1974; Krishan et al., 1975; Misra & Roberts, 1975; Tobey et al., 1978; Kalwinsky et al., 1983) (Section 6).
2. In the few cells which reach mitosis, chromosomes are joined in multiradial conformations and by telomeric fusion (Huang et al., 1973; Deaven et al., 1978) (Section 7).
3. Sister chromatid exchanges in the chromosomes of mitotic cells (Deaven et al., 1978) (Section 7).

These responses clearly provide valuable clues to the nature of the intracellular target of these agents and to their molecular functions.

4.2. Increased Levels of Topoisomerase II Integrated in Chromosomal DNA

DNA purified from cells grown in culture with these agents shows unique properties: It contains strand breaks and covalently bound protein (Burr-Furlong et al., 1978; Ralph, 1980; Zwelling et al., 1981; Ross & Bradley, 1981; Marshall et al., 1983b; Ralph & Hancock, 1985, reviewed in Marshall & Ralph, 1984).

Studies of this phenomenon crystallized at a time when studies of the enzyme topoisomerase II showed that during its action *in vitro*, its DNA substrate acquires the same unique properties, by mechanisms discussed in Section 5.2. The hypothesis was therefore proposed (Zwelling et al., 1981; Filipski, 1983) that elevated levels of topoisomerase II may be present in the DNA of cells exposed to these agents. The first experimental evidence supporting this hypothesis was presented by Marshall et al. (1983a) who showed that while strand breaks are present in the DNA extracted from isolated nuclei incubated with *m*AMSA, their formation is prevented by inhibitors (novobiocin and coumermycin) which block an early step in the topoisomerase II reaction, and the hypothesis has since been well established.

5. EFFECTS ON TOPOISOMERASE II REACTIONS

5.1. Topoisomerase II Reactions

Topoisomerase II passes one double-stranded DNA across a second DNA. It initiates this remarkable reaction by inserting itself covalently into the substrate DNA, forming bonds between tyrosine-OH groups of the enzyme and the 5′-terminus of each DNA strand (reviewed by Wang, 1985; Vosberg, 1985). It then functions as a "molecular gate," allowing passage of a second DNA between its two identical polypeptide chains without disrupting the continuity of the first DNA (Fig. 10-4).

Exposure to protein denaturants while the enzyme is covalently integrated in DNA dissociates its two subunits, and thus effectively cleaves the DNA. The frequency and sites of cleavage therefore reflect the sites of integration of topoisomerase II, and can be studied in *in vitro* systems using an end-labeled DNA substrate and purified enzyme (Liu et al., 1983; Sander & Hsieh, 1983; Tewey et al., 1984; Chen et al., 1984) (Fig. 10-5).

5.2. Effects of Intercalating Agents and Epipodophyllotoxins on Topoisomerase II Reactions *in vitro*

The addition of intercalating agents or epipodophyllotoxins to such model systems in which topoisomerase integrates into a defined DNA substrate increases both the frequency and the number of sites at which topoisomerase II molecules are integrated. This effect is observed at very low concentrations of these agents (Ross et al., 1984; (Tewey et al., 1984; Chen et al., 1984) (Fig. 10-5) which are well within the range of intracellular concentrations measured in studies of their uptake (for example, Allen, 1978; Glisson et al., 1986a; Pommier et al., 1985a). These agents thus block an intermediate step in the enzyme's reaction and cause it to be "trapped" upon integration in the DNA. This phenomenon is not an "inhibition" of the enzyme in a formal sense (although inhibition of enzyme activity *is* observed at higher concentrations: Tewey et al., 1984; Pommier et al., 1985a; Schneider et al., 1988); the term "poisoning" has been employed (Nelson et al., 1984).

This phenomenon explains the properties of the DNA isolated from cells exposed to these agents (Section 4.2): Integrated topoisomerase II molecules are "trapped" in the cell's DNA during their reaction and are denatured during its purification, yielding DNA fragments bearing covalently bound 5′-terminal polypeptides derived from the enzyme (Marshall et al., 1983b; Ralph & Hancock, 1985) (Fig. 10-6).

It should be noted that there is no evidence that breaks exist in the DNA *within* cells exposed to these agents; the "hidden" breaks are revealed and the DNA fragmented only during its purification, as a consequence of denaturation of integrated topoisomerase II molecules.

As discussed, the intercalating agents cannot be regarded as specifically affecting topoisomerase II reactions, because at higher concentrations their intercalative binding affects all DNA functions which require strand separation; they also inhibit topoisomerase I reactions (Pommier et al., 1987). On the other hand, while it has not been formally proved that topoisomerase II is the only intracellular target of the epipodophyllotoxins, all the available evidence supports this conclusion. Notably, certain cell lines resistant to

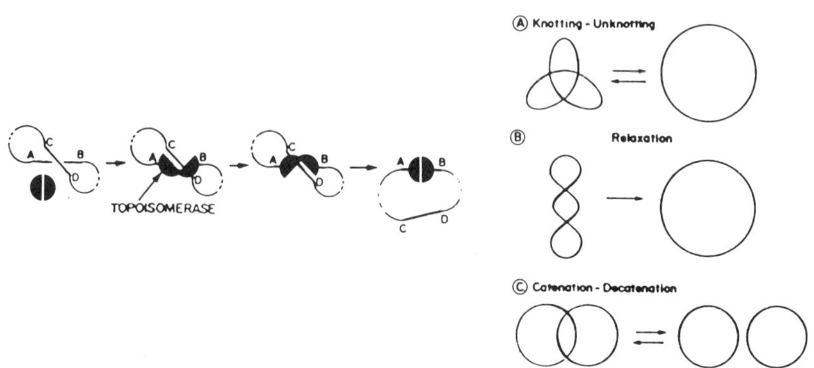

Fig. 10-4. The reaction of topoisomerase II and different conformational changes which its DNA substrate may undergo as a consequence.

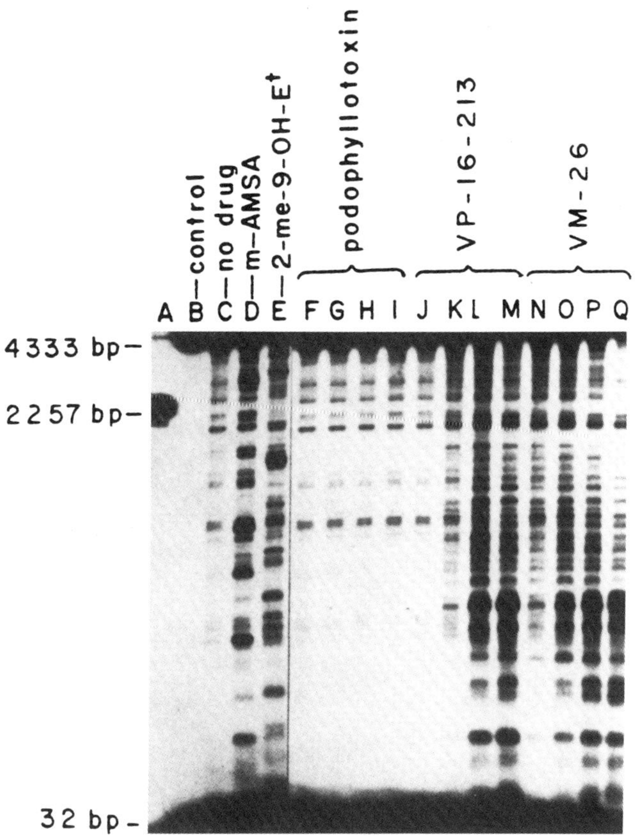

Fig. 10-5. Detection and localization of the sites of integration of topoisomerase II in a linear DNA, and of their modifications by intercalating agents and epipodophyllotoxins (Ross et al., 1984). After its integration into DNA (of plasmid pBR322, with a radioactive label at its 3′-end) the enzyme was denatured with sodium dodecylsulphate and digested proteolytically, and the resulting DNA fragments separated by electrophoresis and revealed by autoradiography. Samples (A) and (B) are the substrate DNA; samples (C) to (Q), DNA and topoisomerase II with (C) no additions; (D) *m*AMSA (0.25 μg/ml); (E) 2-methyl-9-hydroxyellipticinium acetate (0.25 μg/ml); (F) to (I) podophyllotoxin, the parent compound of VP-16 and VM-26, which has no antitumor activity; (J) to (M) VP-16 at 0.04, 0.4, 4, and 40 μg/ml, respectively; (N) to (Q) VM-26 at 0.04, 0.4, 4, and 40 μg/ml, respectively. Bands which migrate faster than the substrate DNA are fragments derived by detergent cleavage of integrated topoisomerase II molecules. Reprinted with permission of Dr. L. F. Liu and the copyright holder, The American Society of Biological Chemists, Inc., Bethesda, MD.

the epipodophyllotoxins show modified topoisomerase II function in nuclear extracts (Section 8.2), although the properties of the purified enzyme have not yet been reported.

5.3. Molecular Mechanisms of Effects on the Topoisomerase II Reaction

Intercalating agents appear to affect topoisomerase II reactions essentially specifically in growing cells when used at minimal growth-inhibitory concentrations, when they show no detectable effects on DNA replication during traverse of the S phase of the cell cycle (Section 6.1). The reason for this selectivity is not yet understood. These agents show preference for binding to certain sequences in DNA (Neidle & Sanderson, 1983; Chen et al., 1986), but this preference may not be meaningful in the situation in the cell, where the conformation of the DNA is constrained in chromatin. A plausible possibility which has not yet been examined is that they may preferentially intercalate in regions of DNA which are distorted at the enzyme's binding site.

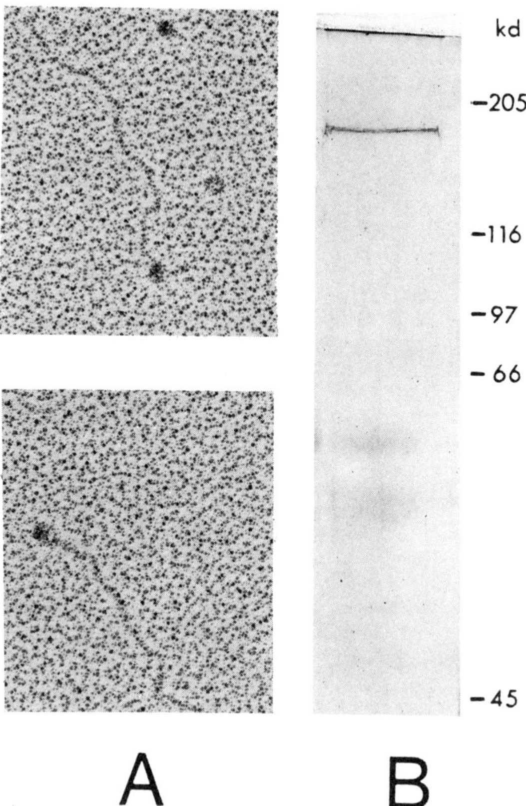

Fig. 10-6. Visualization of topoisomerase II attached to the terminus of DNA fragments from mouse cells exposed to the intercalating agent *m*AMSA. The DNA was purified using detergents but no proteolytic enzymes (Ralph & Hancock, 1985). (A) For electron microscopy, proteins bound to the DNA were visualized by indirect labeling with an electron-dense ferritin marker (bar = 100 nm). (B) Migration of the bound protein in polyacrylamide gel electrophoresis shows a molecular mass identical to that of topoisomerase II.

The epipodophyllotoxins do not bind to DNA according to current evidence (Chen et al., 1984), and it is therefore supposed that they bind directly to the enzyme or to an enzyme–DNA reaction intermediate. The manner and sites of binding have not yet been identified.

There are as yet no detailed models for the molecular events involved in the trapping of topoisomerase II by these agents. The development of such models is clearly a priority in order to understand both their action and the possible mechanisms by which modifications of the enzyme confer resistance (Section 8.2).

6. MOLECULAR BASIS OF CYTOSTATIC AND CYTOCIDAL ACTIONS

It is important to elucidate which, out of the spectrum of effects of these agents on cells growing in culture (Section 4.1), is responsible for the cytostatic and cytocidal effects of the agent and which are epiphenomena. Studies directed at this question have established correlations between the frequency of trapped topoisomerase II molecules, either in growing cells or in *in vitro* systems, and cytotoxicity (Tewey et al., 1984; Pommier et al., 1985b; Long et al., 1986; Rowe et al., 1986; Markovits et al., 1987).

Understanding of this question is also dependent on knowledge of the role of the target enzyme topoisomerase II in the growth of mammalian cells, which is currently not completely clarified.

6.1. Functions of Topoisomerase II in the Growth of Mammalian Cells

Mammalian cells contain of the order of 10^6 molecules of topoisomerase II per cell (Heck & Earnshaw, 1986). The signals which control the enzyme's activity *in vivo* have not been identified; the activity of purified topoisomerase II can be stimulated by phosphorylation (Ackerman et al., 1985) and inhibited by poly(ADP-ribosylation) (Darby et al., 1985), but the role of these modifications in controlling the enzyme's activity *in vivo* is not yet known.

During the replication of small circular DNA chromosomes such as that of SV40 virus (Richter et al., 1987; Yang et al., 1987; Snapka, 1986; Snapka et al., 1988) and of the chromosomes of yeast (DiNardo et al., 1984; Uemura & Yanagida, 1984, 1986; Uemura et al., 1987), all current evidence indicates that the only essential biological role of the topoisomerase II reaction is during the terminal period of chromosome replication and segregation. The bacterial homologue of topoisomerase II, DNA gyrase, plays a similar role in the segregation of bacterial chromosomes (Steck & Drlica, 1984).

The replication of SV40 virus DNA *in vivo* (Yang et al., 1985; Richter et al., 1987; Snapka, 1986; Snapka et al., 1988) or *in vitro* (Yang et al., 1987) represents the simplest model system, and current evidence suggests that topoisomerase II plays a role in the synthesis of the terminal DNA region as well as in the decatenation of the completed daughter DNA molecules (Richter et al., 1987; Snapka et al., 1988). The precise mechanistic analogy of these reactions in the replication of the chromosomes of mammalian cells is not yet clear. These chromosomes are formed of a series of constrained DNA loops each topologically analogous to a circular DNA molecule, but the events at the end of their replication, when they are assembled together into a continuous chromosomal DNA molecule, are not yet understood (Hancock, 1982).

This work has also established clearly that topoisomerase II is not essential during the replication of DNA, where topoisomerase I is responsible for relieving the torsional stress associated with unwinding of the parental DNA during replication.

To analyze the role of topoisomerase II in the growth of mammalian cells, we are studying the effects of agents of which this enzyme is a target on the growth of synchronized Chinese hamster ovary (CHO) cells.

These agents specifically arrest growth of essentially all the cells in the G2 phase of the cell cycle when DNA replication is virtually or completely terminated (Fig. 10-7). This phenomenon was observed in earlier studies of randomly growing cell cultures (Section 4.1). Observation of these cells in the electron microscope shows that the condensation of their chromatin to form mitotic chromosomes has not been initiated (N. Pepin, R. Pankov, and R. Hancock, unpublished observations).

The epipodophyllotoxins, even at very high concentrations, do not arrest but somewhat slow the rate of DNA synthesis during the S phase. This finding correlates with evidence that only topoisomerase I is essential, although topoisomerase II may function facultatively, during DNA replication (Uemura & Yanagida, 1984; Snapka, 1986; Richter et al., 1987; Yang et al., 1987). It may be noted that the effect of intercalating agents and of epipodophyllotoxins in "trapping" cellular topoisomerase II during its reaction not only inactivates this population of enzyme molecules, but will also lead to depletion of the cell's pool of free enzyme molecules.

The observations cited show that topoisomerase II functions are essential only during the period of mitotic chromosome formation in mammalian cells. These functions could, as in the replication of SV40 virus DNA (Snapka et al., 1988), include roles in the terminal replication of DNA and/or in a process mechanistically equivalent to the decatenation reaction in SV40 in which the continuity of each daughter chromosomal DNA molecule is reestablished. A further possibility that should perhaps not be excluded is that topoisomerase II may, like its bacterial homologue DNA gyrase, be capable under conditions which have not yet been identified of actively winding the chromatin of G2 cells into its compact conformation in mitotic chromosomes.

These reactions appear to represent the fundamental target of the epipodophyllotoxins, and of the intercalating agents at low concentrations.

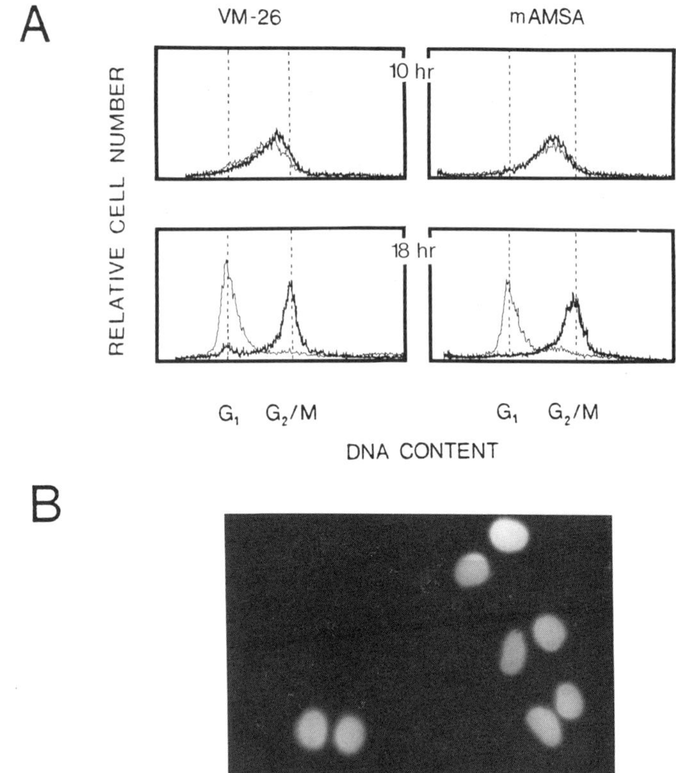

FIG. 10-7. The epipodophyllotoxin VM-26 and the intercalating agent *m*AMSA specifically arrest synchronously growing Chinese hamster ovary fibroblasts in the G2 phase of the cell cycle. (A) Flow cytometric analysis of progression through the cell cycle during synchronous growth of control cells (light trace), and with VM-26 or *m*AMSA at 0.05 μg/ml (heavy trace). (B) Staining of the arrested cells with the DNA stain Hoechst 32558 shows that they are in the G2 phase. Each pair of cells has grown from a single initial mitotic cell until G2 arrest.

The small number of cells which escape the G2 arrest form incompletely condensed or fused mitotic chromosomes (Figs. 10-8A and 10-8B). This effect is seen when the agents are present only during the G2 phase, and thus effects during the S phase do not appear to be involved. These chromosomes cannot be segregated correctly during cell division, and a nuclear membrane is usually reformed around them, producing micronucleated cells which are not viable (Fig. 10-8C).

6.2. Molecular Basis of Cytostatic and Cytocidal Actions

The foregoing observations suggest a plausible hypothesis for the mechanisms of the cytostatic and cytocidal action of these agents. In general, the majority of the cells arrested in the G2 phase appear to be capable of recovery upon their removal, and this arrest may thus be responsible for the *cytostatic* action. On the other hand, the cells which reach mitosis show severely impaired viability, because they cannot segregate their chromosomes successfully; this irreversible phenomenon may thus be responsible for the *cytocidal* action of the agents.

This model suggests that the cytocidal action of the epipodophyllotoxins, and of the intercalating agents at minimal concentrations, is due to a "suicide" process: The segregation of chromosomes at cell division is impaired, but other associated events (spindle function, cytokinesis, and nuclear membrane reformation) proceed, driving the cell irreversibly into a state incompatible with viability. This mechanism is in some ways analogous to that of the cytocidal effect of penicillin on growing bacterial cells.

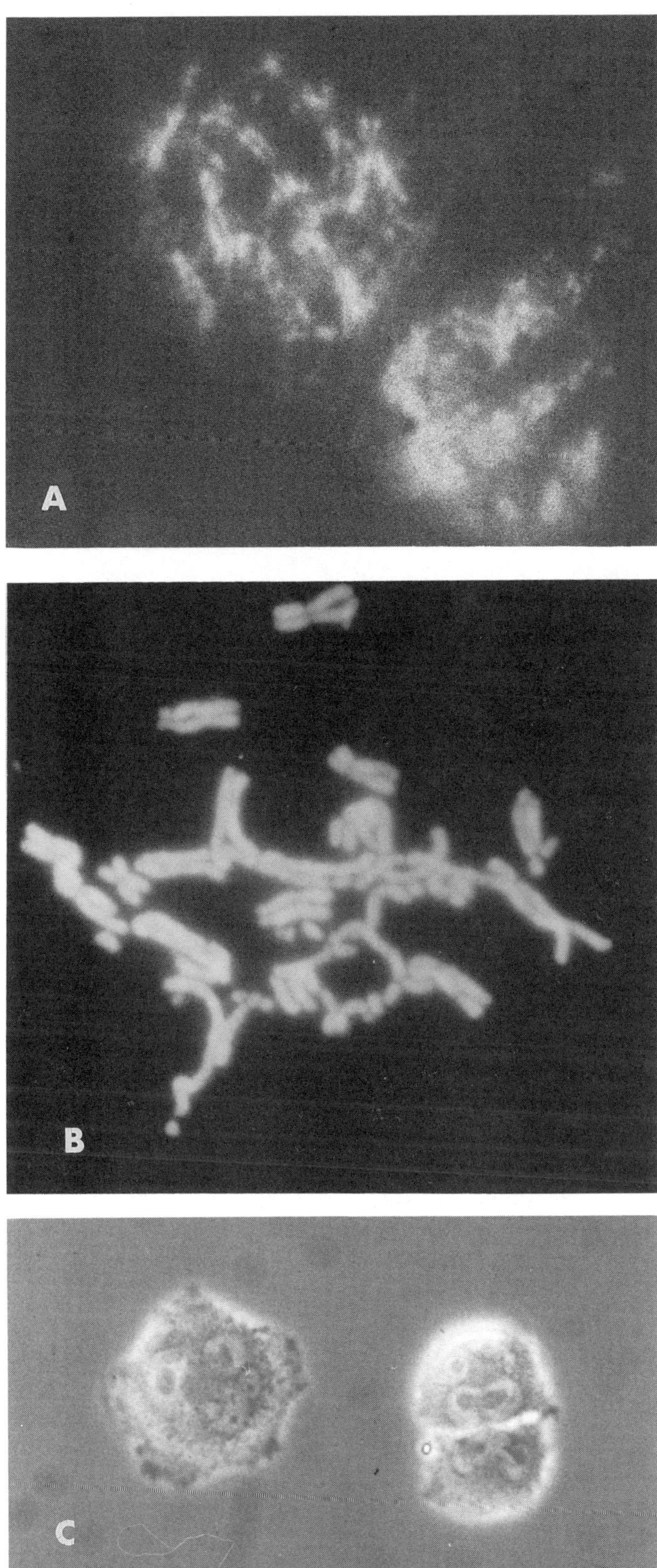

FIG. 10-8. Chromosome abnormalities in cells which reach mitosis after growth for one cell cycle with the epipodophyllotoxin VM-26 as in Fig. 10.7. (A) Incompletely condensed chromosomes; (B) representative multiradial configurations and telomeric fusion, which occur in the majority of mitotic cells; (C) micronucleated cells which are formed after aborted division of mitotic cells which contain chromosomes such as those in (B).

This model can also explain satisfactorily the resistance of noncycling cells to these agents, because these cells do not reach the G2 phase where this cytotoxic effect occurs. This phenomenon appears to be crucially important in tumor chemotherapy (Section 8.3).

7. ABNORMALITIES IN MITOTIC CHROMOSOMES: MOLECULAR MECHANISMS

7.1. Chromosome Abnormalities and Recombination

Mitotic cells from cultures exposed to intercalating agents or epipodophyllotoxins contain a large proportion of their chromosomes in multiradial configurations which result from recombination processes (Kato, 1977; Kuhn & Therman, 1982) and show a high frequency of chromosomes joined by terminal chiasmata (Fig. 10-8A). These effects are seen when the agents are present only during the G2 phase, and thus effects on DNA replication during the S phase do not appear to be involved.

Molecular interpretations of these cytological phenomena have not yet been developed. On the premise that the epipodophyllotoxins target specifically topoisomerase II (Section 5.2), these phenomena suggest that chromosomal recombination occurs when topoisomerase II function is perturbed by these agents.

Topoisomerase II from phage T4 (Ikeda, 1986) and from calf thymus (Bae et al., 1988) shows recombinational activity on DNA *in vitro*. The hypothesis has been proposed that this process results from exchange of polypeptide subunits between two juxtaposed topoisomerase II molecules integrated into DNA (Filipski, 1983). Topoisomerase II molecules integrated into DNA are more abundant in cells exposed to intercalating agents and epipodophyllotoxins, because these agents cause the enzyme to be trapped (Section 5.2), and thus the possibility of subunit exchange would be enhanced. This important hypothesis remains to be tested experimentally.

7.2. Sister Chromatid Exchanges

The agents discussed here induce sister chromatid exchange (SCE) in the chromosomes of mitotic cells (Crossen, 1979). SCE is a manifestation of DNA strand exchanges between the two daughter molecules arising from DNA replication (Kato, 1977), but the underlying molecular mechanisms are not understood, nor is it known if SCE reflects single- or double-strand exchanges. Analysis of this phenomenon is complicated by the observation that the principle of indeterminacy plays a role: The chromosomal DNA must be labeled with bromodeoxyuridine in order to detect exchanged regions by cytological methods, but recent reports show that the presence of this label in DNA in itself increases the SCE frequency (Pinkel et al., 1985; Saffhill & Ockey, 1985; Tsuji et al., 1988). Attempts to demonstrate recombined DNA strands whose formation underlies the cytological phenomenon of SCE have yielded equivocal results (Rommalaere & Miller-Faurès, 1975; Moore & Holliday, 1976; Loveday & Latt, 1981), but by using an improved protocol to detect these strands, we have confirmed that they are formed only when the template DNA strand contains bromodeoxyuridine (M. Charron and R. Hancock, unpublished results). Thus SCE may be a manifestation of a potential defect in DNA replication which only materializes as a strand exchange when the template DNA contains bromodeoxyuridine; it may not occur or be related to the effects of these agents in normal conditions of growth.

Since the epipodophyllotoxins appear to target topoisomerase II specifically, it is logical that this enzyme may be involved in SCE (Heartlein et al., 1987).

8. RESISTANCE IN CELLS AND HUMAN TUMORS

The long-term clinical success of the intercalating agents and the epipodophyllotoxins is severely limited by the emergence of resistant tumor cells, seen especially clearly in single agent trials (Table 10-2). Work on cell lines in culture reveals that resistance is a complex phenomenon which has multiple mechanisms.

8.1. Multidrug Resistance

Work with cell lines or mutants selected for resistance has revealed one well-characterized mechanism of resistance in which the intracellular concentration of several chemotherapeutic agents, including the intercalating agents and the epipodophyllotoxins, is reduced due to an active efflux process. This process is due to the functioning of a membrane protein, the P-glycoprotein, whose level is increased in resistant cells either by amplification or by an increased rate of transcription of its gene (reviewed in Ferro-Luzzi Ames, 1986; Moscow & Cowan, 1988).

The active efflux of chemotherapeutic agents promoted by this protein can be suppressed, and their cytotoxicity increased, in cultured cells by the calcium influx blockers verapamil (Tsuruo et al., 1982; Yalowich & Ross, 1985; Darkin & Ralph, 1986; Willingham et al., 1986) and amiodarone (Chauffert et al., 1987), by calmodulin inhibitors (Ganapathi & Grabowski, 1983), and by isoprenoids (Yamaguchi et al., 1986). These agents have not yet been shown to increase the clinical effectiveness of intercalating agents or epipodophyllotoxins.

Although the multidrug resistance phenotype due to this protein is frequently observed in cell lines, the resistance of many other lines in culture is *not* correlated with modifications of intracellular concentration or efflux rate (Salles et al., 1982; Glisson et al., 1986a,b; Pommier et al., 1986a; Danks et al., 1987; Mirski et al., 1987) or with presence of overexpressed P-glycoprotein mRNA (Beck et al., 1987) which are characteristic of this system (Table 10-3).

8.2. Evidence for Modified Topoisomerase II in Resistant Cell Lines

The plausible hypothesis that the target enzyme topoisomerase II may have modified properties in cell lines resistant to intercalating agents and epipodophyllotoxins, but which do not show the classical multidrug resistance phenotype, has been addressed in several recent reports (Glisson et al., 1986b; Pommier et al., 1986b).

Topoisomerase II activity in nuclear extracts from some resistant cell lines of this type shows characteristically modified properties, but the properties of the purified enzyme have not been reported. The integration of the enzyme to generate "hidden" breaks in the DNA

Table 10-3. *Uptake of Chemotherapeutic Agents and P-Glycoprotein Expression in Some Resistant Cell Lines*

Line and Origin	Factor of Resistance to		Uptake at Plateau	P-Glycoprotein Overexpression	Reference
	Intercalators	VP-16/VM-26			
Human					
Small-cell lung cancer	74 (adriamycin*)	38	–	No	Mirski et al. (1987)
HL-60 (AML)	70 (*m*AMSA*)	11	*m*AMSA normal	–	Odaimi et al. (1986)
CEM/VM1 (leukemia)	80 (adriamycin)	54*	–	No	Beck et al. (1987)
Hamster					
Ovary	5 (adriamycin)	5*	*m*AMSA normal	–	Glisson et al. (1986a)
Ovary	+	20*	VP-16 normal daunomycin 50%	–	Glisson et al. (1986b)
Lung	10 (9-OH ellipticine*)	8	*m*AMSA normal 9-OH ellipticine normal	–	Salles et al. (1982)
Mouse					
Ehrlich	+	6*	VP-16 20%	–	Seeber et al. (1982)

*Agent used for selection of the resistant line.

substrate is resistant to stimulation by VP-16 (Glisson et al., 1986b) or by *m*AMSA (Pommier et al., 1986b), which is characteristic of the enzyme in extracts of sensitive cells and of the purified enzyme (Section 5).

A more detailed study of a cell line resistant to *m*AMSA, derived from P388 leukemia cells, shows the presence of two forms of topoisomerase II which can be identified and distinguished by specific antibodies; their relative levels differ from those in the parent cell line and show a correlation with sensitivity to the cytotoxic action of *m*AMSA (Drake et al., 1987).

8.3. Resistance in Human Tumors

Experimental work on the molecular mechanisms responsible for resistance of human tumors to these agents is in an early stage. Cells expressing the multidrug resistance phenotype have been detected in human tumors, using monoclonal antibodies specific for the gene product, the P-glycoprotein (Ma et al., 1987), or using DNA probes to detect the messenger RNA for this protein (Fojo et al., 1987a). The presence of this protein in some normal tissues (Fojo et al., 1987b) could lead to intrinsic resistance of tumors derived from these tissues. However, some cell lines established from resistant tumors do *not* show a decreased drug accumulation characteristic of the P-glycoprotein system (Fojo et al., 1985).

The observations cited earlier on resistance in cell lines and mutants suggest that the emergence of cells whose topoisomerase II has modified properties is a plausible mechanism for the development of resistance in human tumors. No work has yet been published to address this important question. A major objective for the future is therefore to examine the molecular mechanisms responsible for resistance in human tumors, and especially the possibility that their cells have acquired variant, resistant forms of topoisomerase II.

8.4. Prediction of Tumor Response

Understanding of the molecular mechanisms responsible for resistance should allow predictive tests of tumor sensitivity to be applied to tissue or cells in biopsies.

Peripheral blast cells from patients with acute myelogenous leukemia and exposed to adriamycin in culture show "hidden" breaks in their DNA derived from sites of integrated topoisomerase II, and a higher frequency of these breaks shows some correlation with a successful response of the patient to a chemotherapy protocol containing adriamycin (Schwartz, 1983). This type of predictive test does not appear to have found general application.

Other types of predictive test could be imagined if modification of topoisomerase II is established as a mechanism of resistance in human tumors. Antibodies which can discriminate the modified from the normal enzyme could then provide probes for prediction of response to chemotherapeutic agents. Further, if future studies show that the epipodophyllotoxins bind directly to topoisomerase II and if this binding is modified or suppressed in resistant variants of the enzyme, the determination of epipodophyllotoxin binding in extracts of tumor cells could predict their sensitivity.

8.5. Resistance in Solid Tumors

A further important limitation to the chemotherapeutic success of these agents is that cells which are not traversing the cell cycle are much more resistant (Chow & Ross, 1987; Finally et al., 1987; Zwelling et al., 1987; Schneider et al., 1988); solid tumors contain a central mass of nondividing cells. In nongrowing (contact inhibited) cells, stimulation by *m*AMSA or VP-16 of the trapping of topoisomerase II in DNA is reduced compared with growing cells (Schneider et al., 1988), as it is in resistant cell lines (Section 8).

This resistance of noncycling or stationary phase cells would appear to be a logical consequence of the selective action of these agents on dividing cells (Section 6).

New derivatives of amsacrine designed to be more active against solid tumors are being developed and are undergoing clinical trials (Traganos et al., 1987; Baguley & Finlay, 1988).

9. FUTURE PERSPECTIVES

The observations discussed here establish that the crucial requirement for topoisomerase II function in chromosome formation and segregation in growing mammalian cells makes it potentially a very suitable and sensitive target for antitumor agents. How can this situation be exploited to provide new chemotherapeutic agents and to overcome the problem of resistance?

The property of topoisomerase II which allows it to cleave and religate an internucleotide linkage in double-stranded DNA is an essentially unique enzymic reaction in mammalian cells (possibly shared with the uncharacterized enzymes involved in recombination). Understanding of its reaction could therefore allow the design of new mechanism based on suicide inhibitors. Such understanding is not yet available, but a preliminary model has been proposed of the mechanism of an enzyme which shares features of topoisomerase II and reversibly cleaves and religates the DNA of phage $\phi X174$ during its replication; the model proposes how adjacent tyrosine-OH groups of the enzyme serve as accepter and donor of the 5′-termini of the DNA (van Mansfeld et al., 1986).

It is apparent from the present discussion that many important and fascinating aspects of the action of these agents remain to be elucidated. It appears reasonable that detailed understanding of the molecular details of topoisomerase II and of its reaction, of the manner in which these agents interfere with the reaction, and of possible modifications of the target enzyme in resistant human tumors, will contribute to the rational design of new chemotherapeutic agents.

Acknowledgments—Our work is supported by Medical Research Council of Canada Grant MA-9589. M. Charron is a Scholar of the Fonds de la Recherche en Santé du Québec and N. Pepin a Scholar of the FCAR (Québec). We thank Pierre Paquin and Guy Langlois for photographic work, and Elisabeth Lemay for her help in preparing this review. R.H. is especially grateful to Ray Ralph for his stimulating introduction to this field.

REFERENCES

Ackerman, P., Glover, C. V. C., and Osheroff, N. (1985) Phosphorylation of DNA topoisomerase II by casein kinase: Modulation of topoisomerase II activity *in vitro*. *Proc. Natl. Acad. Sci. USA* **82**: 3164–3168.

Allen, L. M. (1978) Comparison of uptake and binding of two epipodophyllotoxin glucopyranosides, 4′-demethyl epipodophyllotoxin thenylidene-beta-D-glucoside and 4′-demethyl epipodophyllotoxin ethylidene-β-D-glucoside, in the L1210 leukemia cell. *Cancer Res.* 38: 2549–2554.

Amadori, S., Ceci, A., Comelli, A., Madon, E., Masera, G., Nespoli, L., Paolucci, G., Zanesco, L., Covelli, A., and Mandelli, F. (1987) Treatment of acute myelogenous leukemia in children: Results of the Italian cooperative study AIEOP/LAM 8204. *J. Clin. Oncol.* **5**: 1356–1363.

Arcamone, F. (1981) *Doxorubicin, anticancer antibiotics.* New York: Academic Press.

Bae, Y. S., Kawasaki, I., Ikeda, H., and Liu, L. F. (1988) Illegitimate recombination mediated by calf thymus DNA topoisomerase II *in vitro*. *Proc. Natl. Acad. Sci. USA* **85**: 2076–2080.

Baguley, B. C., and Finlay, G. J. (1988) Derivatives of amsacrine: Determinants required for high activity against Lewis lung carcinoma. *J. Natl. Cancer Inst.* **80**: 195–199.

Beck, W. T., Cirtain, M. C., Danks, M. K., Felsted, R. L., Safa, A. R., Wolverton, J. S., Suttle, D. P., and Trent, J. M. (1987) Pharmacological, molecular, and cytogenetic analysis of "atypical" multidrug-resistant human leukemic cells. *Cancer Res.* **47**: 5455–5460.

Bonadonna, G. (1985) Chemotherapy of malignant lymphomas. *Semin. Oncol.* **XII**: 1–14.

Brown, J. R. (1983) New natural, semisynthetic, and synthetic anthracycline derivatives. In *Molecular aspects of anti-cancer drug action*, S. Neidle and M. J. Waring, eds., pp. 57–92. Weinheim: Verlag Chemie.

Burr-Furlong, N., Sato, J., Brown, T., Chavez, F., and Hurlbert, R. B. (1978) Induction of limited DNA damage by the antitumor agent Cain's acridine. *Cancer Res.* **38**: 1329–1335.

Cabanillas, F., Legha, S. S., Bodey, G. P., and Freireich, E. J. (1981) Initial experience with AMSA as single agent treatment against malignant lymphoproliferative disorders. *Blood* **57**: 614–616.

Chauffert, B., Rey, D., Coudert, B., Dumas, M., and Martin, F. (1987) Amiodarone is more efficient than verapamil in reversing resistance to anthracyclines in tumor cells. *Br. J. Cancer* **56**: 109–122.

Chen, G. L., Yang, L., Rowe, T. C., Halligan, B. D., Tewey, K. M., and Liu L. F. (1984) Nonintercalative antitumor drugs interfere with the breakage-reunion reaction of mammalian DNA topoisomerase II. *J. Biol. Chem.* **259**: 13560–13566.

Chen, K. S., Gresh, N., and Pullman, B. (1986) A theoretical investigation on the sequence selective binding of adriamycin to double-stranded polynucleotides. *Nucleic Acids Res.* **14**: 2251–2267.
Chow, K.-C., and Ross, W. E. (1987) Topoisomerase-specific drug sensitivty in relation to cell cycle progression. *Mol. Cell. Biol.* **7**: 3119–3123.
Crossen, P. E. (1979) The effect of acridine compounds on sister-chromatid exchange formation in cultured human lymphocytes. *Mutat. Res.* **68**: 295–299.
Danks, M. K., Yalowich, J. C., and Beck, W. T. (1987) Atypical multiple drug resistance in a human leukemic cell line selected for resistance to teniposide (VM-26). *Cancer Res.* **47**: 1297–1301.
Darby, M. K., Schmitt, B., Jongstra-Bilen, J., and Vosberg, H. P. (1985) Inhibition of calf thymus type II DNA topoisomerase by poly(ADP-ribosylation). *EMBO J.* **4**: 2129–2134.
Darkin, S., and Ralph, R. K. (1986) Potentiation of 4′-[(9-acridinyl)amino]methane sulphon-m-anisidide) action by verapamil. *Cancer Lett.* **30**: 25–33.
Deaven, L. L., Oka, M. S., and Tobey, R. A. (1978) Cell cycle specific chromosome damage following treatment of Chinese hamster cells with 4′-[(9-acridinyl)-amino] methansulphon-m-anisidide-HCl. *J. Natl. Cancer Ins.* **60**: 1155–1161.
Denny, W. A., Baguley, B. C., Cain, B. F., and Waring, M. J. (1983) Antitumor acridines. In *Molecular aspects of anti-cancer drug action*, S. Neidle and M. J. Waring, eds., pp. 1–34. Weinheim: Verlag Chemie.
DiNardo, S., Voelkel, K., and Sternglanz, R. (1984) DNA topoisomerase II mutant of *Saccharomyces cerevisiae*: Topoisomerase II is required for segregation of daughter molecules at the termination of DNA replication. *Proc. Natl. Acad. Sci. USA* **81**: 2616–2620.
Doyle, T. W. (1984) The chemistry of etoposide. In *Etoposide (VP-16). Current status and new developments*, B. F. Issell, F. M. Muggia, and S. K. Carter, eds., pp. 15–32. New York: Academic Press.
Drake, F. H., Zimmerman, J. P., McCabe, F. L., Bartus, H. F., Per, S. R., Sullivan, D. M., Ross, W. E., Mattern, M. R., Johnson, R. K., and Crooke, S. T. (1987) Purification of topoisomerase II from amsacrine-resistant P388 leukemia cells. Evidence for two forms of the enzyme. *J. Biol. Chem.* **262**: 16739–16747.
Ferro-Luzzi Ames, G. (1986) The basis of multidrug resistance in mammalian cells: Homology with bacterial transport. *Cell* **47**: 322–324.
Filipski, J. (1983) Competitive inhibition of nicking-closing enzymes may explain some biological effects of DNA intercalators. *FEBS Lett.* **159**: 6–12.
Finlay, G. J., Wilson, W. R., and Baguley, B. C. (1987) Cytokinetic factors in drug resistance of Lewis lung carcinoma: Comparison of cells freshly isolated from tumors with cells from exponential and plateau-phase cultures. *Br. J. Cancer* **56**: 755–762.
Fojo, A. T., Shen, D.-W., Mickley, L. A., Pastan, I., and Gottesman, M. M. (1987a) Intrinsic drug resistance in human kidney cancer is associated with expression of a human multidrug-resistance gene. *J. Clin. Oncol.* **5**: 1922–1927.
Fojo, A. T., Ueda, K., Slamon, D. J., Poplack, D. G., Gottesman, M. M., and Pastan, I. (1987b) Expression of a multidrug-resistance gene in human tumors and tissues. *Proc. Natl. Acad. Sci. USA* **84**: 265–269.
Fojo, A., Akiyama, S., Gottesman, M. M., and Pastan, I. (1985) Reduced drug accumulation in multiple drug-resistant human KB carcinoma cell lines. *Cancer Res.* **45**: 3002–3007.
Ganapathi, R., and Grabowski, D. (1983) Enhancement of sensitivity to adriamycin in resistant P388 leukemia by the calmodulin inhibitor trifluoperazine. *Cancer Res.* **43**: 3696–3699.
Glisson, B., Gupta, R., Hodges, P., and Ross, W. (1986a) Cross-resistance to intercalating agents in an epipodophyllotoxin-resistant Chinese hamster ovary cell line: Evidence for a common intracellular target. *Cancer Res.* **46**: 1939–1942.
Glisson, B., Gupta, R., Smallwood-Kentro, S., and Ross, W. (1986b) Characterization of acquired epipodophyllotoxin resistance in a Chinese hamster ovary cell line: Loss of drug-stimulated DNA cleavage activtiy. *Cancer Res.* **46**: 1934–1938.
Grieder, A., Maurer, R., and Stähelin, H. (1974) Effect of an epipodophyllotoxin derivative (VP 16-213) on macromolecular synthesis and mitosis in mastocytoma cells in vitro. *Cancer Res.* **34**: 1788–1793.
Hall, D., Swann, D. A., and Waters, T. N. (1974) Crystal and molecular structure of 4′-(acridin-9-ylamino)methane-sulphonanilide hydrochloride, a compound showing antileukemic activity. *J. Chem. Soc. Perkins* **II**: 1334–1337.
Hancock, R. (1982) Topological organisation of interphase DNA: The nuclear matrix and other skeletal structures. *Biol. Cell* **46**: 105–122.
Heartlein, M. W., Tsuji, H., and Latt, S. A. (1987) 5-bromodeoxyuridine-dependent increase in sister chromatid exchange in Bloom's syndrome is associated with reduction in topoisomerase II activity. *Exp. Cell Res.* **169**: 245–254.
Heck, M. M. S., and Earnshaw, W. C. (1986) Topoisomerase II: A specific marker for cell proliferation. *J. Cell Biol.* **103**: 2569–2581.
Huang, C. C., Hou, Y., and Wang, J. J. (1973) Effects of a new antitumor agent, epipodophyllotoxin, on growth and chromosomes in human hematopoietic cell lines. *Cancer Res.* **33**: 3123–3129.
Ikeda, H. (1986) Bacteriophage T4 DNA topoisomerase mediates illegitimate recombination *in vitro. Proc. Natl. Acad. Sci. USA* **83**: 922–926.
Issell, B. F., Muggia, F. M., and Carter, S. K. (eds.) (1984) *Etoposide (VP-16). Current status and new developments.* New York: Academic Press.
Kalwinsky, D. K., Look, A. T., Ducore, J., and Fridland, A. (1983) Effects of the epipodophyllotoxin VP-16-213 on cell cycle traverse, DNA synthesis, and DNA strand size in cultures of human leukemic lymphocytes. *Cancer Res.* **43**: 1592–1597.
Kantarjian, H. M., Keating, M. J., Walters, R. S., Estey, E. H., McCredie, K. B., Smith, T. L., Dalton, W. T., Cork, A., Trujillo, J. M., and Freireich, E. J. (1986) Acute promyelocytic leukemia. *Am. J. Med.* **80**: 789–797.
Kato, H. (1977) Spontaneous and induced sister chromatid exchanges as revealed by the BrdU labeling method. *Int. Rev. Cytol.* **49**: 55–97.

Keating, M. J., Gehan, E. A., Smith, T. L., Estey, E. H., Walters, R. S., Kantarjian, H. M., McCredie, K. B., and Freireich, E. J. (1987) A strategy for evaluation of new treatments in untreated patients: Application to a clinical trial of AMSA for acute leukemia. *J. Clin. Oncol.* **5**: 710–721.

Keating, M. J., Smith, T. L., McCredie, K. B., Bodey, G. P., Hersh, E. M., Gutterman, J. U., Gehan, E., and Freireich, E. J. (1981) A four-year experience wth anthracycline, cytosine arabinoside, vincristine, and prednisone combination therapy in 325 adults with acute leukemia. *Cancer* **47**: 2779–2788.

Krishan, A., Paika, K., and Frei, E. III. (1975) Cytofluorometric studies on the action of podophyllotoxin and epipodophyllotoxins (VM-26, VP-16-213) on the cell cycle traverse of human lymphoblasts. *J. Cell Biol.* **66**: 521–530.

Kuhn, E. M., and Therman, E. (1982) Origin of symmetrical triradial chromosomes in human cells. *Chromosoma (Berl).* **86**: 673–681.

Liu, L. F., Rowe, T. C., Yang, L., Tewey, K. M., and Chen, G. L. (1983) Cleavage of DNA by mammalian DNA topoisomerase II. *J. Biol. Chem.* **258**: 15365–15370.

Long, B. H., Musial, S. T., and Brattain, M. G. (1986) DNA breakage in human lung carcinoma cells and nuclei that are naturally sensitive or resistant to etoposide and teniposide. *Cancer Res.* **46**: 3809–3916.

Loveday, K. S., and Latt, S. A. (1981) A high buoyant density fraction in mammalian DNA. Characterization and impact on the detection of heteroduplex DNA. *Exp. Cell Res.* **136**: 177–187.

Ma, D. D. F., Davey, R. A., Harman, D. H., Isbister, J. P., Scurr, R. D., Mackertich, S. M., Dowden, G., and Bell, D. R. (1987) Detection of a multidrug resistant phenotype in acute non-lymphoblastic leukaemia. *Lancet* 135–137.

Markovits, J., Pommier, Y., Kerrigan, D., Covey, J. M., Tilchen, E. J., and Kohn, K. W. (1987) Topoisomerase II-mediated DNA breaks and cytotoxicity in relation to cell proliferation and the cell cycle in NIH 3T3 fibroblasts and L1210 leukemia cells. *Cancer Res.* **47**: 2050–2055.

Marshall, B., and Ralph, R. K. (1984) The mechanism of action of *m*AMSA. *Adv. Cancer Res.* **44**: 267–294.

Marshall, B., Darkin, S., and Ralph, R. K. (1983a) Evidence that *m*AMSA induces topoisomerase action. *FEBS Lett.* **161**: 75–78.

Marshall, B., Ralph, R. K., and Hancock, R. (1983b) Blocked 5′-termini in the fragments of chromosomal DNA produced in cells exposed to the antitumor drug 4′-[(9-acridinyl)-amino] methansulphon-m-anisidide (*m*AMSA). *Nucl. Acid. Res.* **11**: 4251–4256.

Matsui, Y., Oshima, S., Kado, M., Nakayama, M., Shimokata, K., Sakai, S., Ito, F., Chikata, E., Hara, K., Kanda, T., Shima, K., Takenaka, S., Hokama, S., and Genga, K. (1987) Phase II study of oral VP-16-213 in small cell lung cancer. *Cancer* **60**: 2882–2885.

McElwain, T. J., and Selby, P. (1984) Etoposide in combination for treatment of Hodgkin's disease. In *Etoposide (VP-16). Current status and new developments*, B. F. Issell, F. M. Muggia, and S. K. Carter, eds., pp. 293–299. New York: Academic Press.

Mirski, S. E. L., Gerlach, J. H., and Cole, S. P. C. (1987) Multidrug resistance in a human small cell lung cancer cell line selected in adriamycin. *Cancer Res.* **47**: 2594–2598.

Miser, J. S., Kinsella, T. J., Triche, T. J., Tsokos, M., Jarosinski, P., Forquer, R., Wesley, R., and Margrath, I. (1987) Ifosfamide with mesna uroprotection and etoposide: An effective regimen in the treatment of recurrent sarcomas and other tumors of children and young adults. *J. Clin. Oncol.* **5**: 1191–1198.

Misra, N. C., and Roberts, D. (1975) Inhibition by 4′-demethyl-epipodophyllotoxin 9-(4,6-O-2-thenylidene-beta-D-glucopyranoside) of human lymphoblast cultures in G2 phase of the cell cycle. *Cancer Res.* **35**: 99–105.

Moore, P. D., and Holliday, R. (1976) Evidence for the formation of hybrid DNA during mitotic recombination in Chinese hamster cells. *Cell* **8**: 573–579.

Moscow, J. A., and Cowan, K. H. (1988) Multidrug resistance. *J. Natl. Cancer Inst.* **80**: 14–20.

Neidle, S., and Sanderson, M. R. (1983) The interactions of daunomycin and adriamycin with nucleic acids. In *Molecular aspects of anti-cancer drug action*, S. Neidle and M. J. Waring, eds., pp. 35–55. Weinheim: Verlag Chemie.

Neidle, S., and Waring, M. J. (eds.) (1983) *Molecular aspects of anti-cancer drug action.* Weinheim: Verlag Chemie.

Nelson, E. M., Tewey, K. M., and Liu, L. F. (1984) Mechanism of antitumor drug action: Poisoning of mammalian DNA topoisomerase II on DNA by 4′-[(9-acridinyl)amino] methanesulfon-m-anisidide. *Proc. Natl. Acad. Sci. USA* **81**: 1361–1365.

Odaimi, M., Andersson, B. S., McCredie, K. B., and Beran, M. (1986) Drug sensitivity and cross-resistance of the 4′-[(9-acridinyl)amino]methansulfon-m-anisidide–resistant subline of HL-60 human leukemia. *Cancer Res.* **46**: 3330–3333.

Pinkel, D., Thompson, L. H., Gray, J. W., and Vanderlaan, M. (1985) Measurement of sister chromatid exchanges at very low bromodeoxyuridine substitution levels using a monoclonal antibody in Chinese hamster cells. *Cancer Res.* **45**: 5795–5798.

Pommier, Y., Covey, J. M., Kerrigan, D., Markovits, J., and Pham, R. (1987) DNA unwinding and inhibition of mouse leukemia L1210 DNA topoisomerase I by intercalators. *Nucl. Acid. Res.* **15**: 6713–6731.

Pommier, Y., Kerrigan, D., Schwartz, R. E., Swack, J. A., and McCurdy, A. (1986a) Altered DNA topoisomerase II activity in Chinese hamster cells resistant to topoisomerase II inhibitors. *Cancer Res.* **46**: 3075–3081.

Pommier, Y., Schwartz, R. E., Zwelling, L. A., Kerrigan, D., Mattern, M. R., Charcosset, J. Y., Jacquemin-Sablon, A., and Kohn, K. W. (1986b) Reduced formation of protein-associated DNA strand breaks in Chinese hamster cells resistant to topoisomerase II inhibitors. *Cancer Res.* **46**: 611–616.

Pommier, Y., Minford, J. K., Schwartz, R. E., Zwelling, L. A., and Kohn, K. W. (1985a) Effects of the DNA intercalators 4′(9-acridinylamino)methansulfon-m-anisidide and 2-methyl-9-hydroxyellipticinium on topoisomerase II mediated DNA strand cleavage and strand passage. *Biochemistry* **24**: 6410–6416.

Pommier, Y., Zwelling, L. A., Kao-Shan, C., Whang-Peng, J., and Bradley, M. O. (1985b). Correlations between intercalator-induced DNA strand breaks and sister chromatid exchanges, mutations, and cytotoxicity in Chinese hamster cells. *Cancer Res.* **45**: 3143–3149.

Potmesil, M., and Ross, W. E. (eds.) (1987) First Conference on DNA Topoisomerases in Cancer Chemotherapy. *NCI Monograph* **4**: 1–149.

Quigley, G. J., Wang, A. H. J., Ughetto, G., van der Marel, G., van Boom, J. H., and Rich, A. (1980) Molecular structure of an anticancer drug-DNA complex: Daunomycin plus d(CpGpTpApCpG). *Proc. Natl. Acad. Sci. USA* **77**: 7204–7208.

Ralph, R. K. (1980) On the mechanism of action of 4′-[(9-acridinyl)-amino] methansulphon-m-anisidide. *Eur. J. Cancer.* **16**: 595–600.

Ralph, R. K., and Hancock, R. (1985) Chromosomal DNA fragments from mouse cells exposed to an intercalating agent contain a 175-kdalton terminal polypeptide. *Can. J. Biochem. Cell. Biol.* **63**: 780–783.

Richter, A., Strausfeld, U., and Knippers, R. (1987) Effects of VM26 (teniposide), a specific inhibitor of type II DNA topoisomerase, on SV40 DNA replication *in vivo*. *Nucl. Acid. Res.* **15**: 3455–3468.

Rommalaere, J., and Miller-Faurès, A. (1975) Detection by density equilibrium centrifugation of recombinant-like DNA molecules in somatic mammalian cells. *J. Mol. Biol.* **98**: 195–218.

Ross, W., Rowe, T., Glisson, B., Yalowich, J., and Liu, L. (1984) Role of topoisomerase II in mediating epipodophyllotoxin-induced DNA cleavage. *Cancer Res.* **44**: 5857–5860.

Ross, W. E., and Bradley, M. O. (1981) DNA double-strand breaks in mammalian cells after exposure to intercalating agents. *Biochim. Biophys. Acta* **654**: 129–134.

Rowe, T. C., Chen, G. L., Hsiang, Y.-H., and Liu, L. F. (1986) DNA damage by antitumor acridines mediated by mammalian DNA topoisomerase II. *Cancer Res.* **46**: 2021–2026.

Saffhill, R., and Ockey, C. H. (1985) Strand breaks arising from the repair of the 5-bromodeoxyuridine-substituted template and methyl methanesulphonate-induced lesions can explain the formation of sister chromatid exchanges. *Chromosoma (Berl)* **92**: 218–224.

Salles, B., Charcosset, J.-Y., and Jacquemin-Sablon, A. (1982) Isolation and properties of Chinese hamster lung cells resistant to ellipticine derivatives. *Cancer Treat. Rep.* **66**: 327–338.

Sander, M., and Hsieh, T. (1983) Double-strand DNA cleavage by type II topoisomerase from *Drosophila melanogaster*. *J. Biol. Chem.* **258**: 8421–8428.

Schneider, E., Darkin, S. J., Robbie, M. A., Wilson, W. R., and Ralph, R. K. (1988) Mechanism of resistance of non-cycling mammalian cells to 4′-[(9-acridinyl)-amino]methansulphon-m-anisidide: Role of DNA topoisomerase II in log- and plateau-phase CHO cells. *Biochim. Biophys. Acta* **949**: 264–272.

Schwartz, H. S. (1983) Mechanisms of selective toxicity of adriamycin, daunomycin, and related anthracyclines. In *Molecular aspects of anti-cancer drug action*, S. Neidle and M. J. Waring, eds., pp. 93–125. Weinheim: Verlag Chemie.

Seeber, S., Osieka, R., Schmidt, C. G., Achterrath, W., and Crooke, S. T. (1982) *In vivo* resistance toward anthracyclines, etoposide, and cis-diamminedichloroplatinum (II). *Cancer Res.* **42**: 4719–4725.

Snapka, R. M. (1986) Topoisomerase inhibitors can selectively interfere with different stages of simian virus 40 DNA replication. *Mol. Cell. Biol.* **6**: 4221-4227.

Snapka, R. M., Powelson, M. A., and Strayer, J. M. (1988) Swiveling and decatenation of replicating simian virus 40 genomes *in vivo*. *Mol. Cell. Biol.* **8**: 515–521.

Steck, T. R., and Drlica, K. (1984) Bacterial chromosome segregation: Evidence for DNA gyrase involvement in decatenation. *Cell* **36**: 1081–1088.

Tewey, K. M., Chen, G. L., Nelson, E. M., and Liu, L. F. (1984) Intercalative antitumor drugs interfere with the breakage-reunion reaction of mammalian DNA topoisomerase II. *J. Biol. Chem.* **259**: 9182–9187.

Tobey, R. A., Deaven, L. L., and Oka, M. S. (1978) Kinetic response of cultured Chinese hamster cells to treatment with 4′-[(9-acridinyl)-amino] methanesulphon-m-anisidide-HCl. *J. Natl. Cancer Ins.* **60**: 1147–1152.

Traganos, F., Bueti, C., Darzynkiewicz, Z., and Melamed, M. R. (1987) Effects of a new amsacrine derivative, N-5-dimethyl-9-(2-methoxy-4-methylsulfonylamino)phenylamino-4-acridinecarboxamide, on cultured mammalian cells. *Cancer Res.* **47**: 424–432.

Tsuji, H., Heartlein, M. W., and Latt, S. A. (1988) Disparate effects of 5-bromodeoxyuridine on sister-chromatid exchanges and chromosomal aberrations in Bloom syndrome fibroblasts. *Mutat. Res.* **198**: 241–253.

Tsuruo, T., Iida, H., and Tsukagoshi, S. Y. (1982) Increased accumulation of vincristine and adriamycin in drug-resistant P388 tumor cells following incubation with calcium antagonists and calmodulin inhibitors. *Cancer Res.* **42**: 4730–4733.

Uemura, T., and Yanagida, M. (1984) Isolation of type I and II DNA topoisomerase mutants from fission yeast: Single and double mutants show different phenotypes in cell growth and chromatin organization. *EMBO J.* **3**: 1737–1744.

Uemura, T., and Yanagida, M. (1986) Mitotic spindle pulls but fails to separate chromosomes in type II DNA topoisomerase mutants: Uncoordinated mitosis. *EMBO J.* **5**: 1003–1010.

Uemura, T., Ohkura, H., Adachi, Y., Morino, K., Shiozaki, K., and Yanagida, M. (1987) DNA topoisomerase II is required for condensation and separation of mitotic chromosomes in *S. pombe*. *Cell* **50**: 917–925.

van Mansfeld, A. D. M., van Teeffelen, H. A. A. M., Baas, P. D., and Jansz, H. S. (1986) Two juxtaposed tyrosyl-OH groups participate in ϕX174 gene A protein-catalyzed cleavage and ligation of DNA. *Nucl. Acid Res.* **14**: 4229-4238.

Vosberg, H.-P. (1985) DNA topoisomerases: Enzymes that control DNA conformation. *Curr. Top. Microbiol. Immunol.* **114**: 19–102.

Wang, J. C. (1985) DNA topoisomerases. *Ann. Rev. Biochem.* **54**: 665–697.

Willingham, M. C., Cornwell, M. M., Cardarelli, C. O., Gottesman, M. M., and Pastan, I. (1986) Single cell analysis of daunomycin uptake and efflux in multidrug-resistant and -sensitive KB cells: Effects of verapamil and other drugs. *Cancer Res.* **46**: 5941–5946.

Wong, L. C., Choo, Y. C., and Ma, H. K. (1986) Primary oral etoposide therapy in gestational trophoblastic disease. *Cancer* **58**: 14–17.

Yalowich, J. C., and Ross, W. E. (1985) Verapamil-induced augmentation of etoposide accumulation in L1210 cells *in vitro*. *Cancer Res.* **45**: 1651–1656.

Yamaguchi, T., Nakagawa, M., Shiraishi, N., Yoshida, T., Kiyosue, T., Arita, M., Akiyama, S., and Kuwano, M. (1986) Overcoming drug resistance in cancer cells with synthetic isoprenoids. *J. Natl. Cancer Inst.* **75**: 947–953.

Yang, L., Rowe, T. C., and Liu, L. F. (1985) Identification of DNA topoisomerase II as an intracellular target of antitumor epipodophyllotoxins in simian virus 40–infected monkey cells. *Cancer Res.* **45**: 5872–5876.

Yang, L., Wold, M. S., Li, J. J., Kelly, T. J., and Liu, L. F. (1987) Roles of DNA topoisomerases in simian virus 40 DNA replication *in vitro. Proc. Natl. Acad. Sci. USA* **84**: 950–954.

Young, R. C., Fisher, R. I., Longo, D. L., Bender, R. A., and Devita, V. Y. (1984) Activity of the epipodophyllotoxin VP-16 in diffuse large-cell lymphomas. In *Etoposide (VP-16). Current status and new developments*, B. F. Issell, F. M. Muggia, and S. K. Carter, eds., pp. 301–311. New York: Academic Press.

Zwelling, L. A., Michaels, S., Erickson, L. C., Ungerleider, R. S., Nichols, M., and Kohn, K. W. (1981) Protein-associated DNA strand breaks in L1210 cells treated with the intercalating agents *m*AMSA and adriamycin. *Biochemistry* **20**: 6553–6563.

Zwelling, L. A., Estey, E., Silberman, L., Doyle, S., and Hittelman, W. (1987) Effect of cell proliferation and chromatin conformation on intercalator-induced, protein-associated DNA cleavage in human brain tumor cells and human fibroblasts. *Cancer Res.* **47**: 251–257.

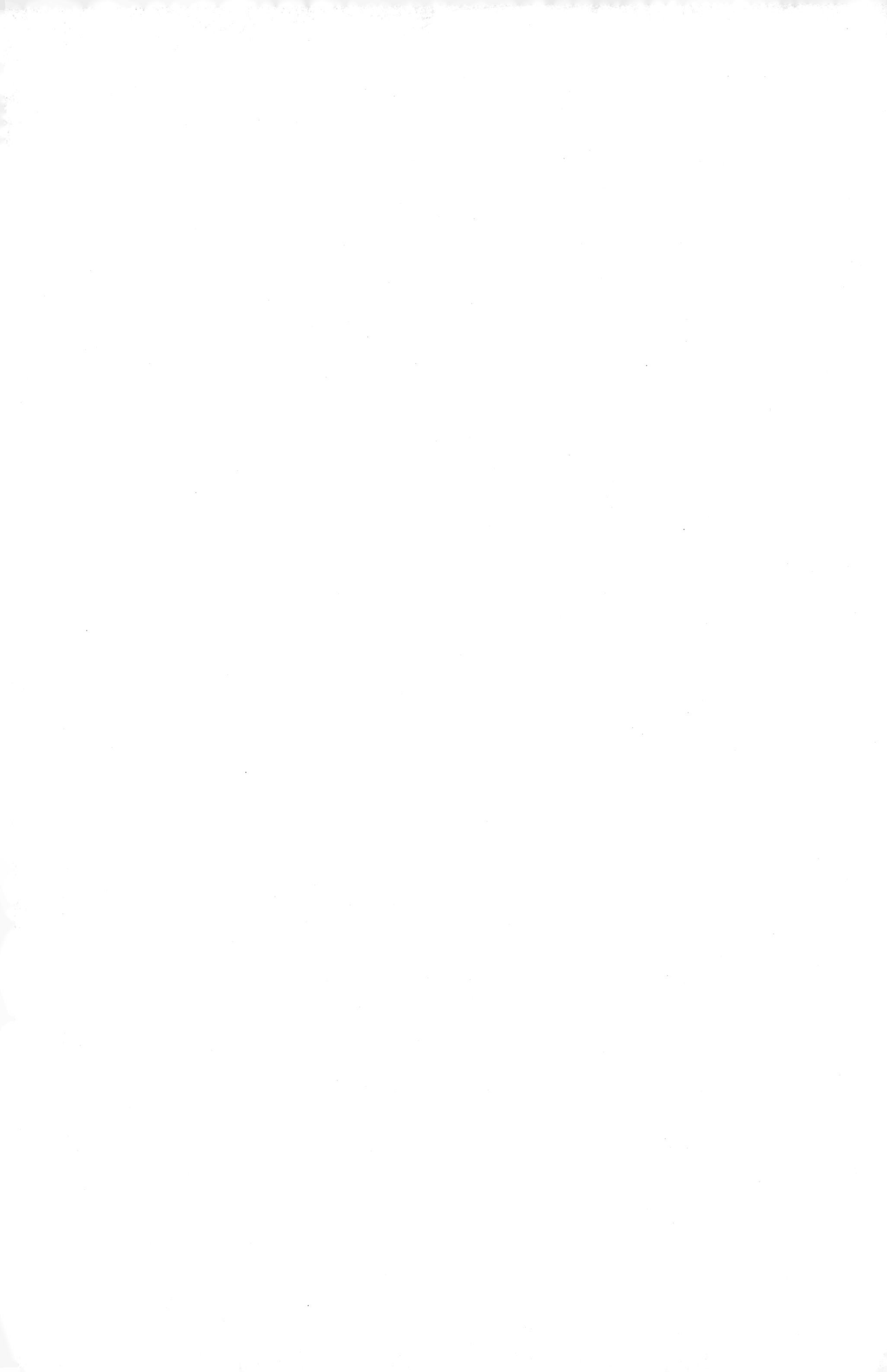

CHAPTER 11

POLYGLUTAMYLATION OF FOLATES AND ANTIFOLATES AS A TARGET OF CHEMOTHERAPY

THOMAS I. KALMAN

State University of New York at Buffalo, Departments of Medicinal Chemistry and Biochemical Pharmacology, Buffalo, New York, United States

Abstract—The functional forms of folic acid coenzymes are tetrahydropteroyl oligo-gamma-glutamates (folate polyglutamates) containing 3–7 glutamic acid residues. Their formation is catalyzed by folylpolyglutamate synthetase (FPGS), an enzyme essential for cellular viability. Selective inhibitors of FPGS are novel folate antagonists of potential utility in cancer chemotherapy. Classical antifolates (e.g., methotrexate) also serve as substrates for FPGS and their polyglutamylated forms are selectively retained in mammalian cells, increasing the potency and duration of action of these drugs. The degradation of the polyglutamate tail of folates and antifolates is catalyzed by gamma-glutamyl hydrolases (GGH). Selective inhibitors of these enzymes also have potential therapeutic applications. Strategies for the design of selective inhibitors of FPGS and GGH have been advanced based on the catalytic mechanisms of these enzymes. Current research in this area is reviewed with a focus on approaches developed in the author's laboratory.

1. INTRODUCTION

Folic acid, an important member of the vitamin B group, occurs in nature predominantly as oligo-γ-glutamate conjugates (polyglutamates) containing 3–7 or even more glutamic acid residues (see Fig. 11-1). The occurrence of folate polyglutamates is universal; they have been identified in all species and animal tissues so far examined. The metabolically functional forms of the vitamin are polyglutamylated tetrahydrofolates, serving as cofactors for a variety of enzyme-catalyzed reactions inside the cell.

The essential role of folate polyglutamylation is not fully understood. Polyglutamylation appears to contribute significantly to the intracellular retention of folate cofactors. In addition, most folate-requiring enzymes have higher affinity (Matthews et al., 1985) to their polyglutamylated cofactors than to the corresponding monoglutamates. It is of special interest that many cytotoxic folate analogs, after entering cells, become polyglutamated, which may affect their enzyme inhibitory activities, selectivity, toxicity, and duration of action (Baugh et al., 1973; Brown et al., 1974; Whitehead, 1977; Rosenblatt et al., 1978; Fry et al., 1982; Allegra et al., 1985). Reviews on various aspects of folate and antifolate polyglutamates have appeared (Cichowicz et al., 1981; Covey, 1980; Goldman, 1985; Goldman et al., 1983; Kisliuk, 1981; McGuire & Bertino, 1981; McGuire & Coward, 1984; Shane & Stockstad, 1985).

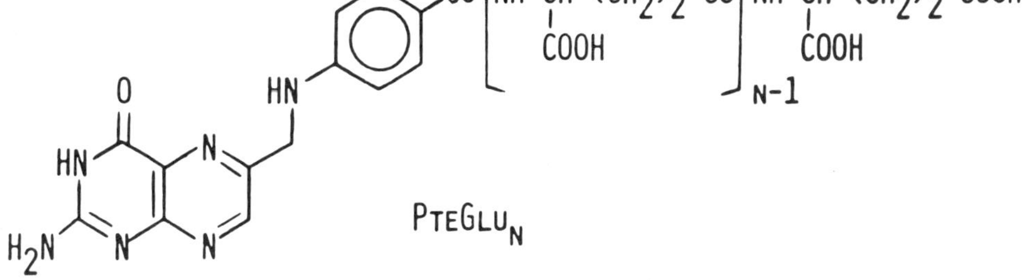

$$\text{PteGlu}_N:\ \text{pteridine–CH}_2\text{–NH–C}_6\text{H}_4\text{–CO}\left[\text{NH–CH(COOH)–(CH}_2)_2\text{–CO}\right]_{N-1}\text{NH–CH(COOH)–(CH}_2)_2\text{–COOH}$$

FIG. 11-1. Structure of folate polyglutamates. PteGlu, pteroylglutamic acid (folic acid); N, number of glutamic acid residues.

In this chapter, folate and antifolate polyglutamylation is examined as a target in cancer chemotherapy. The potential therapeutic applications of the inhibition of *both* the synthesis and the degradation of polyglutamates are discussed, and current strategies toward the design of selective inhibitors of these enzymatic reactions are reviewed with the main emphasis on approaches developed in the author's laboratory.

2. FOLATE POLYGLUTAMATE METABOLISM

The enzyme responsible for the formation of poly-γ-glutamates of folates is folylpolyglutamate synthetase discovered by Griffin and Brown (1964) in *Escherichia coli* extracts. Although the specificity of FPGS from different sources may vary with respect to the oxidation level and the one-carbon unit substitution of the folate substrates, the products of the enzyme accumulate in the cell predominantly as pentaglutamates or higher-chain-length polyglutamates.

Most of the nutritional folate is highly polyglutamylated and requires the enzymatic hydrolysis of the polyglutamate chain for the uptake of the vitamin. Intestinal brush border conjugases play an important role in dietary folate absorption, and a decrease in their activity may lead to certain folate deficiency syndromes. The distribution of gamma-glutamyl hydrolases varies in different species (McGuire & Coward, 1984). In mammalian cells they are localized primarily in the lysosomes. Other hydrolytic activities in the cytoplasm may be involved in polyglutamate chain length regulation. Whitehead and Rosenblatt (1985) suggested that folate polyglutamates may exist in a dynamic state within cells, being hydrolyzed by conjugases (GGH) and then resynthesized by FPGS (see Fig. 11-2).

3. POLYGLUTAMYLATION AND THE THYMIDYLATE SYNTHASE CYCLE

3.1. Inhibition of Thymidylate Synthesis by Folate, Folate Analogs, and Their Polyglutamates in Permeabilized L1210 Cells

While the L1210 cellular thymidylate synthase (TS) assay (Yalowich & Kalman, 1985) has been extremely useful for the study of a variety of drug effects on thymidylate biosynthesis (Kalman & Yalowich, 1979; Yalowich & Kalman, 1985), polyglutamates had negligible effect in this system due to their inability to enter the cell. Further development of the method to include partially permeabilized cells (Kalman & Hsiao, 1984) greatly extended the scope of the cellular enzyme assay system. The absence of a membrane bar-

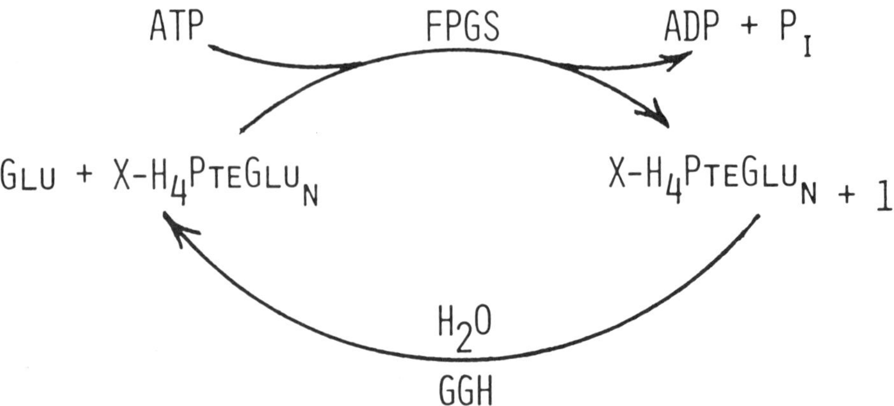

FIG. 11-2. Folate polyglutamate metabolism. FPGS, folylpolyglutamate synthetase; GGH, gamma-glutamate hydrolase; X, coenzyme substituent (one-carbon unit). In the case of tetrahydrofolate (H_4PteGlu), there is no X-substituent.

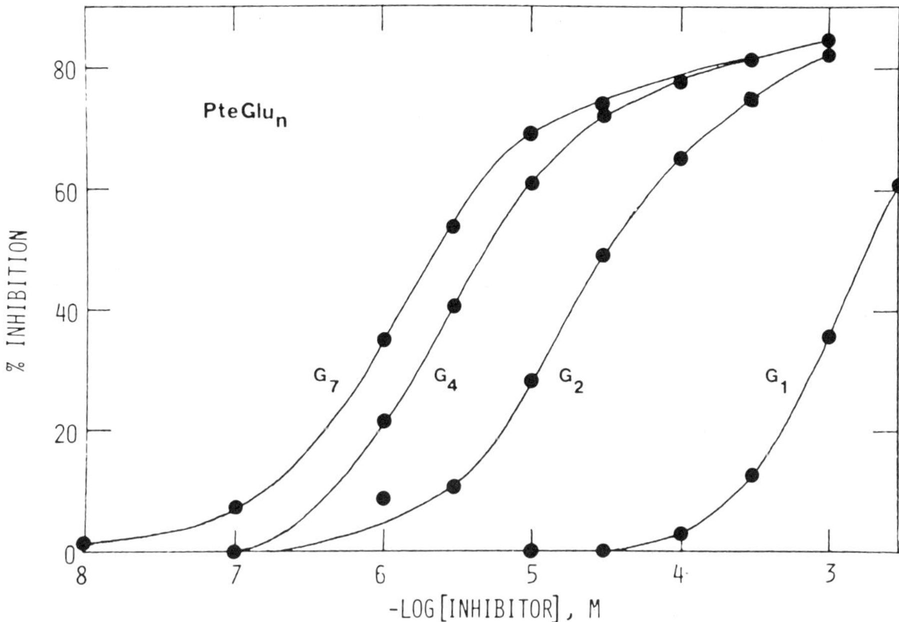

FIG. 11-3. Inhibition of thymidylate synthase by folic acid and its polyglutamates in permeabilized L1210 cells. G_1: folic acid ($n = 1$).

rier in L1210 cells permeabilized by dextran sulfate (Kucera & Paulus, 1982) permitted the study of folate polyglutamates as inhibitors of thymidylate synthase (see Fig. 11-3). The inhibition increased with increasing number of glutamic acid residues by three orders of magnitude from folate (G_1) to pteroylheptaglutamate (G_7). The increase in potency of methotrexate was much less pronounced as the glutamate residues were increased from 1 to 7. Maximum inhibition ($IC_{50} = 1$–2 μM) was achieved by the tetraglutamate, and no further increase was observed (see Table 11-1). A similar study was performed with CB3717, 5,8-dideaza-10-propargylfolic acid, the potent quinazoline thymidylate synthase inhibitor (Jones et al., 1981), and its polyglutamylated derivatives (Kisliuk et al., 1985; Nair et al., 1986). It was discovered that the triglutamate derivative of CB3717 behaved like a stoichiometric inhibitor ($IC_{50} = 2$ μM) of thymidylate synthase, therefore further addition of glutamate residues could not enhance the observed inhibition (Nair et al., 1986).

Purified thymidylate synthase from various sources has shown higher affinities to polyglutamylated substrates and inhibitors (Dolnick & Cheng, 1978; Kisliuk et al., 1979; Lu et al., 1984).

TABLE 11-1. *Inhibition of Thymidylate Synthase by Polyglutamates of Methotrexate in Permeabilized L1210 Cells*

n	4-NH_2-10-CH_3-PteGlu$_n$,* IC_{50} μM
1	60
2	13
3	2.7
4	1.1
5	1.2
6	2.4
7	1.3

*4-Amino-4-deoxy-10-methylpteroylglutamates (methotrexate, $n = 1$).

3.2. Dependence of the Thymidylate Synthase Cycle on the Polyglutamylation of Folate Cofactors

The effects of the extent of cofactor polyglutamylation in permeabilized L1210 cells on the functioning of the TS cycle (see Fig. 11-4) were investigated (Kalman, 1986). Figure 11-5 shows the effects of varying the chain length from 1 to 7 glutamic acid residues at different concentrations of cofactors. A typical pattern is seen at 1 μM concentration. A steady increase in the rate is observed up to 4 glutamate residues without a significant further change at longer chain length. Kinetic analysis of the data showed that the apparent overall K_m values decrease as the glutamate tail is lengthened. However, identical maximum velocities were obtained for all polyglutamates containing 2 to 7 glu residues. From these data, cofactor efficiencies of the pteroylglutamates were calculated as the apparent V_{max} divided by the apparent K_m. The second and third glutamate residue contribute to an efficiency increase of 14-fold and 40-fold, respectively, whereas at chain lengths of 4 to 7 residues, the cofactor efficiency is increased by 50- to 60-fold over that of the monoglutamate (Kalman, 1986). When folic acid was compared with its hexaglutamate form at the physiologically relevant concentration range of 1–3 μM, maximum activity was achieved using the hexaglutamate, whereas the monoglutamate gave only negligible activity (Kalman, 1986), suggesting that *in vivo* the monoglutamate forms of the cofactor could not support the operation of the TS cycle (and DNA synthesis). These results demonstrated a significant dependence of the thymidylate synthase metabolic cycle on the polyglutamate chain length of folate cofactors.

4. FOLYLPOLYGLUTAMATE SYNTHETASE AS A CHEMOTHERAPEUTIC TARGET

4.1. The Essential Role of Folylpolyglutamate Synthetase in Cellular Metabolism

Folylpolyglutamate synthetase is required for cellular viability. Mutant mammalian cells lacking FPGS activity are auxotrophic for thymidine, glycine, and purines, products of folate requiring metabolic pathways, and cannot survive in the absence of these metabolites

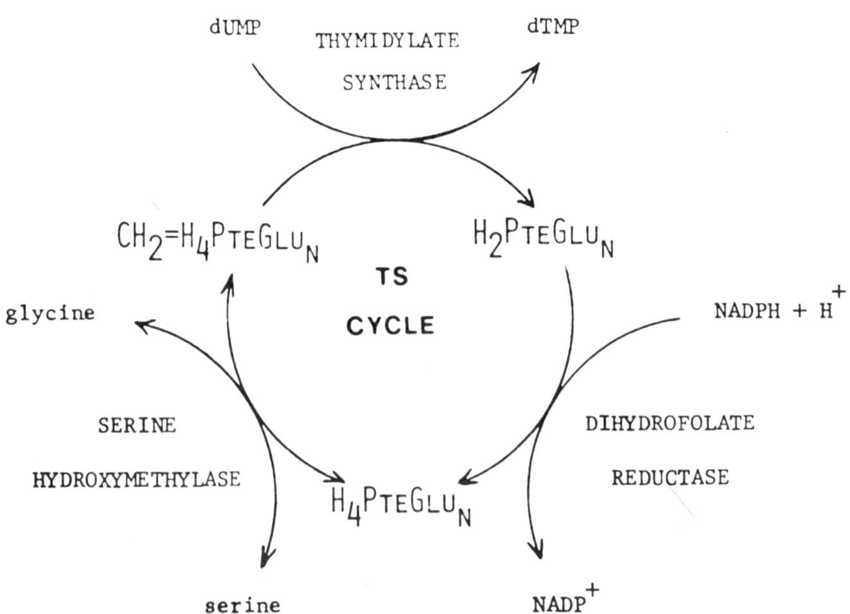

Fig. 11-4. The thymidylate synthase cycle. $CH_2{=}H_4PteGlu_n$, polyglutamates of 5,10-methylenetetrahydrofolate.

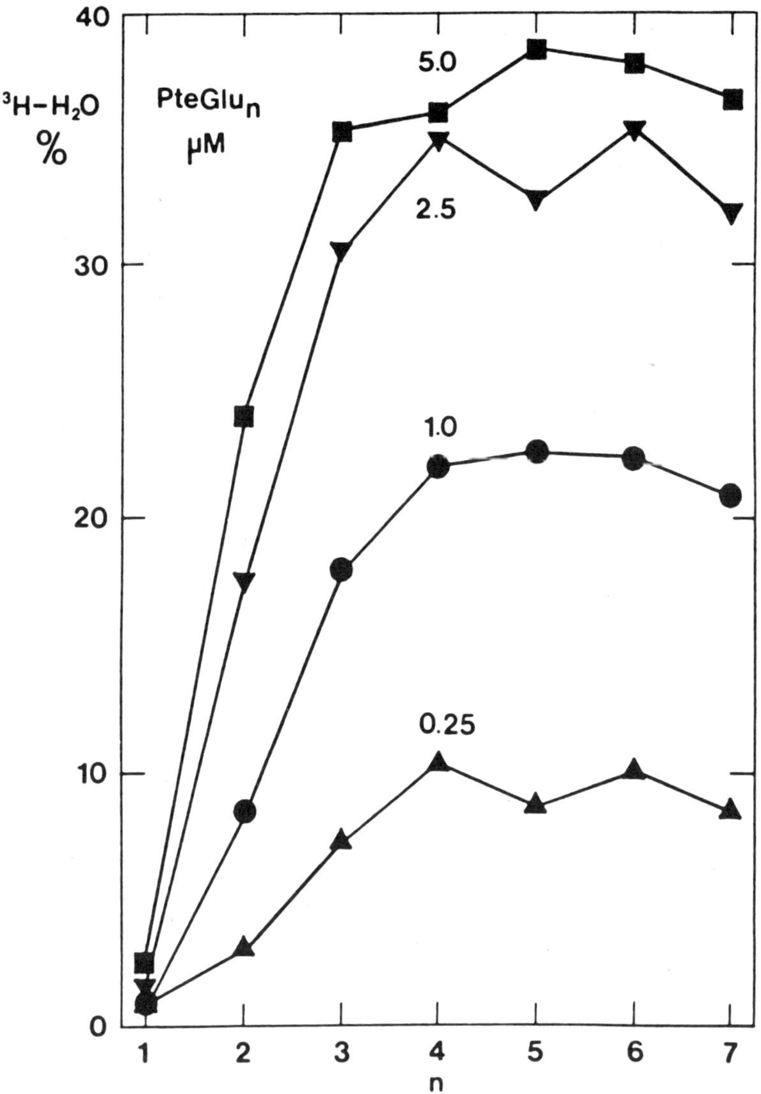

FIG. 11-5. Polyglutamate chain length dependence of folate cofactor activity in the TS cycle of permeabilized L1210 cells. Thymidylate synthase activity is expressed as the percentage of tritium released into water from the substrate, 5-^{3}H-dUMP.

(McBurney & Whitemore, 1974a,b; Taylor & Hanna, 1979; Foo & Shane, 1982). These mutants have greatly reduced intracellular levels of folates and lack their polyglutamylated derivatives. Thus, the reason for the auxotrophy for products of one-carbon metabolism in these mutants is the consequence of both the loss of folate from the cells and the inability of the monoglutamate cofactors to function effectively in the folate dependent metabolic pathways, the latter likely to be the more critical factor (see Section 3). It is of special interest that folate polyglutamates are accumulated to a greater extent in SV-40 transformed cells than normal cells (Hoffman et al., 1981) suggesting that cells transformed by the virus may have a greater requirement for polyglutamates. Such a requirement can result in selective toxicity of FPGS inhibitors.

On the basis of these considerations, it is anticipated that selective inhibitors of FPGS should be effective cytotoxic agents and therefore would find useful applications in cancer chemotherapy. The action of these novel antimetabolites would not be limited to the S phase of the cell cycle, broadening the scope of the therapeutic utility of the antifolate drugs.

4.2. Design of Folylpolyglutamate Synthetase Inhibitors

Folylpolyglutamate synthetase (McGuire & Coward, 1984; Cichowicz & Shane, 1987a,b) belongs to the group of gamma-glutamyl transferase enzymes which catalyze γ-glutamylation of amino groups. These reactions generally proceed by activation of the γ-COOH group using ATP to form a phosphoric acid mixed anhydride, which subsequently becomes aminolyzed, yielding the amide product.

The best studied gamma-glutamyl transferases are glutamine synthetase (GS) and γ-glutamylcysteine synthetase (GCS). Both enzymes are strongly inhibited by methionine sulfoximine (and its S-alkyl homologs) (Meister, 1978; Griffith & Meister, 1979) via the enzyme-catalyzed formation of the corresponding sulfoximine phosphate (Rowe et al., 1969; Meister, 1978). The phosphorylated inhibitor remains strongly bound to the enzyme, which may be considered an enzyme-generated transition-state analog (Kalman, 1985) resembling the tetrahedral intermediate formed from glutamyl phosphate and the γ-glutamyl acceptor.

On the basis of the analogy between the mechanism of FPGS and that of the other gamma-glutamyl transferases, particularly γ-glutamylcysteine synthetase, we designed and synthesized a series of pteroyl-*S*-alkylhomocysteine sulfoximines (see Fig. 11-6) as potential inhibitors of FPGS (Kalman & Harvison, 1983; Moran et al., 1988). None of these folate analogs showed any inhibitory activity against mouse liver FPGS (Moran et al., 1988), although they served as substrates for dihydrofolate reductase and the reduced folate analogs could substitute for H_4folate in the TS cycle of L1210 cells *in vitro* (Kalman & Harvison, 1983).

The lack of activity of this series could be explained by the absence of a negative charge at the γ-position. Extensive structure–activity studies (Moran et al., 1985a,b; Cichowicz et al., 1981; Cichowicz & Shane, 1987b; George et al., 1987) of substrates and inhibitors of FPGS indicated that donor substrates or their analogs must have a negative charge at the γ-position for initial binding to the enzyme. This requirement was not apparent, however, in the use of the ornithine analogs of H_4folate (Cichowicz et al., 1981), methotrexate (Piper et al., 1985; McGuire et al., 1986), and aminopterin (Rosowsky et al., 1986). The last is the most potent inhibitor of FPGS ($K_i = 15\ \mu M$) found so far. It appears that the ornithine derivatives bearing a positively charged protonated amino group act as multisubstrate analogs by partially occupying both the donor and the acceptor substrate binding sites, which may overcompensate for the absence of the negative charge at the γ-position (see Fig. 11-7). It should be noted that the ornithine analogs of aminopterin and methotrexate are potent inhibitors of dihydrofolate reductase, but lack cytotoxicity apparently due to their inability to enter cells.

Our current efforts are directed toward the design of second-generation FPGS inhibitors based on the recognized binding interactions outlined in Fig. 11-7. Thus, new struc-

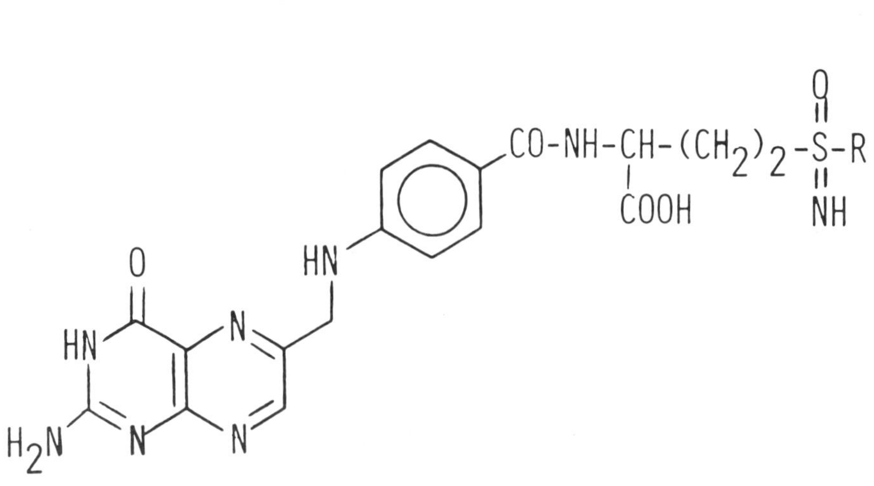

Fig. 11-6. Pteroyl-S-alkylhomocysteine sulfoximines. R = methyl, ethyl, *n*-propyl, *n*-butyl.

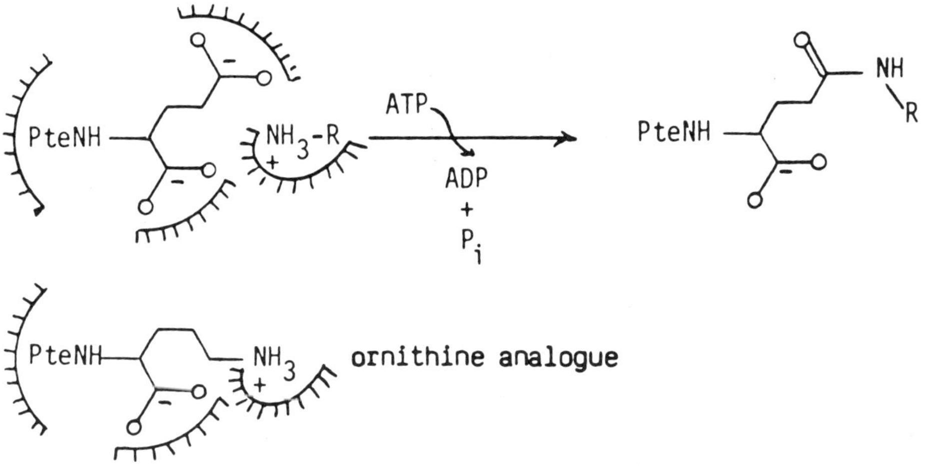

FIG. 11-7. Hypothetical binding interactions at the active site of folylpolyglutamate synthetase.

tures with retention of the negative charge at the γ-position are considered, as well as transition-state analogs designed on the basis of computer modeling of the tetrahedral intermediate of the enzyme-catalyzed reaction.

5. GAMMA-GLUTAMYL HYDROLASE AS A CHEMOTHERAPEUTIC TARGET

5.1. The Role of Gamma-Glutamyl Hydrolase in Cellular Metabolism

The occurrence of gamma-glutamyl hydrolases or conjugases is ubiquitous in nature (McGuire & Coward, 1984). Their substrate specificities vary depending on their source and physiological function. Both endopeptidase and exopeptidase activities were demonstrated for many conjugase preparations. However, we hypothesized that if an extralysosomal cytoplasmic hydrolase were involved in folylpolyglutamate chain length regulation, it should behave primarily as a carboxypeptidase. This would permit the stepwise shortening of the polyglutamate tails of folate cofactors, more desirable for an effective metabolic control mechanism than random cleavage along the chain. Such an enzyme would fulfill the metabolic role of GGH indicated in Fig. 11-2.

5.2. Design of Gamma-Glutamyl Hydrolase Inhibitors

Rational design of carboxypeptidase inhibitors has been a very successful approach in the development of selective enzyme inhibitors and has contributed significantly to contemporary drug discoveries. The pioneering work in Wolfenden's laboratory on transition-state analogs (Byers & Wolfenden, 1972; Wolfenden, 1976, 1978) led to the rational development of selective angiotensin-converting enzyme inhibitors of major therapeutic utility by Ondetti's group (Ondetti et al., 1979). The most potent inhibitor developed by Ondetti against carboxypeptidase A, an enzyme specific for peptide substrates with C-terminal phenylalanine, is a simple derivative of phenylalanine in which the $-NH_2$ group is replaced by the $-HSCH_2$ group. Similarly, potent and selective inhibition of the C-terminal arginine-specific carboxypeptidase B was achieved by the corresponding mercaptomethyl analog of arginine. Each inhibitor was selective toward its own target enzyme (Ondetti et al., 1979). The salient features of these inhibitor molecules involve (1) the $-COOH$ group mimicking the C-terminal $-COOH$ of the substrate, (2) the amino acid side chain providing specificity, and (3) the $HSCH_2-$ group which is coordinated *via* the sulfur to the Zn ion at the enzyme active site.

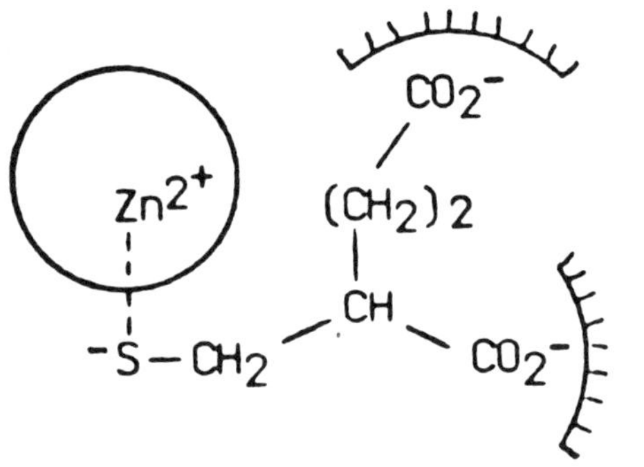

FIG. 11-8. The structure of 2-mercaptomethylglutaric acid and its binding interactions with gamma-glutamyl hydrolase.

Based on this precedent, we designed and synthesized 2-mercaptomethylglutaric acid (MMGA) as a prototype of glutamate side chain–specific carboxypeptidase inhibitors (Kalman et al., 1986, 1988). The structure of MMGA and its interaction with the hypothetical active site of GGH are illustrated in Fig. 11-8.

5.3. BIOLOGICAL ACTIVITY OF 2-MERCAPTOMETHYLGLUTARIC ACID

5.3.1. *Enzyme Inhibition*

A partially purified conjugase preparation from chicken pancreas was found to be strongly inhibited by 2-mercaptomethylglutaric acid, whereas lysosomal hog kidney conjugase was not inhibited by MMGA (Kalman et al., 1986).

Carboxypeptidase G_1 (McCullough et al., 1971) and carboxypeptidase G_2 (Minton et al., 1983), two similar enzymes capable of catalyzing the hydrolytic cleavage of the glutamate moiety of folic acid, were strongly inhibited by MMGA, with K_i values of 0.23 and 0.21 μM, respectively. In contrast, carboxypeptidases A and B were much less inhibited (see Table 11-2), showing the importance of the carboxyethyl side chain in determining substratelike specificity of binding. Replacement of the $HSCH_2$— group of MMGA by HOOC— or CH_3— group resulted in complete loss of enzyme inhibitory activity, demonstrating that the postulated interaction between the active site Zn atom and the SH— group is essential for activity.

5.3.2. *Effects on Cellular Polyglutamate Metabolism*

Following a 24-hr incubation of human fibroblasts or transformed human lymphocytes in culture with radioisotope-labeled methotrexate (MTX), during further growth for 24 and 48 hr, longer-chain MTX polyglutamates accumulate and are preferentially retained. It was observed that in the presence of 0.1–0.4 mM MMGA, the ratio of the longer- to shorter-

TABLE 11-2. *Inhibition of Carboxypeptidases by 2-Mercaptomethylglutamic Acid (MMGA)*

Enzyme	K_i (MMGA), μM
Carboxypeptidase A	100
Carboxypeptidase B	190
Carboxypeptidase G_1	0.23
Carboxypeptidase G_2	0.21

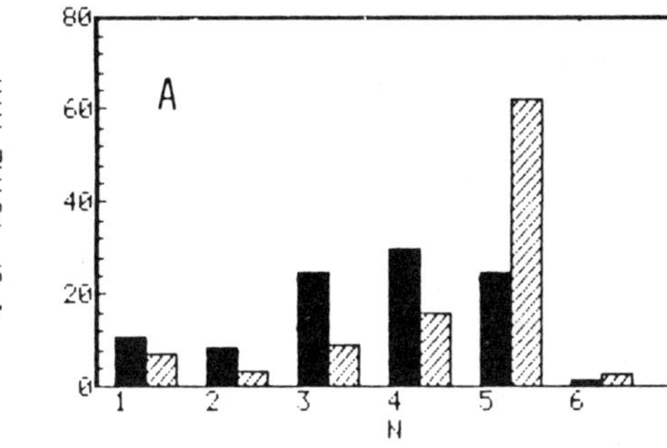

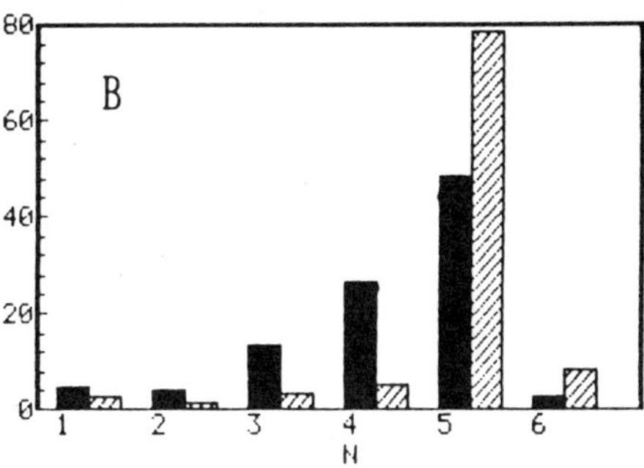

FIG. 11-9. The effects of 2-mercaptomethylglutaric acid on the retention of methotrexate polyglutamates in human transformed lymphocytes (A) and in normal human fibroblasts (B) in culture. Filled bars, no MMGA added; hatched bars, 0.1 mM (A) and 0.4 mM (B) of MMGA added after 24 hr incubation of the cells with 1 μM MTX. Polyglutamate distribution was determined 48 hr after the extracellular MTX was removed. N, number of glutamic acid residues in polyglutamates of MTX (MTX, $N = 1$).

chain polyglutamates greatly increased with the pentaglutamate predominating (Whitehead et al., 1987). These results are illustrated in Fig. 11-9, showing the distribution of MTX polyglutamates (from 1 to 6 glutamate residues) in lymphocytes (A) and in fibroblasts (B) 48 hr after removal of MTX from the medium, in the presence and absence of MMGA. It should be noted that in cultured L1210 murine leukemia cells, MMGA did not show significant cytotoxicity at 0.1 mM, and it had no effect on the growth of transformed human lymphocytes at up to 0.4 mM.

Recently, GGH activity modulating the polyglutamylation pattern of MTX in lymphoblasts and myeloblasts obtained from leukemic children was demonstrated with the aid of MMGA (Whitehead et al., 1988). Myeloblasts from acute nonlymphoblastic leukemia patients generally refractory to MTX treatment accumulate predominantly triglutamates of MTX, in contrast to lymphoblasts from the MTX responsive acute lymphoblastic leukemias, which accumulate predominantly MTX pentaglutamates. In the presence of MMGA, both lymphoblasts and myeloblasts accumulate predominantly the longer-chain-length MTX pentaglutamates (Whitehead et al., 1988), and after a 24-hr efflux period, the patterns of MTX polyglutamate distribution are very similar in the two cell types. The results suggest that inhibition of cellular GGH may render the otherwise refractory acute nonlymphoblastic leukemias susceptible to MTX treatment. The validity of this prediction remains to be determined.

6. CONCLUSIONS

Polyglutamylation of folates and antifolates provides two potential chemotherapeutic targets: (1) folylpolyglutamate synthetase, the enzyme responsible for the formation of the polyglutamate metabolites, and (2) gamma-glutamyl hydrolase, the enzyme responsible for the breakdown of the polyglutamate chains. FPGS inhibitors are potential cytotoxic agents with the unique ability to block all pathways of folate-dependent one-carbon metabolism interfering with *de novo* purine and DNA-thymine biosynthesis and amino acid metabolism, without affecting dihydrofolate reductase, the target of currently used antifolate drugs. Selective inhibitors of GGH may extend the usefulness of folate analogs as anticancer agents and lead to new approaches in combination chemotherapy. The future success of the rational design of these two types of enzyme inhibitors greatly depends on our increasing knowledge about the structure and function of their respective targets.

Acknowledgments—This work was supported by a grant (CA35212) from the National Cancer Institute, NIH, DHHS.

REFERENCES

Allegra, C. J., Chabner, B. A., Drake, J. C., Lutz, R., Rodbard, D., and Jolivet, J. (1985) Enhanced inhibition of thymidylate synthase by methotrexate polyglutamates. *J. Biol. Chem.* **260**: 9720–9726.

Baugh, C. M., Krumdieck, C. L., and Nair, M. G. (1973) Polygammaglutamyl metabolites of methotrexate. *Biochem. Biophys. Res. Commun.* **52**: 27–34.

Brown, J. P., Davidson, G. E., Weir, D. G., and Scott, J. M. (1974) Specificity of folate-γ-L-glutamate ligase in rat liver and kidney. Biosynthesis of poly-γ-L-glutamates of unreduced methotrexate and the effect of methotrexate on folate polyglutamate biosynthesis. *Internat. J. Biochem.* **5**: 727–733.

Byers, L. D., and Wolfenden, R. (1972) A potent reversible inhibitor of carboxypeptidase A. *J. Biol. Chem.* **247**: 606–608.

Cichowicz, D. J., and Shane, B. (1987a) Mammalian folylpoly-γ-glutamate synthetase. 1. Purification and general properties of the hog liver enzyme. *Biochemistry* **26**: 504–512.

Cichowicz, D. J., and Shane, B. (1987b) Mammalian folylpoly-γ-glutamate synthetase. 2. Substrate specificity and kinetic properties. *Biochemistry* **26**: 513–521.

Cichowicz, D. J., Foo, S. K., and Shane, B. (1981) Folylpoly-γ-glutamate synthesis in bacteria and mammalian cells. *Mol. Cell. Biochemistry* **39**: 209–228.

Covey, J. M. (1980) Polyglutamate derivatives of folic acid coenzymes and methotrexate. *Life Sci.* **26**: 665–678.

Dolnick, B. J., and Cheng, Y.-C. (1978) Human thymidylate synthetase. II. Derivatives of pteroylmono- and polyglutamates as substrates and inhibitors. *J. Biol. Chem.* **253**: 3563–3567.

Foo, S. K., and Shane, B. (1982) Regulation of folylpolyglutamate synthesis in mammalian cells. *J. Biol. Chem.* **257**: 13587–13592.

Fry, D. W., Yalowich, J. C., and Goldman, I. D. (1982) Rapid formation of poly-γ-glutamyl derivatives of methotrexate and their association with dihydrofolate reductase as assessed by high-pressure liquid chromatography in the Ehrlich ascites tumor cell *in vitro*. *J. Biol. Chem.* **257**: 1890–1896.

George, S., Cichowicz, D. J., and Shane, B. (1987) Mammalian folylpoly-γ-glutamate synthetase. 3. Specificity of folate analogues. *Biochemistry* **26**: 522–529.

Goldman, I. D. (ed.). (1985) *Proceedings of the second workshop on folyl and antifolyl polyglutamates.* New York: Praeger.

Goldman, I. D., Chabner, B. A., and Bertino, J. R. (eds.) (1983) *Folyl and antifolyl polyglutamates.* New York: Plenum.

Griffin, M. J., and Brown, G. M. (1964) The biosynthesis of folic acid. III. Enzymatic formation of dihydrofolic acid from dihydropteroic acid and of tetrahydropteroylpolyglutamic acid compounds from tetrahydrofolic acid. *J. Biol. Chem.* **239**: 310–316.

Griffith, O. W., and Meister, A. (1979) Potent and specific inhibition of glutathione synthesis by buthionine sulfoximine (S-n-butyl homocysteine sulfoximine). *J. Biol. Chem.* **254**: 7558-7560.

Hoffman, R. M., Coalson, D. W., Jacobsen, S. J., and Erbe, R. W. (1981) Folate polyglutamate and monoglutamate accumulation in normal and SV-40 transformed human fibroblasts. *J. Cell Physiol.* **109**: 497–505.

Jones, T. R., Calvert, A. H., Jackman, A. L., Brown, S. J., Jones, M., and Harrap, K. R. (1981) A potent antitumor quinazoline inhibitor of thymidylate synthetase: Synthesis, biological properties, and therapeutic results in mice. *Eur. J. Cancer* **17**: 11–19.

Kalman, T. I. (1986) Effects of polyglutamylation on folate cofactor and antifolate activity in the thymidylate synthase cycle of permeabilized murine leukemia L1210 cells. In *Chemistry and biology of pteridines*, B. A. Cooper and V. M. Whitehead, eds., pp. 763-766. Berlin: W. de Gruyter.

Kalman, T. I. (1985) Enzyme generated transition state analogues. *Acta Pharm. Suecica*, Suppl. 2: 279–301.

Kalman, T. I., Nayak, V. K., and Reddy, A. R. V. (1988) Selective inhibition of carboxypeptidases with C-terminal glutamate specificity. *14th Internat. Congr. Biochemistry*, Abstract TH: 070.

Kalman, T. I., Nayak, V. K., and Reddy, A. R. V. (1986) Selective inhibition of bacterial carboxypeptidase G and pancreatic conjugase by 2-mercaptomethylglutaric acid. In *Chemistry and biology of pteridines*, B. A. Cooper and V. M. Whitehead, eds., pp. 583–586. Berlin: W. de Gruyter.

Kalman, T. I., and Hsiao, M. C. (1984) Inhibition of thymidylate synthesis by antifolates in permeabilized murine leukemia L1210 cells. *Proc. Amer. Assoc. Cancer Res.* **25**: 311.

Kalman, T. I., and Harvison, P. J. (1983) Novel folic acid analogs: Pteroyl S-alkylhomocysteine sulfoximines. *Proc. Amer. Assoc. Cancer Res.* **24**: 278.

Kalman, T. I., and Yalowich, J. C. (1979) Studies of the effects of folic acid antagonists on thymidylate synthetase activity in intact mammalian cells. In *Chemistry and biology of pteridines*, R. L. Kisliuk and G. M. Brown, eds., pp. 671–682. New York: Elsevier.

Kisliuk, R. L. (1981) Pteroylpolyglutamates. *Mol. Cell. Biochemistry* **39**: 331–345.

Kisliuk, R. L., Gaumont, Y., Kumar, P., Coutts, M., Nair, M. G., Nanavati, N. T., and Kalman, T. I. (1985) The effect of polyglutamylation on the inhibitory activity of folate analogs. In *Proceedings of the second workshop on folyl and antifolyl polyglutamates*, I. D. Goldman, ed., pp. 319–328. New York: Praeger.

Kisliuk, R. L., Gaumont, Y., Baugh, C. M., Galivan, J. H., Maley, G. F., and Maley, F. (1979) Inhibition of thymidylate synthetase by poly-glutamyl derivatives of folate and methotrexate. In *Chemistry and biology of pteridines*, R. L. Kisliuk and G. M. Brown, eds., pp. 431–435. New York: Elsevier.

Kucera, R., and Paulus, H. (1982) Studies on ribonucleoside-diphosphate reductase in permeable animal cells. 1. Reversible permeabilization of mouse L cells with dextran sulfate. *Arch. Biochem. Biophys.* **214**: 102–113.

Lu, Y.-Z., Aiello, P. D., and Matthews, R. G. (1984) Studies on the polyglutamate specificity of thymidylate synthase from fetal pig liver. *Biochemistry* **23**: 6870–6876.

Matthews, R. G., Lu, Y., Green, J. M., and MacKenzie, R. E. (1985) The polyglutamate specificities of four folate-dependent enzymes from pig liver. In *Proceedings of the second workshop on folyl and antifolyl polyglutamates*, I. D. Goldman, ed., pp. 65–75. New York: Praeger.

McBurney, M. W., and Whitmore, G. F. (1974a) Isolation and biochemical characterization of folate deficient mutants of Chinese hamster cells. *Cell* **2**: 173–182.

McBurney, M. W., and Whitmore, G. F. (1974b) Characterization of a Chinese hamster cell with a temperature-sensitive mutation in folate metabolism. *Cell* **2**: 183–188.

McCullough, J. L., Chabner, B. A., and Bertino, J. R. (1971) Purification and properties of carboxypeptidase G_1. *J. Biol. Chem.* **246**: 7207–7213.

McGuire, J. J., Hsieh, P., and Franco, C. T. (1986) Folylpolyglutamate synthetase inhibition and cytotoxic effects of methotrexate analogs containing 2-ω-diaminoalkanoic acids. *Biochem. Pharmacol.* **35**: 2607–2613.

McGuire, J. J., and Coward, J. K. (1984) Pteroylpolyglutamates: Biosynthesis, degradation, and function. In *Folates and pterines*, R. L. Blakely and S. J. Benkovic, eds., Vol. 1, pp. 135–190. New York: John Wiley.

McGuire, J. J., and Bertino, J. R. (1981) Enzymatic synthesis and function of folylpolyglutamates. *Mol. Cell. Biochemistry* **38**: 19–49.

Meister, A. (1978) Inhibition of glutamine synthetase and γ-glutamylcysteine synthetase by methionine sulfoximine and related compounds. In *Enzyme-activated irreversible inhibitors*, N. Seiler, M. J. Jung, and J. Koch-Weser, eds., pp. 187–210. New York: Elsevier.

Minton, N. P., Atkinson, T., and Sherwood, R. F. (1983) Molecular cloning of the pseudomonas carboxypeptidase G_2 gene and its expression in *Escherichia coli* and *Pseudomonas putida*. *J. Bacteriol.* **156**: 1222–1227.

Moran, R. G., Colman, P. D., Harvison, P. J., and Kalman, T. I. (1988) Evaluation of pteroyl-S-alkylhomocysteine sulfoximines as inhibitors of mammalian folylpolyglutamate synthetase. *Biochem. Pharmacol.* **37**: 1997–2003.

Moran, R. G., Colman, P. D., Rosowsky, A., Forsch, R. A., and Chan, K. K. (1985a) Structural features of 4-amino antifolates required for substrate activity with mammalian folylpolyglutamate synthetase. *Mol. Pharmacol.* **27**: 156–166.

Moran, R. G., Rosowsky, A., Colman, P., Forsch, R. Solan, V., Bader, H., Harvision, P., and Kalman, T. I. (1985b) Structural features of folate analogs that determine substrate or inhibitor activity for mammalian folylpolyglutamate synthetase. In *Proceedings of the second workshop on folyl and antifolyl polyglutamates*, I. D. Goldman, ed., pp. 51–64. New York: Praeger.

Nair, M. G., Nanavati, N. T., Nair, I. G., Kisliuk, R. L., Gaumont, Y., Hsiao, M. C., and Kalman, T. I. (1986) Folate analogues. 26. Syntheses and antifolate activity of 10-substituted derivatives of 5,8-dideazafolic acid and of the poly-γ-glutamyl metabolites of N^{10}-propargyl-5,8-dideazafolic acid (PDDF). *J. Med. Chem.* **29**: 1754–1760.

Ondetti, M. A., Cushman, D. W., Sabo, E. F., and Cheung, H. S. (1979) The design of active-site-directed reversible inhibitors of carboxypeptidases. In *Drug action and design: Mechanism-based enzyme inhibitors*, T. I. Kalman, ed., pp. 271–283. New York: Elsevier.

Piper, J. R., McCaleb, G. S., Montgomery, F. A., Schmid, F. A., and Sirotnak, F. M. (1985) Syntheses and evaluation as antifolates of MTX analogues derived from 2,ω-diaminoalkanoic acids. *J. Med. Chem.* **28**: 1016–1025.

Rosenblatt, D. S., Whitehead, V. M., Dupont, M. M., Vuchich, M. J., and Vera, N. (1978) Synthesis of methotrexate polyglutamates in cultured human cells. *Mol. Pharmacol.* **14**: 210–214.

Rosowsky, A., Freisheim, J. H., Moran, R. G., Solan, V. C., Bader, H., Wright, J. E., and Radlike-Smith, M. (1986). Methotrexate analogues. 26. Inhibition of dihydrofolate reductase and folylpolyglutamate synthetase activity and *in vitro* tumor cell growth by methotrexate and aminopterin analogues containing a basic amino acid side chain. *J. Med. Chem.* **29**: 655–660.

Rowe, W. B., Ronzio, R. A., and Meister, A. (1969) Inhibition of glutamine synthetase by methionine sulfoximine. Studies on methionine sulfoximine phosphate. *Biochemistry* **8**: 2674–2680.

Shane, B., and Stockstad, E. L. R. (1985) Vitamin B_{12}–folate interrelationships. *Ann. Rev. Nutr.* **5**: 115–141.

Taylor, T. R., and Hanna, L. M. (1979) Folate-dependent enzymes in cultured Chinese hamster ovary cells: Evidence for mutant forms of folylpolyglutamate synthetase. *Arch. Biochem. Biophys.* **197**: 36–43.

Whitehead, V. M. (1977) Synthesis of methotrexate polyglutamates in L1210 murine leukemia cells. *Cancer Res.* **37**: 408–412.

Whitehead, V. M., and Rosenblatt, D. S. (1985) Metabolism of methotrexate (MTX) and folates in transformed human lymphocytes. *Proc. Amer. Assoc. Cancer Res.* **26**: 232.

Whitehead, V. M., Kalman, T. I., and Vuchich, M.-J. (1987) Inhibition of gamma-glutamyl hydrolases in human cells by 2-mercaptomethylglutaric acid. *Biochem. Biophys. Res. Commun.* **144**: 292–297.

Whitehead, V. M., Kalman, T. I., Rosenblatt, D. S., Vuchich, M.-J. and Payment, C. (1988) Regulation of methotrexate polyglutamate (MTXPG) formation in human leukemic cells. *Proc. Amer. Assoc. Cancer Res.* **29**: 287.

Wolfenden, R. (1976) Transition-state analog inhibitors and enzyme catalysis. *Ann. Rev. Biophys. Bioeng.* **5**: 271–306.

Wolfenden, R. (1978) Transition-state affinity as a basis for the design of enzyme inhibitors. In *Transition states of biochemical processes*, R. D. Gandour and R. L. Schowen, eds., pp. 555–578. New York: Plenum Press.

Yalowich, J. C., and Kalman, T. I. (1985) Rapid determination of thymidylate synthase activity and its inhibition in intact L1210 leukemia cells *in vitro*. *Biochem. Pharmacol.* **34**: 2319–2324.

CHAPTER 12

ANTITUMOR, CYTOTOXIC, AND ENZYME INHIBITORY PROPERTIES OF HOMOFOLATES

ROY L. KISLIUK,* YVETTE GAUMONT,* JANET THORNDIKE,* FRANZ A. SCHMID,** FRANCIS M. SIROTNAK,** JAMES R. PIPER,† B. RAMA MURTHY,‡ AND MADHAVAN G. NAIR‡

*Department of Biochemistry, Tufts University, Boston, Massachusetts, United States
**Laboratory for Molecular Therapeutics, Memorial Sloan-Kettering Cancer Center, New York, New York, United States
†Drug Synthesis Section, Southern Research Institute, Birmingham, Alabama, United States
‡Department of Biochemistry, University of South Alabama, Mobile, Alabama, United States

Abstract—To elucidate further the mechanism of the antitumor and cytotoxic action of homofolates, appropriate homofolate and tetrahydrohomofolate derivatives were synthesized and tested for their antitumor, cytotoxic, and enzyme inhibitory properties. Our results support the view that homofolates are active intracellularly in the form of tetrahydrohomofolate polyglutamates which inhibit glycinamide ribonucleotide formyltransferase, an enzyme on the pathway of purine biosynthesis. (1) The dihydrofolate reductase inhibitor trimetrexate partially blocks cytotoxicity of homofolate for human lymphoma cells but does not block the cytotoxicity of 5-methyltetrahydrohomofolate. (2) The cytoxicity of both inhibitors is prevented by inosine. (3) Tetrahydrohomofolate polyglutamates are potent and specific inhibitors of glycinamide ribonucleotide formyltransferase *in vitro*, whereas monoglutamates and the corresponding homofolate polyglutamates are much weaker inhibitors. (4) Both antitumor activity and glycinamide ribonucleotide formyltransferase inhibition in L1210 murine leukemia systems show a surprising lack of stereospecificity with respect to carbon 6 of tetrahydrohomofolate. Enzymes from *Lactobacillus casei* show much greater stereospecificity, with the stereoisomer having the unnatural configuration showing the greater inhibition.

1. INTRODUCTION

Homofolate is an analog of folate that possesses an additional methylene group between the 9 carbon and 10 nitrogen of folate (Fig. 12-1). Its synthesis and some biological tests with bacteria and bacterial enzymes were first reported in 1964 (Goodman et al., 1964). The close structural analogy between folate and homofolate made it an excellent candidate to test an earlier suggestion (Kisliuk, 1960) that folate antagonists be prepared as their 5,6,7,8-tetrahydro derivatives with the hope that they would act as inhibitors of enzymes requiring tetrahydrofolate coenzymes (Kisliuk, 1984). Prime examples are the enzymes of the thymidylate cycle, thymidylate synthase, dihydrofolate reductase, and serine hydroxymethyltransferase as well as the enzymes on the *de novo* pathway of purine biosynthesis, glycinamide ribonucleotide formyltransferase, and aminoimidazolecarboxamide ribonucleotide formyltransferase.

Homofolate was also of interest because its 7,8-dihydro form (Fig. 12-1) is a substrate for dihydrofolate reductase. It was envisioned that homofolate or dihydrohomofolate might be converted to a cytotoxic tetrahydro form (Fig. 12-1) by tumors which were resistant to methotrexate due to enhanced levels of dihydrofolate reductase, leading to selective toxicity of the methotrexate-resistant cells (Goodman et al., 1964; Friedkin et al., 1971).

It therefore aroused a great deal of interest when it was found that not only does (6RS)-tetrahydrohomofolate show superior antitumor activity to homofolate in the L1210 system, it is significantly more active in a strain of L1210 resistant to methotrexate which has high levels of dihydrofolate reductase (Mead et al., 1966). It appeared likely that oxidation of tetrahydrohomofolate to dihydrohomofolate, either spontaneously or through metabolism via thymidylate synthase [5,11-methylenetetrahydrohomofolate turned out to be a slow substrate for most thymidylate synthases (Kisliuk & Gaumont, 1970; Dwivedi et al., 1983)], was reversed by the action of dihydrofolate reductase. Literature describing the development of the stable derivative (6RS)-5-methyltetrahydrohomofolate (NSC 139490,

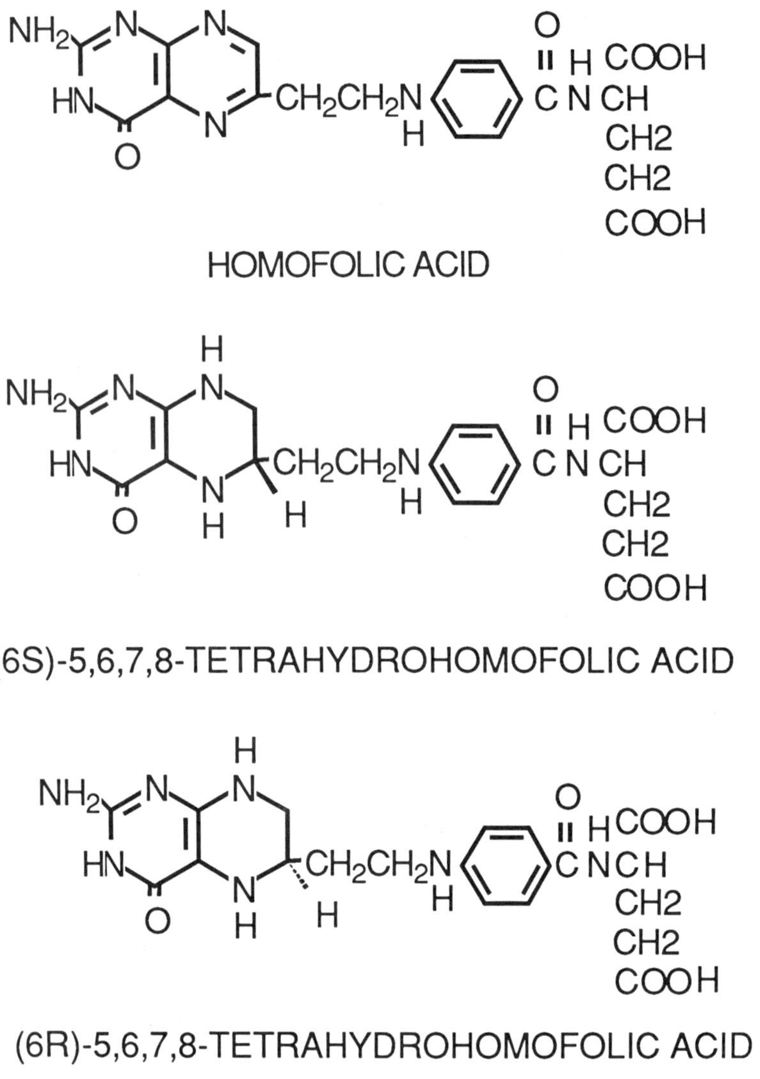

HOMOFOLIC ACID

(6S)-5,6,7,8-TETRAHYDROHOMOFOLIC ACID

(6R)-5,6,7,8-TETRAHYDROHOMOFOLIC ACID

FIG. 12-1. Structures of homofolates.

Fig. 12-1) and its antitumor activity in experimental systems has been reviewed (Kisliuk, 1982). Its clinical pharmacokinetics and a phase I trial have been reported (Cohen et al., 1982; Loo et al., 1983). Although plans for further clinical trials of this compound are not active at this time, homofolates are important because they were the first antifolates not possessing the 2,4-diamino structure to show activity as antitumor agents.

Early results in bacterial systems indicated that thymidylate synthase is the target enzyme for homofolates. (6RS)-Tetrahydrohomofolate is an inhibitor of *Escherichia coli* (Goodman et al., 1964) and *Lactobacillus casei* (Crusberg et al., 1970) thymidylate synthases, and its inhibition of the growth of folate-requiring bacteria is prevented by the addition of thymidine (Goodman et al., 1964). However, studies of the reversal of homofolate toxicity in sarcoma 180 cells by purines and pyrimidines provided strong evidence for a block at the glycinamide ribonucleotide formyltransferase step (Divekar & Hakala, 1975).

Figure 12-2 outlines some potential metabolites and inhibitory sites of homofolates. After entering the cell, homofolate (HPteGlu) could be polyglutamated directly. Our work described here shows that homofolate polyglutamates do show some inhibition of thymidylate synthase and aminoimidazaolecarboxamide ribonucleotide formyltransferase. However, our evidence indicates that the cytotoxicity of homofolate involves its reduction to

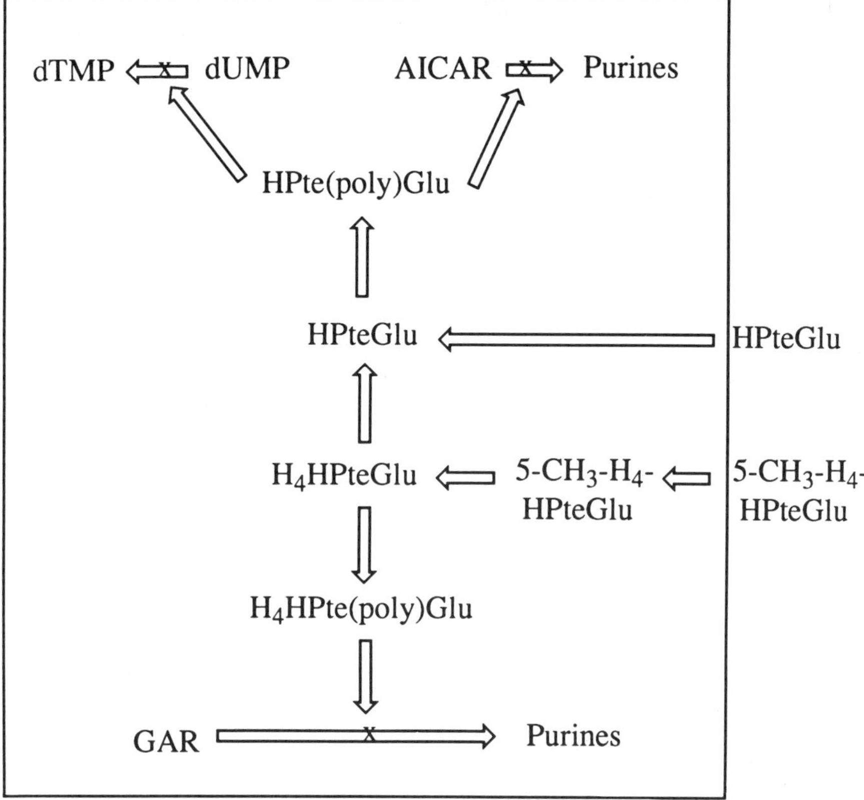

FIG. 12-2. Potential metabolites and potential inhibitory sites of homofolates.

tetrahydrohomofolate (H_4HPteGlu) as well as its polyglutamation with glycinamide ribonucleotide formyltransferase as the primary target. 5-Methyltetrahydrohomofolate (5-CH_3-H_4HPteGlu) may be metabolically demethylated to tetrahydrohomofolate (Taylor & Hanna, 1974) as shown or could be converted directly to polyglutamate forms. The ultimate target of 5-methyltetrahydrohomofolate is assumed to be glycinamide ribonucleotide formyltransferase.

We here review new evidence on the mechanism of the antitumor and cytotoxic activity of homofolates as well as the inhibition of folate enzymes by homofolate polyglutamates. Special emphasis will be placed on stereochemical aspects related to the configuration at carbon 6 of tetrahydrohomofolates. We will also discuss the chemotherapeutic potential of homofolates in relation to other developments in the antifolate field.

2. ANTITUMOR ACTIVITY OF HOMOFOLATES

The inhibition of the growth of folate-requiring bacteria by (6RS)-tetrahydrohomofolate was shown to be caused by the compound with the (6R) (unnatural) configuration at carbon 6 (Fig. 12-1) (Kisliuk & Gaumont, 1970, 1971). The (6S) (natural) form served as a growth factor for these organisms in place of folate. To determine the effect of stereochemical configuration on antitumor activity, the individual diastereoisomers of 5-methyltetrahydrohomofolate were prepared and tested against a methotrexate-resistant variant of L1210, L1210/FR8 (Mead et al., 1966) known to have elevated dihydrofolate reductase activity. Recent experiments showed that both the R and S diastereoisomers of 5-methyltetrahydrohomofolate are transported into L1210 cells (Sirotnak et al., 1987). The results of Table 12-1 show that, in contrast to the bacterial system, both diastereoisomers show antitumor activity.

TABLE 12-1. *Evaluation of the Antitumor Activity of Diastereoisomers of 5-Methyltetrahydrohomofolate Against L1210/FR8 Murine Leukemia*

Compound (mg/kg)	Increase in lifespan (%)
Methotrexate	
0.75	5
1.5	<0
3.0	<0
Tetrahydrohomofolate	
(6RS) 200	29
(6R)* 200	49
(6S)† 200	60

*Unnatural diastereomer.
†Natural diastereomer.

BDF 1 mice, 19–21 g, eight mice for each dose, were inoculated IP with 6×10^6 L1210/FR8 cells on day 1. Drugs in saline given daily IP for eight days. L1210/FR8 is a methotrexate-resistant strain of L1210 with high dihydrofolate reductase levels.

2.1. CYTOTOXICITY OF HOMOFOLATES AGAINST HUMAN LYMPHOMA CELLS

From the foregoing it would be anticipated that the growth of tissue culture cells incubated with homofolate would be inhibited because the homofolate would be expected to be reduced to (6S)-tetrahydrohomofolate intracellularly, catalyzed by dihydrofolate reductase. Homofolate is known to inhibit the growth of sarcoma 180 cells (Divekar & Hakala, 1975). We show here (Fig. 12-3A) that homofolate also inhibits the growth of Manca human lymphoma cells (Nishikori et al., 1984) where the IC_{50} for homofolate is 6 μM. The inhibitory effect of homofolate is completely prevented by addition of inosine, indicating a block in purine biosynthesis.

The inhibitory effect of homofolate is partially blocked by the addition of low levels of the dihydrofolate reductase inhibitor trimetrexate, which when added alone causes no growth inhibition. These results are consistent with the view that homofolate must be reduced before it becomes cytotoxic.

As expected, (6RS)-5-methyltetrahydrohomofolate also inhibits the growth of cultured Manca cells ($IC_{50} = 8$ μM), an effect also prevented by inosine (Fig. 12-3B). However, in this case, the addition of subinhibitory levels of trimetrexate enhances growth inhibition. Although it was anticipated that trimetrexate would not diminish the growth inhibition caused by 5-methyltetrahydrohomofolate, since the latter is already at the tetrahydro level, it was not anticipated that trimetrexate would enhance growth inhibition. However, other examples of enhanced growth inhibition when an inhibitor of glycinamide ribonucleotide formyltransferase, 5,10-dideazatetrahydrofolate, is combined with a dihydrofolate reductase inhibitor have recently been reported and will be discussed shortly.

3. INHIBITION OF FOLATE ENZYMES BY HOMOFOLATE POLYGLUTAMATES

From our present knowledge of the metabolism of folates and antifolates, it would be anticipated that homofolate and tetrahydrohomofolate would be converted to polyglutamate forms (Fig. 12-4) in cells and that these polyglutamate forms would show enhanced inhibition of folate enzymes as compared with the monoglutamate forms (Kisliuk, 1984). It is known that homofolates are substrates for mammalian folylpolyglutamate synthetase (McGuire et al., 1980; Cook et al., 1987). We therefore undertook the synthesis of homofolate and tetrahydrohomofolate polyglutamates and determined their inhibition of folate enzymes.

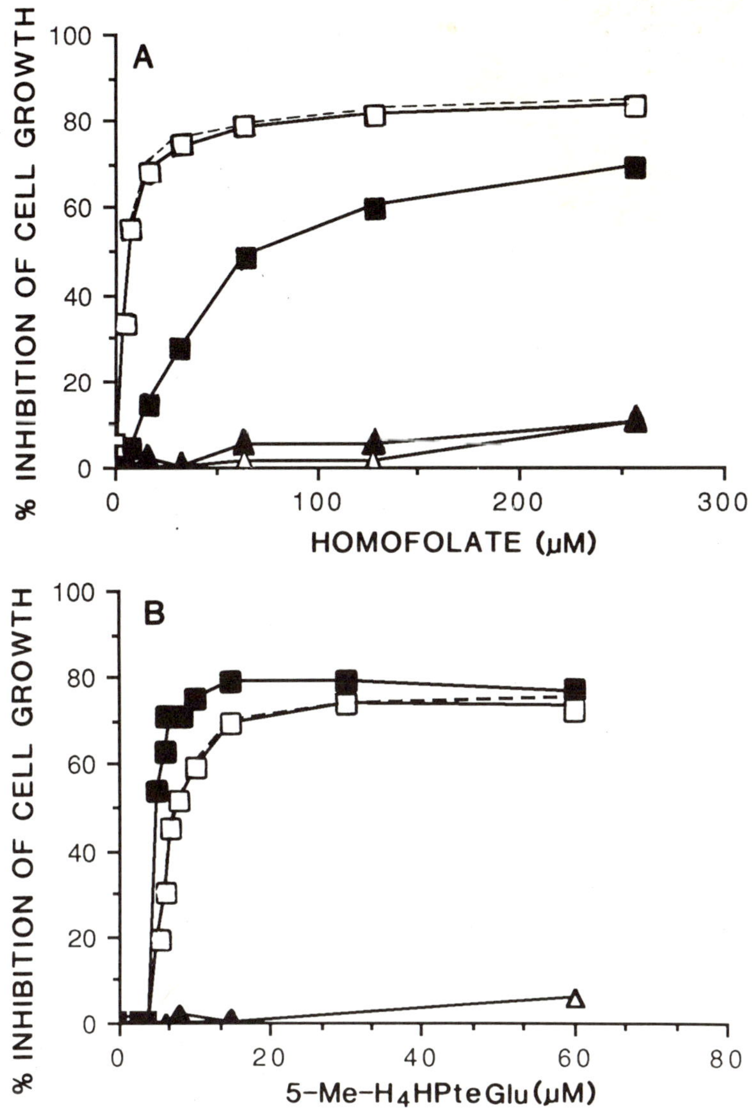

FIG. 12-3. Effect of combinations of homofolate (HPteGlu) or (RS)-5-methyltetrahydrohomofolate ($5\text{-}CH_3\text{-}H_4PteGlu$) with trimetrexate on the growth of cultured Manca human lymphoma cells. (A) Cultures were grown 72 hr in 96-well microtiter plates starting with 7000 cells per well, and growth was estimated by tetrazolium reduction. (□ — □) HPteGlu alone, (■ — ■) plus 10 nM trimetrexate (TMTX), (△ — △) plus 0.1 mM inosine, (▲ — ▲) plus 10 nM TMTX plus 0.1 mM inosine. (B) Same as (A) except that homofolate was replaced with (6RS)-5-methyltetrahydrohomofolate.

The most striking inhibition was found against glycinamide ribonucleotide formyltransferase derived either from Manca cells or L1210 cells (Table 12-2). While homofolate and tetrahydrohomofolate monoglutamates as well as homofolate polyglutamates were not inhibitory, tetrahydrohomofolate polyglutamates were strong inhibitors. In Manca cell extracts, inhibition by the (6RS) Glu_6 is competitive with the substrate, 10-formyltetrahydrofolate, with a K_i value of 0.3 μM (data not shown). As shown in Fig. 12-5, inhibition generally increases with increasing glutamate chain length. In addition, the dihydrohexaglutamate is somewhat less inhibitory than the (6RS)-tetrahydrohexaglutamate.

The individual diastereoisomers at carbon 6 of tetrahydrohomofolate hexaglutamate were tested for inhibition of glycinamide ribonucleotide formyltransferase in Manca cell and L1210 cell extracts (Table 12-2). In Manca cell extracts the (6S) form is four times more inhibitory than the (6R) form, whereas in the L1210 extracts the situation is reversed,

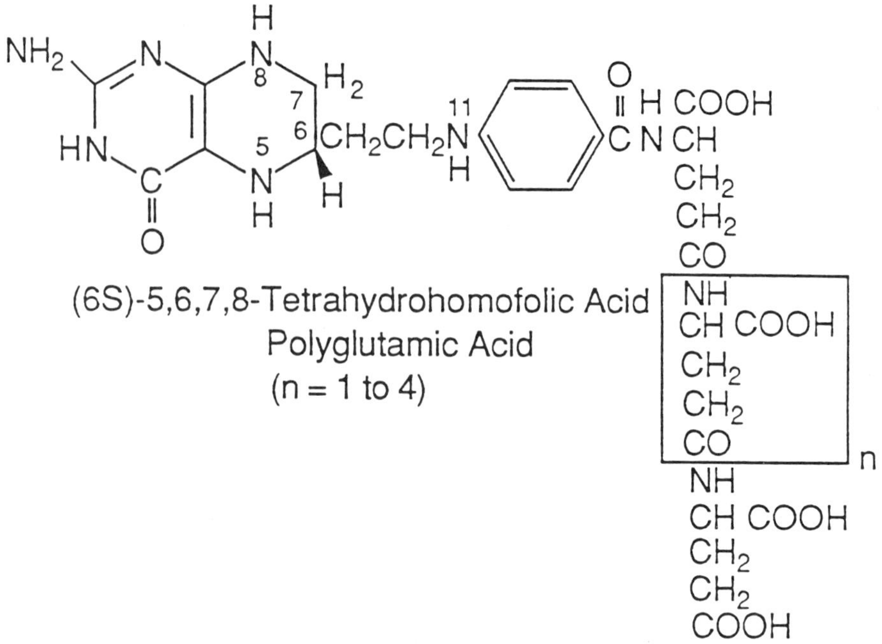

(6S)-5,6,7,8-Tetrahydrohomofolic Acid Polyglutamic Acid (n = 1 to 4)

FIG. 12-4. The structure of tetrahydrohomofolate polyglutamate.

the (6R) form being twice as inhibitory as the (6S) form. These differences are further illustrated in Fig. 12-6AB which compares inhibition by the individual diastereoisomers with the (6RS) mixture. The similar potency of the 6S and 6R hexaglutamate forms in inhibiting glycinamide ribonucleotide formyltransferase in L1210 cell extracts is consistent with the similar antitumor activity against L1210 shown by the 6S and 6R forms of 5-methyltetrahydrohomofolate (Table 12-1).

Additional folate enzymes tested for inhibition by homofolates in Manca cell extracts were aminoimidazolecarboxamide ribonucleotide formyltransferase, thymidylate synthase, and serine hydroxymethyltransferase (Table 12-3). Inhibition of these enzymes is much weaker than for glycinamide ribonucleotide formyltransferase, especially for the tetrahydrohomofolate hexaglutamate, the likely intracellular form. It is conceivable, however, that tetrahydrohomofolate polyglutamates are metabolized to 5 or 10-formyl, 5,10-methylene, or 5-methyltetrahydrohomofolates which could be more effective enzyme inhibitors.

TABLE 12-2. *Inhibition of Glycinamide Ribonucleotide Formyltransferase* from Manca Human Lymphoma Cells and L1210 Murine Leukemia Cells by Homofolate (HPteGlu) Derivatives*

	IC_{50} μM	
Compound	Manca	L1210
$HPteGlu_1$	>20	>20
$HPteGlu_6$	>20	>20
(6RS)-$H_4HPteGlu_1$	>20	>20
(6RS)-$H_4HPteGlu_6$	0.5	0.6
(6S)-$H_4HPteGlu_6$	0.37	0.74
(6R)-$H_4HPteGlu_6$	1.5	0.33

*Assayed by the method of Smith et al. (1981).

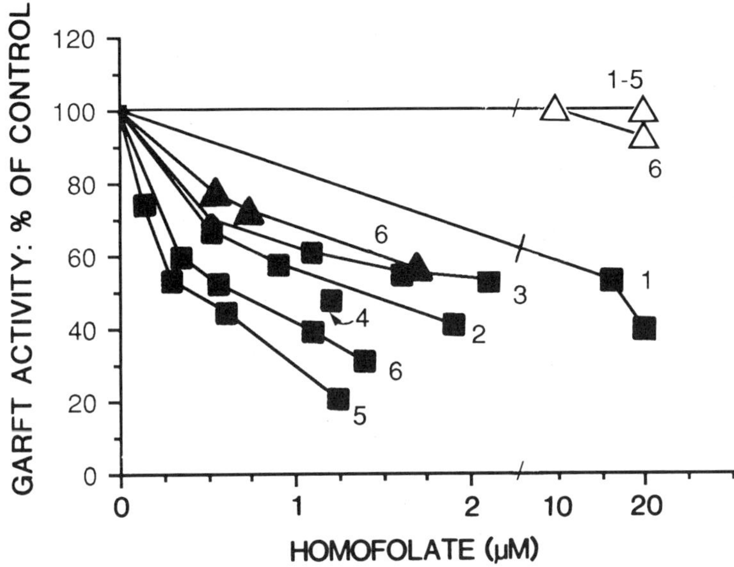

FIG. 12-5. The effect of polyglutamate chain length on the inhibition of glycinamide ribonucleotide formyltransferase derived from Manca human lymphoma cells. The total number of glutamate residues is indicated on each curve: (△ — △) homofolate, (▲ — ▲) dihydrohomofolate, (■ — ■) (6RS)-tetrahydrohomofolate. Assay as described by Smith et al. (1981).

3.1. Inhibition of Bacterial Folate Enzymes by Homofolates

The inhibition of *Lactobacillus casei* glycinamide ribonucleotide formyltransferase shows some similarities as well as striking differences when compared to the mammalian enzymes. In both systems the tetrahydrohomofolates are more inhibitory than homofolates. However, with the *L. casei* enzyme, tetrahydrohomofolate is a potent inhibitor even without polyglutamation. The addition of five glutamate residues increases inhibition only twofold (Table 12-4). Another striking difference between the mammalian and *L. casei* enzymes is that the latter shows a much greater differential inhibition between diastereoisomers. The tetrahydrohomofolate Glu_6 derivative with the 6R (unnatural) configuration is 40 times more inhibitory than the 6S (natural) form. The differential inhibition between diastereoisomers is even greater with 11-deazatetrahydrohomofolate derivatives where the 6R form is at least 100 times more potent than the 6S form.

TABLE 12-3. *Inhibition of Folate Enzymes from Manca Human Lymphoma Cells by Homofolate (HPteGlu) Derivatives*

	IC_{50} μM		
Compound	AICAR formyltransferase*	Thymidylate synthase†	Serine hydroxymethyltransferase‡
$HPteGlu_1$	>20	>20	>20
$HPteGlu_6$	2.1	9	>20
(6RS)-$H_4HPteGlu_1$	>20	>20	>20
(6RS)-$H_4HPteGlu_6$	10	>20	>20

*Assayed by the method of Baggott & Krumdieck (1979).
†Assayed by the method of Herzfeld & Raper (1980).
‡Assayed by the method of Thorndike et al. (1979).

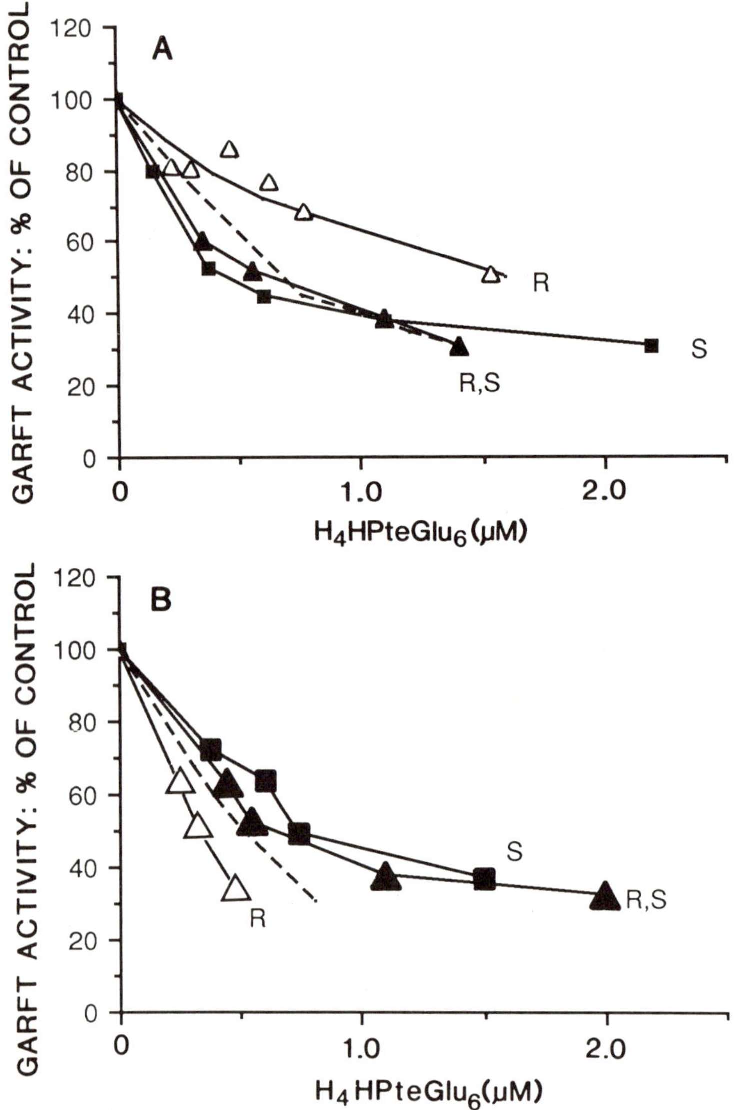

FIG. 12-6. The effect of diastereoisomers of tetrahydrohomofolate hexaglutamate (H_4HPteGlu$_6$) on glycinamide ribonucleotide formyltransferase activity. (A) Manca cell extracts. (B) L1210 cell extracts. S represents the natural diastereoisomer, R the unnatural diastereoisomer, and RS the equimolar mixture of diastereoisomers at carbon 6. The dashed lines represent the additive values expected for the RS mixture calculated from the values obtained for R and S individually by the fractional inhibition method (Harvey, 1982).

L. casei thymidylate synthase is at least 28 times more susceptible to inhibition by (6RS) tetrahydrohomofolate hexaglutamate than the corresponding Manca cell enzyme (Table 12-5, Table 12-3). Experiments with the individual diastereoisomers of tetrahydrohomofolate pentaglutamate (Table 12-5) show that the 6R form is about 5 times more inhibitory than the 6S form. These results suggest that bacterial growth inhibition by (6R)-tetrahydrohomofolate (Kisliuk & Gaumont, 1970, 1971) is due to its conversion to polyglutamates which inhibit thymidylate synthase. This is consistent with the reversal of *L. casei* growth inhibition by thymidine (Goodman et al., 1964). Since the bacterial growth medium used contained purines, inhibition of glycinamide ribonucleotide formyltransferase by tetrahydrohomofolate polyglutamates would not be expected to inhibit growth.

TABLE 12-4. *Inhibition of Glycinamide Ribonucleotide Formyltransferase* from* Lactobacillus casei *by Homofolate (HPteGlu) Derivatives*

Compound	IC_{50} μM
$HPteGlu_1$	>20
$HPteGlu_6$	>20
(6RS)-$H_4HPteGlu_1$	0.9
(6RS)-$H_4HPteGlu_6$	0.4
(6S)-$H_4HPteGlu_6$	4.0
(6R)-$H_4HPteGlu_6$	0.1
(6RS)-11-Deaza-$H_4HPteGlu_1$	0.05**
(6S)-11-Deaza-$H_4HPteGlu_1$	>5.0**
(6RS)-8-Deaza-$H_4HPteGlu_1$	>20†

*Assayed as described by Smith et al. (1981).
**Nair et al. (1989).
†DeGraw et al. (1988).

TABLE 12-5. *Inhibition of* Lactobacillus casei *Thymidylate Synthase* by Homofolate (HPteGlu) Derivatives*

Compound	IC_{50} μM
$HPteGlu_1$	>20
$HPteGlu_6$	6.4
(6RS)-$H_4HPteGlu_1$	>20
(6RS)-$H_4HPteGlu_6$	0.7
(6S)-$H_4HPteGlu_5$	5
(6R)-$H_4HPteGlu_5$	1

*Assayed by the method of Wahba & Friedkin (1962).

4. CHEMOTHERAPEUTIC POTENTIAL OF HOMOFOLATES

A limited phase I clinical trial of (6RS)-5-methyltetrahydrohomofolate (Cohen et al., 1982) did not show antitumor activity and the low potency of the compound limits its utility. Its potency is most likely restricted because (1) it is relatively poorly transported (Sirotnak et al., 1987), (2) it is a relatively poor substrate for folylpolyglutamate synthetase (McGuire et al., 1980; Cook et al., 1987), and (3) compared to the powerful inhibition of dihydrofolate reductase by methotrexate, tetrahydrohomofolate is a modest inhibitor of glycinamide ribonucleotide formyltransferase even after polyglutamylation (Table 12-2). None of the congeners of homofolate, 11-thiohomofolate (Nair et al., 1979), 11-oxohomofolate (Nair et al., 1980), 1′,2′,3′,4′,5′,6′-hexahydrohomofolate (Nair et al., 1983), 8-deazahomofolic acid (DeGraw et al., 1988), or their tetrahydro forms have shown outstanding biological activity. Nonetheless, work with homofolates established that antitumor activity is possible with glycinamide ribonucleotide formyltransferase as the target enzyme.

5,10-Dideazatetrahydrofolate (Fig. 12-7) (Beardsley et al., 1986) is an inhibitor of glycinamide ribonucleotide formyltransferase which shows promising antitumor activity in experimental systems. Both 5,10-dideazatetrahydrofolate (Shih et al., 1988) and 5-methyltetrahydrohomofolate show low stereospecificity at carbon 6 toward growth inhibition of cells in culture and both compounds also show synergistic inhibition of the growth of human lymphoma cells when combined with the dihydrofolate reductase inhibitor trimetrexate (Fig. 12-3B, Fig. 12-8). The combination of 5,10-dideazatetrahydrofolate and trimetrexate also shows synergistic inhibition of the growth of rat hepatoma cells (Galivan et al., 1988) and combination of 5,10-dideazatetrahydrofolate and trimethoprim shows synergistic inhibition of the growth of *L. casei* (Thorndike et al., 1988). Thus, combination of an inhibitor of dihydrofolate reductase with an inhibitor of glycinamide ribonucleotide

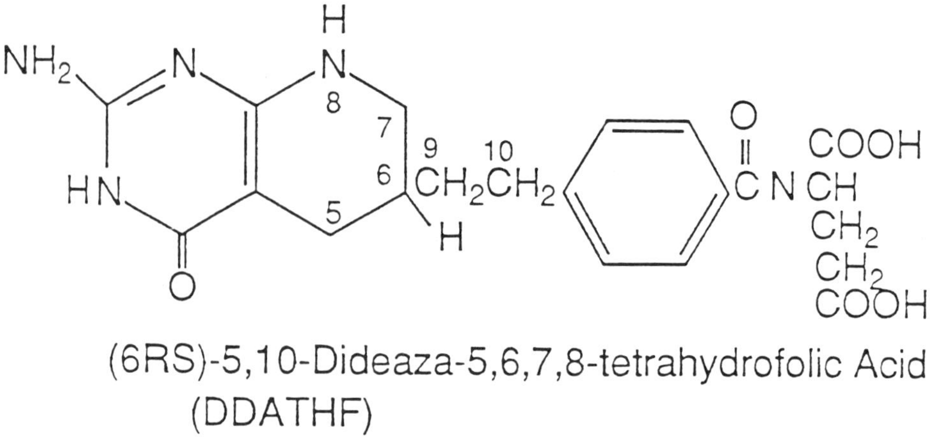

(6RS)-5,10-Dideaza-5,6,7,8-tetrahydrofolic Acid (DDATHF)

FIG. 12-7. The structure of 5,10-dideazatetrahydrofolic acid.

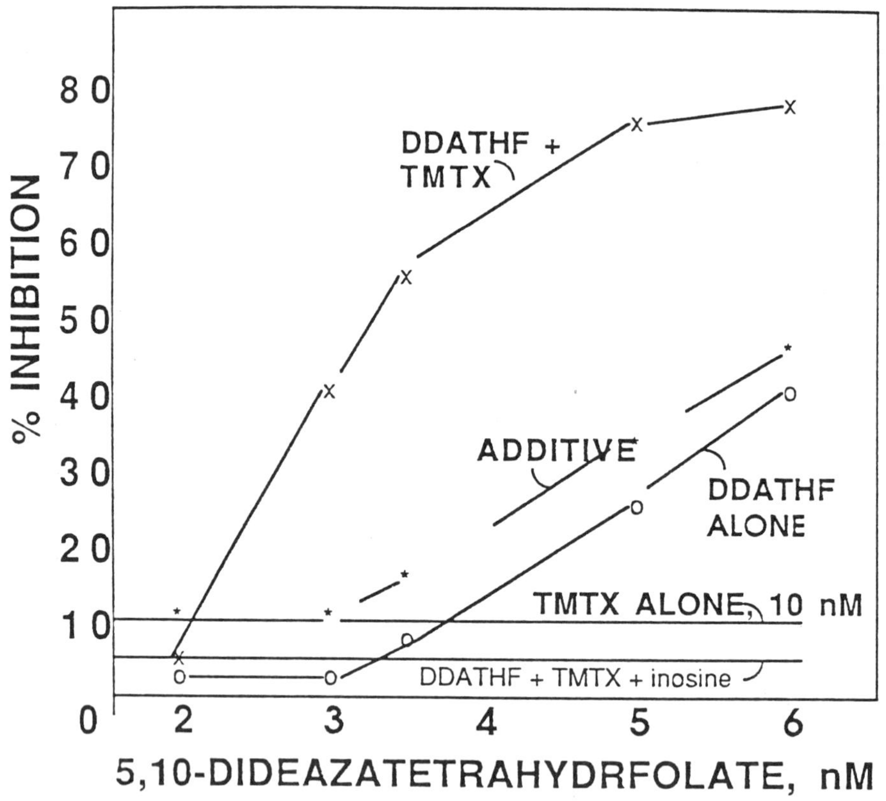

FIG. 12-8. Inhibition of the growth of Manca human lymphoma cells by combination of 5,10-dideazatetrahydrofolate (DDATHF) and trimetrexate (TMTX). Conditions as described in the Fig. 12-3 legend.

formyltransferase is potentially useful in antibacterial as well as antitumor chemotherapy.

It is noteworthy in this connection that the combination of dihydrofolate reductase inhibitors with a specific inhibitor of thymidylate synthase, 10-propargyl-5,8-dideazafolate, also leads to synergistic inhibition of *L. casei* (Kisliuk et al., 1985), Manca human lymphoma (Y. Gaumont, J. Thorndike, and R. L. Kisliuk, unpublished work), and rat hepatoma (Galivan et al., 1987) cell growth. These results illustrate instances where growth inhibition by prevention of either purine or thymidylate biosynthesis can be selectively enhanced by combination with a dihydrofolate reductase inhibitor.

An intriguing aspect of work with tetrahydrohomofolates is the selective inhibition of bacterial systems by compounds having the unnatural configuration at carbon 6. Inhibition of *L. casei* glycinamide ribonucleotide formyltransferase by (6R)-tetrahydrohomofolate hexaglutamate and (6R)11-deazatetrahydrohomofolate (Table 12-4) as well as the selective inhibition of *L. casei* thymidylate synthase by (6R)-tetrahydrohomofolate pentaglutamate (Table 12-5) suggest that useful chemotherapeutic agents containing the 6R configuration found in tetrahydrohomofolate might be developed.

Acknowledgments—Homofolate and (6RS)-5-methyltetrahydrohomofolate (NSC 139490) were kindly supplied by Dr. J. A. R. Mead from the National Cancer Institute. This work was supported by National Cancer Institute grants CA 10914 (RK), CA 22764, CA 08748, CA 18856 (FMS), CA 32687 (MGN), and CA 25236 (JRP).

REFERENCES

Baggott, J. E., and Krumdieck, C. L. (1979) Folyl-gamma-glutamates as cosubstrates of 10-formyltetrahydrofolate: 5′phosphoribosyl-5-amino-4-imidazolecarboxamide formyltransferase. *Biochemistry* **18**: 1036–1041.

Beardsley, G. P., Taylor, E. C., Grindey, G. B., and Moran, R. G. (1986) Deaza derivatives of tetrahydrofolic acid. A new class of folate antimetabolites. In *Chemistry and biology of pteridines*, B. A. Cooper and V. M. Whitehead, eds., pp. 953–957. Berlin: W. de Gruyter.

Cohen, G. I., Parker, L. M., Rosowsky, A., Ervin, T. J., Modest, E. J., and Frei, E., III. (1982) 5-Methyltetrahydrohomofolate (MTHHF): Phase 1 trial and pharmacology in man. *Proc. Am. Soc. Clin. Oncol.* **1**: 14.

Cook, J. D., Cichowicz, D. J., Sabu, G., Lawler, A., and Shane, B. (1987) Mammalian folyl-gamma-glutamate synthetase. 4. In vitro and in vivo metabolism of folates and analogues and regulation of folate homeostasis. *Biochemistry* **26**: 530–539.

Crusberg, T. C., Leary, R. P., and Kisliuk, R. L. (1970) Properties of thymidylate synthetase from dichloromethotrexate-resistant Lactobacillus casei. *J. Biol. Chem.* **245**: 5292–5296.

DeGraw, J. I., Colwell, W. T., Brown, V. H., Sato, M., Kisliuk, R. L., Gaumont, Y., Thorndike, J., and Sirotnak, F. M. (1988) Synthesis and biological evaluation of 8-deazahomofolic acid and its tetrahydro derivative. *J. Med. Chem.* **31**: 150–153.

Divekar, A. Y., and Hakala, M. T. (1975) Inhibition of the biosynthesis of 5′-phosphoribosyl-N-formylglycinamide in sarcoma 180 cells by homofolate. *Mol. Pharmacol.* **11**: 319–325.

Dwivedi, C. M., Kisliuk, R. L., and Baugh, C. M. (1983) The interaction of pteroylpolyglutamates with calf thymus thymidylate synthase. In: *Folyl and antifolyl polyglutamates*, I. D., Goldman, B. A. Chabner, J. R. Bertino, eds., pp. 65–70. New York: Plenum Press.

Friedkin, M., Crawford, E. J., and Plante, L. T. (1971) Empirical vs. rational approaches in cancer chemotherapy. *Ann. N.Y. Acad. Sci.* **186**: 209–213.

Galivan, J., Nimec, Z., Rhee, M., Boschelli, D., Oronsky, A. L., and Kerwar, S. S. (1988) Antifolate drug interactions: Enhancement of growth inhibition due to the antipurine 5,10-dideazatetrahydrofolic acid by the lipophilic dihydrofolate reductase inhibitors metoprine and trimetrexate. *Cancer Res.* **48**: 2421–2425.

Galivan, J., Nimec, Z., and Rhee, M. (1987) Synergistic inhibition of rat hepatoma cells exposed in vitro to N10-propargyl-5,8-dideazafolate with methotrexate or the lipophilic antifolates trimetrexate or metoprine. *Cancer Res.* **47**: 5256–5260.

Goodman, L., DeGraw, J. I., Kisliuk, R. L., Friedkin, M., Pastore, E. J., Crawford, E. J., Plante, L. T., Al-Nahas, A., Morningstar, J. R., Kwok, G., Wilson, L., Donovan, E., and Ratzan, J. (1964) Tetrahydrohomofolate, a specific inhibitor of thymidylate synthetase. *J. Am. Chem. Soc.* **86**: 808–809.

Harvey, R. J. (1982) Synergism in the folate pathway. *Rev. Infect. Dis.* **4**: 255–260.

Herzfeld, A., and Raper, S. M. (1980) Relative activities of thymidylate synthetase and thymidine kinase in rat tissues. *Cancer Res.* **40**: 744–750.

Kisliuk, R. L. (1984) The biochemistry of folates. In *Folate antagonists as chemotherapeutic agents*, F. M., Sirotnak, J. J. Burchall, W. B. Ensminger, and J. Montgomery, eds., Vol. 1, pp. 1–68. Orlando, FL: Academic Press.

Kisliuk, R. L. (1982) Homofolates and other 2-NH_2-4-oxy antifolates. In *New approaches to the design of antineoplastic agents*, T. J. Bardos, and T. I. Kalman, eds., pp. 201–214. New York: Elsevier Biomedical.

Kisliuk, R. L. (1960) Reduced folic acid analogs as antimetabolites. *Nature* **188**: 584–585.

Kisliuk, R. L., Gaumont, Y., Kumar, P., Coutts, M., Nair, M. G., Nanavati, N. T., and Kalman, T. I. (1985) The effect of polyglutamylation on the inhibitory activity of folate analogs. In *Folyl and antifolyl polyglutamates*, I. D. Goldman, ed., Vol. 2, pp. 319–328. New York: Praeger.

Kisliuk, R. L., and Gaumont, Y. (1971) Action of diastereoisomers of tetrahydrohomofolate on the growth of *Lactobacillus casei*. *Ann. N.Y. Acad. Sci.* **186**: 438–440.

Kisliuk, R. L., and Gaumont, Y. (1970) Tetrahydrohomofolate, an inhibitor of folate transport in *Streptococcus faecium*. In *Chemistry and biology of pteridines*, K. Iwai, M. Akino, M. Goto, and Y. Iwanami, eds., pp. 357–364. Tokyo: International Academic Printing.

Loo, T. L., Juishi, L., Lu, K., and Savara, N. (1983) Clinical pharmacology of 5-methyltetrahydrohomofolate. *Cancer Res.* **43**: 921–924.

McGuire, J. J., Hsieh, P., Coward, J. K., and Bertino, J. R. (1980) Enzymatic synthesis of folyl polyglutamates: Characterization of the reaction and its products. *J. Biol. Chem.* **255**: 5776–5778.

Mead, J. A. R., Goldin, A., Kisliuk, R. L., Friedkin, M., Plante, L., Crawford, E. J., and Kwok, G. (1966) Pharmacological aspects of homofolate derivatives in relation to amethopterin-resistant murine leukemia. *Cancer Res.* **26**: 2374–2379.

Nair, M. G., Murthy, B. R., Patil, S. D., Kisliuk, R. L., Thorndike, J., Gaumont, Y., Ferone, R., Duch, D. S., and Edelstein, M. P. (1989) Folate analogues. 31. Synthesis of the reduced derivatives of 11-deazahomofolic acid, 10-methyl-11-deazahomofolic acid, and their evaluation as inhibitors of glycinamide ribonucleotide formyltransferase. *J. Med. Chem.* **32**: 1277–1283.

Nair, M. G., Otis, E. B., Kisliuk, R. L., and Gaumont, Y. (1983) Folate analogues. 20. Synthesis and antifolate activity of 1′,2′,3′,4′,5′,6′-hexahydrohomofolic acid. *J. Med. Chem.* **26**: 135–140.

Nair, M. G., Saunders, C., Chen, S.-Y., Kisliuk, R. L., and Gaumont, Y. (1980) Folate analogues altered in the C9-N10 bridge region. 14. 11-Oxahomofolic acid, a potential antitumor agent. *J. Med. Chem.* **23**: 59–65.

Nair, M. G., Chen, Y.-C., Kisliuk, R. L., Gaumont, Y., and Strumpf, D. (1979) Folate analogues altered in the C^9-N^{10} bridge region: 11-thiohomofolic acid. *J. Med. Chem.* **22**: 850–855.

Nishikori, M., Hansen, H., Jhanwar, S., Fried, J., Sordillo, P., Koziner, B., Lloyd, K., and Clarkson, B. (1984) Establishment of a near-tetraploid B-cell lymphoma line with duplication of the 8,14 translocation. *Cancer Genetics and Cytogenetics* **12**: 39–50.

Shih, C., Grindey, G. B., Houghton, P. J., and Houghton, J. A. (1988) In vivo antitumor activity of 5,10-dideazatetrahydrofolic acid (DDATHF) and its diastereomeric isomers. *Proc. Am. Assoc. Cancer Research* **29**: 283.

Sirotnak, F. M., Goutas, L., Jacobsen, D. M., Mines, L., Barruecco, J. R., Gaumont, Y., and Kisliuk, R. L. (1987) Carrier-mediated transport of folate compounds in L1210 cells. Initial rate kinetics and extent of duality of entry routes for folic acid and diastereoisomers of 5-methyltetrahydrohomofolate in the presence of physiological anions. *Biochem. Pharmacol.* **36**: 1659–1667.

Smith, G. K., Benkovic, P. A., and Benkovic, S. J. (1981) L-(-)-10-Formyltetrahydrofolate is the cofactor for glycinamide ribonucleotide transformylase from chicken liver. *Biochemistry* **20**: 4034–4036.

Taylor, R. T., and Hanna, M. L. (1974) 5-Methyltetrahydrohomofolate: A substrate for cobalamin methyltransferase and an inhibitor of cell growth. *Arch. Biochem. Biophys.* **163**: 122–132.

Thorndike, J., Gaumont, Y., Powers, J., Kisliuk, R. L., and Piper, J. R. (1988) Synergistic growth inhibition of human lymphoma cells by combination of trimetrexate with 5,10-dideazatetrahydrofolate. *Proc. Am. Assoc. Cancer Research* **29**: 285.

Thorndike, J., Pelliniemi, T. P., and Beck, W. S. (1979) Serine transhydroxymethylase and serine incorporation in leukocytes. *Cancer Res.* **39**: 3435–3440.

Wahba, A. J., and Friedkin, M. (1962) The enzymatic synthesis of thymidylate. 1. Early steps in the purification of thymidylate synthetase of *Escherichia coli*. *J. Biol. Chem.* **237**: 3794–3801.

CHAPTER 13

ANTIFUNGAL DRUGS: CURRENT PROBLEMS, FUTURE PROSPECTS

David Kerridge
Department of Biochemistry, Cambridge University, Cambridge, United Kingdom

1. INTRODUCTION

In recent years fungi have assumed much greater importance as human pathogens. This has resulted from changes in medical practice and in the diseases to which man is exposed. Many fungi, not normally pathogenic to humans, can give rise to severe life-threatening infections in compromised hosts (Table 13-1). The problem is further exacerbated by the difficulties associated with diagnosis of systemic infections and by the lack of nontoxic drugs suitable for prophylactic administration and for treating patients with systemic mycoses. There are innumerable compounds which inhibit growth of pathogenic fungi *in vitro* (Ryley et al., 1981), but the majority are too toxic to be used clinically. The underlying reason for this is that pathogenic fungi like their human hosts are eukaryotic organisms, and since their metabolism is fundamentally similar, the number of suitable targets for therapeutic attack is limited (Table 13-1).

The research which heralded the current era of antifungal therapy was the isolation and characterization of griseofulvin by Oxford et al. (1939). The clinical use of this compound did not occur until the late 1950s when it was shown to eradicate recalcitrant dermatophytic infections from humans. Griseofulvin is one of the few antifungal drugs that can be administered orally, and it is unfortunate that its use is restricted to dermatophytic fungi (Davies, 1980). Since 1950 when the first polyene macrolide antibiotic was isolated (Hazen & Brown, 1950), a number of other antifungal drugs have been introduced into clinical practice, but only amphotericin B, 5-fluorocytosine, and certain azole derivatives are suitable for treating patients suffering from systemic mycoses.

A number of comprehensive reviews on the molecular basis of action of antifungal drugs are available (Kerridge, 1986; Bolard, 1986; Vanden Bossche et al., 1987b; Kerridge, 1988), and this chapter is intended to highlight both the deficiencies in our knowledge of the mode of action of antifungal drugs and the areas of research which might prove fruitful in the search for more effective antifungal agents.

Table 13-1. *Fungal Infections of Man*

Site of infection	Disease	Causative organism	Antifungal drugs used in therapy
Lung	Aspergillosis*	*Aspergillus fumigatus**	Amphotericin B (itraconazole, fluconazole)
	Blastomycoses	*Blastomyces dermatidis*	Amphotericin B
	Coccidioidomycosis	*Coccidioides immitis*	Amphotericin B
	Cryptococcosis	*Cryptococcus neoformans*	Amphotericin B + 5-fluorocytosine
	Histoplasmosis	*Histoplasma capsulatum*	Amphotericin B
Wounds	Chromomycoses	*Cladosporium carrionii* *Phialophora spp*	Amphotericin B
	Mycetoma	Sixteen spp	Amphotericin B
	Sporotrichosis	*Sporothrix schenkii*	Amphotericin B
Skin and mucous membranes	Candidosis*	*Candida albicans**	Polyene macrolide antibiotics Synthetic azole drugs
	Dermatophytosis	*Epidermophyton* spp *Microsporum* spp *Trichophyton* spp	Azole derivatives Allylamines Thiocarbamates

*Opportunistic infections.

2. MOLECULAR BASIS OF DRUG ACTION

An understanding of the interaction of any antifungal drug with its cellular target(s) is essential to explain its selectivity, that is, drug resistance in the host, and to provide a basis for the development of new compounds affecting the same or similar targets. In this section we shall examine the mechanisms of action of the major clinically important antifungal drugs, consider how well they explain selectivity and drug resistance, and whether our knowledge of their modes of action has advanced to the stage where this information, coupled with a knowledge of the metabolism of both host and pathogen, can be used as a firm foundation for future drug development.

2.1. Drugs Interfering with the Functioning of Cellular Organelles

2.1.1. *Griseofulvin*

Griseofulvin was first studied as a possible systemic antibiotic for controlling plant pathogens (Brian, 1952). This potential was not realized, and its importance as an oral antifungal drug arose from the findings of Gentles (1958) and Williams and colleagues (1958) that it could be used to eradicate dermatophytic infections from both guinea pigs and humans. Many derivatives have been synthesized and examined for biological activity (Crosse et al., 1964), but none has replaced the parent compound in clinical practice.

Griseofulvin induces gross hyphal abnormalities in sensitive fungi and was referred to as a "curling factor" (Brian et al., 1946). It was subsequently shown to block mitosis in both *Vicia faba* and rats (Paget & Walpole, 1958, 1960). It was these observations that initiated studies of the interaction of the antibiotic with cellular microtubules and led to our understanding of its mode of action. At first it was not clear if griseofulvin interacted with tubulin or microtubule associated protein, but studies by Sloboda et al. (1982) resolved this problem. The antibiotic reacts with tubulin in the ratio of 1 mole drug per mole tubulin dimer and in doing so prevents tubule extension. Griseofulvin interacts with tubulin from a wide variety of sources, and selectivity does not result from differences in the affinities of various tubulins for the drug but rather from an inability of the drug to reach its target.

Selectivity, at least among the fungi, apparently results from a failure of the antibiotic to enter the cell (El-Nakeeb & Lampen, 1965), yet nothing is known of the mechanism(s) by which griseofulvin crosses the cell envelope. It is, however, probably another example of "illicit" transport. This is clearly one area worthy of detailed study if this compound is to retain its role as an effective oral drug in the treatment of patients suffering from dermatophytic infections and to undergo further development.

An alternative explanation was offered by Yu and Blank (1973) for its action *in vivo*. These authors observed that the association of griseofulvin with keratin rendered this protein less susceptible to proteolytic attack. If this occurs *in vivo* after oral administration of griseofulvin, then the availability of nutrient for the dermatophyte may be reduced resulting in a lower growth rate and elimination of the fungus through normal skin growth. These studies have not been followed up, and it would be of interest to investigate the relative importance of these two effects in mediating the elimination of the fungus from the skin. However, the major unresolved problem is: Why can a drug which induces mitotic damage be used effectively to treat patients suffering from recalcitrant dermatophytic infections with few apparent side effects?

2.1.2. *The Polyene Macrolide Antibiotics*

The first polyene macrolide antibiotic was isolated in 1950 by Hazen and Brown, and since then some 200 drugs in this class have been characterized. Although they are effective against a variety of pathogenic fungi, the majority are too toxic to be used clinically. Amphotericin B, in spite of its toxicity, is still the drug of choice for treating patients suffering from systemic mycoses. The polyene macrolide antibiotics have been reviewed on a number of occasions (Bolard, 1986; Kerridge, 1986, 1988), and we shall therefore highlight areas of interest and controversy.

Amphotericin B interacts reversibly with the plasma membrane of sensitive organisms causing impairment of membrane function, cessation of growth, and ultimately cell death. Selectivity results from the antibiotic having a greater affinity for the ergosterol-containing fungal plasma membrane than for the cholesterol-containing mammalian membrane. The primary effect of amphotericin B is to render the plasma membrane permeable to protons (Palacios & Serrano, 1978). There are two important questions to be asked, namely: What is the molecular mechanism by which amphotericin B induces proton permeability in the plasma membrane of sensitive cells? and, Does the enhanced proton permeability of the plasma membrane account for all biological effects observed on addition of the antibiotic to cultures of sensitive fungi?

It has been proposed that the interaction of amphotericin B with the plasma membrane results in the formation of polyene-bounded aqueous pores which render the membrane permeable to protons. Molecular models have been proposed for these pores (Andreoli, 1974; De Kruijff & Demel, 1974; Marty & Finkelstein, 1975). These comprise annuli of polyene molecules in which the hydrophobic face of the amphotericin interacts with membrane lipids (sterols), and the hydrophilic aspect of the molecule faces inward, so producing an aqueous channel through which protons and other ions can pass. Originally, it was thought that two opposing annuli would be required to span the lipid bilayer, but since the drug molecule cannot cross the plasma membrane (Aracava et al., 1981), more recent models have assumed that the pores comprise single annuli of drug molecules, possibly in association with the membrane sterols, and that the lipid bilayer is distorted in the vicinity of the pore (reviewed Kerridge, 1988).

But what is the evidence for such aqueous pores? The interaction of amphotericin B with lipid bilayers is reversible, and any pore formed will be transient. Their size, predicted from molecular models, is such that they will be difficult to demonstrate directly by electron microscopy, and for this reason it is not surprising that there is no direct microscopical evidence for their existence. Morphological changes do occur which involve a clustering of intramembranous particles, and may result from localized changes in membrane fluidity induced by amphotericin B molecules dissociating the membrane sterols from the phospholipids (Pesti et al., 1981). In *Schizosaccharomyces pombe* these morphological changes are restricted to the growing regions of the cell, suggesting that components of the cell envelope other than membrane sterols may be involved in the interaction of the drug with the plasma membrane (Takeo & Arai, 1987).

Other evidence for the presence of polyene-induced aqueous pores has come largely from physical studies of the effects of these drugs on ion permeability in, and electrical conductance through, artificial lipid bilayers (reviewed in Bolard, 1986; Kerridge, 1988). When added to one side of a bilayer only, a situation analogous to adding the drug to a suspension of cells, amphotericin B induces cation permeability, whereas when added to both sides, the membrane becomes permeable to anions. It has been assumed that this difference in ion specificity results from differences in the structures of pores comprising either a single or a double annulus of polyene molecules. Tetraethylammonium effectively blocks amphotericin B-induced ion leakage, and this together with the ion specificity has been considered as good evidence for the presence of polyene-induced aqueous pores. The polyene-induced changes in solute permeability are both time and concentration dependent, and it has been proposed that two types of pore are formed, those formed initially are small and are blocked by tetraethylammonium, whereas those formed later are not and assumed to be larger (Cohen, 1986).

Diagnostic evidence for aqueous pores in lipid bilayers can also be obtained from electrical conductance measurements (reviews Gale et al., 1981; Bolard, 1986). When amphotericin B is added to both sides of a lipid bilayer, discrete current fluctuations, indicative of aqueous pores, occur; such current fluctuations do not occur when the drug is added to one side only. Discrete current fluctuations across lipid bilayers have also been observed in the absence of polyene macrolide antibiotics at the phase transition temperature (Antonov et al., 1980). An explanation for this is that interactions between different lipid domains result in the formation of aqueous pores. If this is so, there is no need to postulate the formation of discrete pores comprising annuli of polyene molecules to explain drug-induced changes in membrane permeability. Spectrophotometric analysis of the interactions between polyene macrolide antibiotics and membrane lipids has provided information on the specificity and stoichiometry of the interactions and on the conformational changes that occur in the antibiotic and the organizational changes in the membrane lipids. Unfortunately such investigations have not produced direct evidence for the presence of polyene-bounded pores in lipid bilayers. Although such structures were first postulated in 1974 (Andreoli, 1974; De Kruijff & Demel, 1974), there is still no definitive proof of their existence.

But are there other possible molecular mechanisms for drug-induced proton permeability? Thomas (1986) proposed that a polyene-induced alteration in the lipid environment of the plasma membrane ATPase could be responsible for the dissipation of the proton gradient, and subsequently Surarit and Shepherd (1987) observed that at the MGIC (minimum growth inhibitory concentration), amphotericin B inhibited (by greater than 70%) a number of plasma membrane associated enzymes, including ATPase. It is perhaps surprising that four decades after the first isolation of a polyene macrolide antibiotic, the mechanism by which amphotericin B affects the functioning of the plasma membrane is still unknown. If amphotericin B or a derivative is to retain its role in the treatment of patients suffering from systemic mycoses, then it is essential that we should understand the precise molecular mechanism by which it interferes with membrane functions.

But is a single primary event, that is, induction of proton permeability, sufficient to account for all the observed biological effects? At concentrations below the MGIC, amphotericin B enhances the plating efficiency of *Candida albicans*. In the absence of the drug it is 60 to 70%, whereas in its presence it is 80 to 95% (Brajtburg et al., 1981). The mycelial form of *Candida albicans* is more sensitive to the drug than is the yeast form, and transient exposure to the drug inhibits both mycelial initiation and development (Nugent et al., 1987). Rast and Bartnicki-Garcia (1981) observed that, at concentrations in excess of the MGIC, amphotericin B and nystatin inhibited chitin synthase in chitosomal preparations from filamentous fungi. More recently Al-Bassam et al. (1985) found that growth in the presence of amphotericin B at concentrations below the MGIC resulted in changes in the composition and antigenicity of the cell wall of *Candida albicans*. Surarit and Shepherd (1987) reported that a number of antifungal drugs which interfere with membrane functions also affect the activity of a number of membrane enzymes, and amphotericin B was no exception. However, it was not clear from their data whether inhibition resulted from a direct effect on the protein or was indirect, resulting from a polyene-induced alteration of the lipid environment of the enzymes. Finally, it has been known for some time that amphotericin B can reversibly affect the permeability of the plasma membrane to a number of substances ranging from inorganic ions to DNA (Cass & Dalmark, 1973; Kumar et al., 1974), a phenomenon which has important implications in the development of combined drug therapy (Medoff, 1988).

It is difficult to explain all these biological effects on the basis of a polyene-induced enhancement of proton leakage across the plasma membrane. This effect may be of great importance in mediating the fungistatic effects of this drug, but polyene-induced alterations in the lipid environment of membrane enzymes may well be responsible for other biological effects.

The fungicidal effects of the polyene macrolide antibiotics were originally thought to result from acidification of the cell contents resulting from proton uptake associated with potassium ion leakage (Lampen, 1966). The first indication that this was not necessarily so came from the findings by Chen et al. (1978) that it was possible to disassociate potassium leakage from the fungicidal effects of the polyenes, and more recently Sokol-Anderson et al. (1986) provided evidence that the fungicidal effects result from a polyene-induced oxidation of the membrane lipids.

Originally polyene-induced potassium leakage was considered sufficient to account for all the effects of these compounds on sensitive fungi, but it is quite clear that a single target is no longer satisfactory to account for all the observable effects on sensitive fungi and that inhibition of cell growth may well result from not only a drug-induced proton leakage but also from impairment of the functioning of a number of membrane enzymes associated with polyene-induced alteration in the lipid fluidity.

2.2. Drugs Affecting Anabolic Reactions Within Sensitive Cells

2.2.1. *5-Fluorocytosine*

As with griseofulvin, the clinical use of 5-fluorocytosine is restricted since it inhibits growth of a limited number of pathogenic fungi. It is well tolerated by humans and can be administered in relatively large doses for prolonged periods with few adverse side effects (Scholer, 1980). It is the one antifungal drug where the mechanism of action is understood and our knowledge of its mode of action owes much to studies on anticancer and antiviral therapy (reviewed in Kerridge, 1986). 5-Fluorocytosine was synthesized as a potential antineoplastic drug (Duschinsky et al., 1957) and subsequently shown to be effective in treating patients suffering from candidosis and cryptococcosis.

5-Fluorocytosine is transported into sensitive fungi by a cytosine permease and converted to 5-fluorouracil by a cytosine deaminase. The 5-fluorouracil is metabolized by enzymes of the pyrimidine salvage pathway to 5-fluorouridine triphosphate, a precursor of aberrant RNA and to 5-fluorodeoxyuridylate, a potent inhibitor of thymidylate synthase and hence DNA synthesis (Polak & Scholer, 1980). Incorporation of 5-fluorouridylate into RNA affects its processing and hence its functioning within the cell. 5-Fluorodeoxyuridylate forms a complex with tetrahydrofolate at the active site of thymidylate synthase which is responsible for its inhibitory effect. The relative importance of these effects in inhibiting growth of sensitive fungi is not known since either would be sufficient to prevent fungal growth.

The selective use of this drug in treating patients with systemic mycoses results from the fact that humans lack cytosine deaminase and cannot convert 5-fluorocytosine to 5-fluorouracil, and although 5-fluorocytosine enters mammalian cells, it is not further metabolized. Unfortunately this relatively nontoxic drug suffers from two serious drawbacks: the first, already alluded to, is the limited number of fungal species inhibited, and the second is the frequent occurrence of resistant strains of *Candida albicans* during therapy. In two clinical surveys (Stiller et al., 1982; Defever et al., 1982), it was found that while some 5% of the isolates tested were completely resistant, approximately 40% were partially resistant to this drug. These partially resistant strains can give rise by UV-induced mitotic segregation to both resistant and sensitive progeny (Whelan et al., 1981).

Resistance to 5-fluorocytosine in yeast can result from the loss of any one of a number of enzymes of the pyrimidine salvage pathway or from a defect in the feedback control of pyrimidine synthesis (Jund & Lacroute, 1970, 1974). However, partial resistance in clinical isolates of *Candida albicans* results predominantly from heterozygosity at the locus coding for the UMP-pyrophosphate phosphoribosyl transferase and defects at other loci are comparatively rare. There is a good gene dosage effect with the enzyme in cell-free extracts of the homozygous sensitive organisms having twice the specific activity of that in extracts of the heterozygous partially resistant strains. The homozygous resistant strain has little or no enzyme activity (Whelan & Kerridge, 1984). *Candida albicans* is diploid (Olaiya & Sogin, 1979), lacking a sexual stage in its life cycle, and one question that must be answered is: Why are 40% of all clinical isolates heterozygous at this locus? Resistance can result from defects in other enzymes of the pyrimidine salvage pathway without affecting either growth or pathogenicity of *Candida albicans*. Are there particular features of this gene which render it more susceptible to mutation? One final question is: Are all resistant isolates related, that is, derived ultimately from a single or few parental strains, or have they arisen independently? In this context it is of interest to note that with the haploid yeast *Candida glabrata*, selection of 5-fluorocytosine-resistant mutants in the laboratory also results predominantly in the appearance of strains lacking UMP-pyrophosphate phosphoribosyl transferase (Fasoli & Kerridge, 1988).

2.2.2. *The Synthetic Azole Derivatives*

Since the first synthetic imidazole derivative (clotrimazole) was introduced into clinical practice (Plempel et al., 1969), many more have been synthesized, and a number are now used clinically. The early derivatives proved too toxic for systemic administration, and currently two triazole derivatives, itraconazole and fluconazole, are being evaluated for systemic use (see Chapter 16). The azole antifungal drugs are important not only in clinical practice but also in agriculture where they are used to control fungal infections of plants and our understanding of their mode of action owes much to studies on plant pathogens (Trinci & Ryley, 1984).

The interactions of the synthetic azole drugs with sensitive organisms are complex and during the past two decades there have been reports of these compounds inhibiting a number of membrane-associated enzymes. Unlike the polyene macrolide antibiotics, these drugs cross the plasma membrane to affect proteins associated with the endoplasmic reticulum and mitochondria. The mechanism(s) by which the azole derivatives traverse the plasma membrane is (are) not known. Brasseur et al. (1983) devised models for the interaction of miconazole and ketoconazole with lipid bilayers but did not propose a mechanism for their uptake. Resistance in certain strains of *Candida albicans* has been shown by Ryley and colleagues (1984) to be associated with the failure of the cells to take up these drugs, suggesting that specific uptake mechanism(s) is (are) involved. If this is so, then it may well be another example of illicit transport. The one feature these compounds have in common is the nitrogen heterocyclic ring. They differ considerably in the other substituent groups, and it would be surprising if the uptake specificity resided solely with the azole moiety of the molecule. It would certainly be of considerable interest to compare, for example, the uptake of the very water-soluble fluconazole with that of the insoluble itraconazole. Not only do these compounds have to cross the plasma membrane to reach their intracellular targets, but they also traverse the cell wall and modifications, both genotypic (Kerridge et al., 1987) and phenotypic (Cope, 1980), occur which prevent this. However, we know even less of the mechanisms by which these drugs cross this structure and of the changes which can occur to prevent it. In the development of further azole derivatives, it would be advantageous to understand the mechanisms by which these compounds cross the cell envelope to reach their intracellular targets.

The azole-induced inhibition of cytochrome P450 sterol demethylase occurs at concentrations of the drug lower than those required to inhibit completely growth of sensitive fungi. And there are two questions to be asked: the first, Is cytochrome P450 sterol demethylase the primary target for drug action and its inhibition responsible for cessation of growth? and if so, Is it the depletion of the membrane ergosterol or the accumulation of the methylated sterols which is responsible for growth inhibition? Cultures of *Saccharomyces cerevisiae* have an absolute requirement for sterols when grown under strictly anaerobic conditions and lanosterol will not satisfy this requirement (Nes et al., 1978), a finding which would support the hypothesis that accumulation of methylated derivatives is responsible for cessation of growth. However, the sterols which accumulate in *Candida albicans* after prolonged incubation in the presence of the azole derivatives are the 3-β-6-α diols (Vanden Bossche et al., 1987a). The authors suggested that by making the sterols less lipophilic, the cells were attempting to eliminate these membrane disturbing compounds and the depletion of ergosterol was more important in mediating their growth inhibitory effects.

Cytochrome P 450 sterol demethylase is not the only membrane-associated enzyme inhibited by azole derivatives, and both mitochondrial ATPase (Portillo & Gancedo, 1984, 1985) and cytochrome oxidase (Shigematsu et al., 1982) have been implicated as primary targets for these drugs. The azole antimycotics inhibit a number of enzymes either directly as in the case of cytochrome P450 sterol demethylase or indirectly (e.g., chitin synthase, Vanden Bossche et al., 1984). More recently, Surarit and Shepherd (1987) have reported that, at the MGIC, miconazole, and ketoconazole inhibit a number of plasma membrane associated enzymes including ATPase, adenylyl cyclase, 5′-nucleotidase. It is not clear from their data if these inhibitory effects were direct or indirect via a modification of the lipid environment in which these enzymes function. The relative importance of these inhibitory effects will depend on the organism, the specific drug, and the environmental conditions. A knowledge of the interactions of these factors is of considerable importance in the development of new and more effective azole antimycotics.

But are the interactions of the azole drugs with these enzymes important in mediating the growth inhibitory effects of these compounds *in vivo*? For topical infections, where the drug is applied as a cream, there will be a high local concentration, and under these conditions it is likely that inhibition of fungal growth results from an impairment of the barrier function of the plasma membrane. For systemic infections, the concentration of drug attainable at the site of infection will be low, and here the indirect effect on yeast mycelial transformation (at least in *Candida albicans*) may well be of prime importance, given that the host's defense mechanisms are more effective against the yeast than against the mycelial form (Borgers et al., 1979).

But as with the polyene macrolide antibiotics, we still lack a complete understanding of the molecular basis of action of the azole antimycotics. There are a number of important questions to be answered concerning the transport of these compounds across the fungal cell envelope and their interaction with membrane-associated proteins before we can attempt a completely rational design of the next generation of azole derivatives.

2.2.3. *Allylamines and Thiocarbamates*

The remaining two groups of antimycotics are the allylamines, naftifine and terbinafine (Stutz, 1987), and the thiocarbamates, tolnaftate and tolciclate (Ryder et al., 1986; Barrett-Bee et al., 1986). These compounds are used as topical drugs to treat patient with superficial fungal infections. Apart from terbinafine, which is being considered as a potential orally administered drug, the others are too toxic for systemic use. The target for both groups of compounds is squalene epoxidase, one of the first enzymes in the sterol biosynthesis pathway. Selectivity results from the differences in the affinity of these drugs for the enzyme, and as yet there is no evidence for the occurrence of resistant strains of fungi in clinical practice.

3. THE FUTURE

Since the discovery of griseofulvin, considerable advances have been made in the treatment of patients with mycotic infections and in our understanding of the modes of action of clinically important antifungal drugs. Unfortunately, however, the range of such drugs is limited, and as yet there are no nontoxic drugs available suitable for treating patients with systemic infections. The first part of this chapter outlined the deficiencies in our knowledge of the molecular mechanisms of action of the antifungal drugs, here we consider possible future developments in antifungal chemotherapy.

In the past, drugs have been discovered largely as a result of random screening of either natural products or synthetic chemicals produced in the laboratory, and given its success, this approach should not be abandoned. However, there are significant problems with screening methods and the difficulties associated with extrapolating from *in vitro* experiments to the infected animal or human. A number of compounds, for example, ketoconazole and itraconazole, are more effective *in vivo* than could be predicted from laboratory observations on the interaction of the drug with target fungi. The chemical modifications of existing drugs (Table 13-2) has proved particularly successful with the synthetic azole and allylamine derivatives, resulting in the development of orally active drugs suitable for treating patients with systemic or topical fungal infections (Chapters 16 and 17). But this approach has not yet proved fruitful with the polyene macrolide antibiotics. A considerable number of derivatives of amphotericin B have been synthesized (e.g., Cheron et al., 1988), but so far none has been introduced into clinical practice.

Formulation of antifungal drugs is important especially if the drugs are toxic or insoluble as in the case of amphotericin B and certain azole derivatives. One approach that has been

TABLE 13-2. *Chemical Modifications of Antifungal Drugs*

Drug	Laboratory modifications	Introduction into clinical practice
Griseofulvin	Yes	No
Polyene macrolide antibiotics	Yes	No
5-Fluorocytosine	Yes	No
Synthetic azole drugs	Yes	Yes
Allylamines	Yes	Yes

tried but as yet not introduced into clinical practice has been the incorporation of the drugs into liposomal vesicles. This method of drug delivery can be used to reduce the toxicity of the compound or to increase the total amount of the drug that can be administered without adversely affecting the host (Lopez-Berestein et al., 1985). Combination therapy has proved successful with antibacterial antibiotics, but apart from the combined use of amphotericin B and 5-fluorocytosine in the treatment of patients suffering from cryptococcosis, this technique has not been widely exploited clinically. Unfortunately not all combinations of antifungal drugs act synergistically or even additively, and ketoconazole and amphotericin B (Sud & Feingold, 1983) and miconazole and 5-fluorocytosine (D. Kerridge, unpublished observations) are antagonistic. So far all these proposals for the future are merely extensions of our current knowledge of antifungal drugs, and if we are to develop more effective agents, then we must consider other (novel) targets and different approaches to this difficult clinical problem.

Chemotherapy is an "essay in comparative biochemistry," and to proceed to a rational drug design, it is important that we have a detailed knowledge of the metabolism of both host and pathogen. It will then be possible to select suitable targets and either use them to select for specific inhibitors or to attempt a rational design of novel inhibitors. Unfortunately, we are far from this ideal stage at present. However, our knowledge of *Candida albicans* (possibly the most studied pathogenic fungus) although still rudimentary is sufficient to enable us to select possible targets for therapeutic attack.

One feature of particular interest is the importance of sterol metabolism in mediating the action of antifungal drugs. It ranges from the relative affinities of sterol-containing membranes for polyene macrolide antibiotics to specific inhibition of any one of a number of enzymes involved in sterol biosynthesis by allylamines, thiocarbamates, azoles, and morpholine derivatives. Sterol biosynthesis in fungi is complex, many of the anabolic enzymes are membrane-associated, and the end product is an essential component of cellular membranes. Selectivity in most cases is associated with differences in the relative affinities of the target enzyme in humans and the fungal pathogen for the antifungal drugs. But it is difficult to see why this particular anabolic pathway has provided such good targets for antimycotic drugs. Further studies on the basic biochemistry of sterol biosynthesis in both humans and their fungal pathogens should provide an explanation for this phenomenon and also a basis for future development of drugs which specifically inhibit enzymes associated with sterol biosynthesis.

The most obvious differences between humans and fungi reside in the fungal cell wall. Chitin is invariably present as one of the structural polysaccharides in pathogenic fungi, in addition beta glucans and mannoproteins are also present in *Candida albicans*. Many of the fungal polysaccharides are absent from humans, and the biosynthetic enzymes involved in the formation of these macromolecules should provide suitable targets for selective attack. By analogy with bacteria it might be expected that cell wall biosynthesis in fungi would be an important target for antifungal drugs, but this has not proved to be the case. There is, however, one important and possibly significant difference between the two systems in that the active sites on the synthetic enzymes for fungal wall synthesis are within the cell, whereas the penicillin binding sites on the bacterial plasma membrane are on the outside and the beta lactam antibiotics do not cross the plasma membrane, a factor of some significance in the design of novel drugs. There are, however, a number of antibiotics which inhibit polysaccharide synthesis (Table 13-3), yet none is used clinically to treat patients with fungal infections. The synthesis and incorporation of polysaccharides into the fungal cell wall involves not only biosynthetic enzymes but also hydrolytic enzymes which allow the insertion of new constituents into the cell wall. There are a number of antibiotics which inhibit oligosaccharide processing (Fuhrman et al., 1985) and/or act as inhibitors of chitinase (see Chapter 14). These compounds could provide models for the development of antimycotic drugs whose target is exterior to the fungal membrane. Beta glucan synthase is specifically inhibited by a number of antifungal antibiotics, including echinocandin (Sawistowska-Schroder et al., 1984). This antibiotic has been considered as a potential anti-*Candida* drug. Chitin synthase is inhibited by both polyoxins and nikkomycins, and the latter compounds have been shown to prolong the survival time of mice infected systemically with *Candida albicans* (Becker et al., 1988).

There are a number of enzyme inhibitors which could provide the basis for a rational approach to the development of the next generation of antifungal drugs. The targets in all cases involve cellular anabolic reactions. For compounds which inhibit sterol biosynthesis, selectivity depends upon differences in the relative affinities of a specific enzyme for the drug with the host enzyme having a lower affinity than the fungal enzyme. For cell wall biosynthesis certain of the cellular macromolecules are absent for the host and specificity results from the absence of specific biosynthetic enzymes. One might expect that the latter would be more effective as antifungal compounds, and it is therefore surprising that none of the antimycotic drugs in current clinical use have as their target an enzyme involved in cell wall biogenesis. In the search for novel antifungal drugs we should not restrict our search to targets which are absent from humans. Selectivity can result from a number of other factors, for example, failure of the drug to reach the target, failure to be metabolized to an active compound, differences in the affinity of the drug for its target, or differences in the relative importance of the product of the inhibited reaction in the host and pathogen (Milewski et al., 1986) As our knowledge of the biochemistry of humans and their fungal pathogens increases, we will no doubt become aware of many, often subtle, differences which will provide the stimulus for the development of new antimycotic drugs.

One major problem in the control of fungal infections is the absence of drugs suitable for administration to patients at risk from fungal infections. None of the currently used drugs can be administered prophylactically, and there is an undoubted need for nontoxic drugs suitable for prolonged administration to immunocompromised patients. Here the search should be for drugs to prevent establishment of infection (Smith, 1985) rather than for drugs to eliminate the fungus from an already infected patient.

It is only by far reaching and multidisciplinary research that significant advances will be made in the development of new drugs. It will require a deep understanding of the metabolism of both host and pathogen and combine an imaginative approach to the selection of possible targets with persistence and attention to detail in the synthesis and subsequent modification of these inhibitors.

TABLE 13.3. *Inhibitors of Cell Wall Biosynthesis*

Polysaccharide	Enzyme	Inhibitor
β-Glucan	β-Glucan synthase	Echinocandin
	β-Glucanase	Nojirimycin, etc.
Mannoproteins	Multiple enzymes	Tunicamycin
	Oligosaccharide processing enzymes	Nojirimycin, etc.
Chitin	Chitin synthase	Polyoxins, nikkomycins
	Chitinase	Allosamidin

4. SUMMARY

There are no entirely satisfactory antifungal drugs. 5-Fluorocytosine is nontoxic, but has limited use and occurrence of resistant strains is a problem. Amphotericin B is toxic, but is still the drug of choice for treating patients with systemic mycoses. It renders the membrane permeable to protons, but the molecular mechanism is not understood. The most recent development has been the introduction of synthetic azole derivatives. These compounds have multiple effects on cellular metabolism ranging from an impairment of membrane function to inhibition of sterol biosynthesis. Enzymes of the sterol biosynthetic pathway are also targets for allylamine, thiocarbamate, and morpholine derivatives. Apart from 5-fluorocytosine, drug resistance is not a clinical problem. Developments are possible with the polyenes and the azole derivatives, but the most fruitful area will be in drugs that interfere with cell wall synthesis. As knowledge of fungal metabolism increases, other potential targets will be revealed and novel drugs designed to exploit them.

REFERENCES

Al-Bassam, T., Poulain, D., Giummally, B., Lemaître, J., and Bonaly, R. (1985) Chemical and antigenic alterations of *Candida albicans* cell walls related to the action of amphotericin B sub-inhibitory concentrations. *J. Antimicrob. Chemother.* **15**: 263–269.

Andreoli, T. E. (1974) The structure and function of amphotericin B-cholesterol pores in lipid bilayer membranes. *Ann. N.Y. Acad. Sci.* **235**: 448–469.

Antonov, V. F., Petrov, V. V., Molnar, A. A., Predvodifelev, D. A., and Ivanov, A. S. (1980) The appearance of single ion channels in unmodified lipid bilayer membranes at the phase transition temperature. *Nature* **283**: 585–586.

Aracava, I., Schreier, S., Phadke, R., Deslauriers, L., and Smith, I. C. P. (1981) Effects of amphotericin B on membrane permeability—kinetics of spin probe reduction. *Biophys. Chem.* **14**: 325–332.

Barrett-Bee, K. J., Lane, A. Ç., and Turner, R. W. (1986) The mode of antifungal action of tolnaftate. *J. Med. Vet. Mycol.* **24**: 155–160.

Becker, J. M., Marcus, S., Tullock, J., Miller, D., Kraner, E., Khare, R. K., and Naider F. (1988) Use of the chitin-synthesis inhibitor nikkomycin to treat disseminated candidiasis in mice. *J. Infect. Dis.* **117**: 212–214.

Bolard, J. (1986) How do the polyene macrolide antibiotics affect the cellular membrane properties? *Biochim. Biophys. Acta.* **864**: 257–304.

Borgers, M., De Brabander, M., Vanden Bossche, H., and Van Cutsem, J. (1979) Promotion of pseudomycelial formation in *Candida albicans*, a morphological study of the effect of miconazole and ketoconazole. *Postgrad. Med. J.* **55**: 687–691.

Brajtburg, J., Elberg, S., Medoff, G., and Kobayashi, G. S. (1981) Increase in colony-forming units of *Candida albicans* after treatment with polyene antibiotics. *Antimicrob. Agents & Chemother.* **19**: 199–200.

Brasseur, R., De Brabander, M., Vanden Bossche, H., and Ruysschaert, J. M. (1983) Mode of insertion of miconazole, ketoconazole, and deacylated ketoconazole into lipid bilayers, a conformational analysis. *Biochem. Pharmacol.* **32**: 2175–2180.

Brian, P. W. (1952) Antibiotics as systemic fungicides and bacteriocides. *Ann. Appl. Biol.* **39**: 434–438.

Brian, P. W., Curtis, P. V., and Fleming, H. G. (1946) A substance causing abnormal development of fungal hyphase produced by *Penicillium janczewsji* Z.A.L. *Trans. Brit. Mycol. Soc.* **32**: 30–33.

Cass, A., and Dalmark, H. (1973) Equilibrium dialysis of ions in nystatin treated red cells. *Nature* (London) **244**: 47–49.

Chen, W. C., Chou, D. O., and Feingold, D. S. (1978) Dissociation between ion permeability and the lethal action of polyene antibiotics in *Candida albicans. Antimicrob. Agents & Chemother.* **13**: 914–917.

Cheron, M., Cybulşka, B., Mazerski, J., Grzybowska, J., Czerwinski, A., and Borowski, E. (1988) Quantitative structure-activity relationships in amphotericin B derivatives. *Biochem. Pharmacol.* **37**: 827–836.

Cohen, B. E. (1986) Concentration and time dependence of amphotericin B induced permeability changes across ergosterol-containing liposomes. *Biochim. Biophys. Acta.* **857**: 117–122.

Cope, J. E. (1980) The mode of action of miconazole on *Candida albicans*. The effect on growth viability and K^+ release. *J. Gen. Microbiol.* **119**: 245–251.

Crosse, R., McWilliam, R., and Rhodes, A. (1964) Some relations between chemical structure and antifungal effects of griseofulvin analogues. *J. Gen. Microbiol.* **34**: 51–65.

Davies, R. R. (1980) Griseofulvin. In *Antifungal chemotherapy*, D. Speller, ed., pp. 149–182. Chichester, England: John Wiley.

Defever, K. S., Whelan, W. L., Rogers, A. L., Beneke, E. S., Veselanak, J. M., and Soll, D. R. (1982) *Candida albicans* resistant to 5-fluorocytosine: Frequency of partially resistant strains among clinical isolates. *Antimicrob. Agents & Chemother.* **22**: 810–815.

De Kruijff, B., and Demel, R. A. (1974) Polyene antibiotic-sterol interactions in membranes of *Acholeplasma laidlawii* and lecithin liposomes: III. Molecular structure of the polyene antibiotic-cholesterol complexes. *Biochim. Biophys. Acta.* **339**: 57–70.

Duschinsky, R., Pleven, E., and Heidelberger, C. (1957) The synthesis of 5-fluoropyrimidines. *J. Am. Chem. Soc.* **79**: 4599.

El-Nakeeb, M. A., and Lampen, J. O. (1965) Uptake of ^{3}H-griseofulvin by microorganisms and its correlation with sensitivity to griseofulvin. *J. Gen. Microbiol.* **39**: 285–294.

Fasoli, M., and Kerridge, D. (1988) Isolation and characterization of fluoropyrimidine-resistant mutants in two *Candida* species. *Ann. N.Y. Acad. Sci.* in press.

Fuhrmann, U., Bause, E., and Ploegh, M. (1985) Inhibitors of oligosaccharide processing. *Biochim. Biophys. Acta.* **825**: 95–110.

Gale, E. F., Cundliffe, E., Reynolds, P. E., Richmond, M. H., and Waring, M. J. (1981) *The molecular basis of antibiotic action*, 2nd ed. New York: John Wiley.

Gentles, J. C. (1958) Experimental ringworm in guinea pigs: Oral treatment with griseofulvin. *Nature* **182**: 476–477.

Hazen, E. L., and Brown, R. (1950) Two antibiotics produced by a soil actinomycete. *Science* **112**: 423.

Jund, R., and Lacroute, F. (1974) Génétique et Physiologie de la Résistance aux 5-Fluoropyrimidines chez *Saccharomyces cerevisiae. Bull. Sco. Fr. Mycol. Med.* **3**: 5-6.

Jund, R., and Lacroute, F. (1970) Genetic and physiological aspects of resistance to 5-fluoropyrimidines in *Saccharomyces cerevisiae. J. Bacteriol.* **102**: 607-615.

Kerridge, D. (1988) Polyene macrolide antibiotics. In *Aspergillus and aspergillosis*, H. Vanden Bossche, D. W. R. Mackenzie, and G. Cauwenbergh, eds., pp. 147-160. New York and London: Plenum Press.

Kerridge, D. (1986) Mode of action of clinically important antifungal drugs. *Adv. Microbiol. Physiol.* **27**: 1-72.

Kerridge, D., Nicholas, R. O., and Wayman, F. J. (1987) Resistance to clinically important antimycotic drugs in *Candida* spp. *Ann. Ist. Super. Sanita.* **23**: 827-834.

Kumar, B. V., Medoff, G., Kobayashi, G. S., and Schlessinger, D. (1974) Uptake of *Escherichia coli* DNA into HeLa cells enhanced by amphotericin B. *Nature* **250**: 323-325.

Lampen, J. O. (1966) Interference by polyenic antifungal antibiotics (especially nystatin and filipin) with specific membrane functions. *Symp. Soc. Gen. Microbiol.* **16**: 111-130.

Lopez-Berestein, G., Fainstein, V., Hopfer, R. L., Mehta, K., Sullivan, M. P., Keating, M., Rosenblum, W. G., Mehta, R., Luna, M., Herseh, E. M., Reuben, J., Juliano, R. L., and Bodey, G. P. (1985) Liposomal amphotericin B for the treatment of systemic fungal infections in patients with cancer: A preliminary study. *J. Infect. Dis.* **151**: 704-710.

Marty, A., and Finkelstein, A. (1975) Pores formed in lipid bilayers by nystatin: Differences in one-sided and two-sided action. *J. Gen. Physiol.* **65**: 515-526.

Medoff, G. (1988) The mechanisms of action of amphotericin. In *Aspergillus and aspergillosis*, H. Vanden Bossche, D. W. R. Mackenzie, and G. Cauwenbergh, eds., pp. 161-164. New York and London: Plenum Press.

Milewski, S., Chmara, H., and Borowski, E. (1986) Anticapsin: An active site directed inhibitor of glucosamine-6-phosphate synthetase from *Candida albicans. Drugs Exp. Clin. Res.* **12**: 577-583.

Nes, W. R., Sekula, B. C., Nes, W. D., and Adler, J. H. (1978) The functional importance of structural features of ergosterol in yeast. *J. Biol. Chem.* **253**: 6218-6225.

Nugent, K. M., Couchot, K. R., and Gray, L. D. (1987) Effect of *Candida* morphology of amphotericin B susceptibility. *Antimicrob. Agents & Chemother.* **31**: 335-336.

Olaiya, A. F., and Sogin, S. J. (1979) Ploidy determination of *Candida albicans J. Bacteriol.* **140**: 1043-1409.

Oxford, A. E., Raistrick, M., and Simonart, P. (1939) Studies in biochemistry of microorganisms LX griseofulvin $C_{17}H_{16}O_6Cl$ metabolic product of *Penicillium griseo-fulvin* Dierckx. *Biochem. J.* **33**: 240-248.

Palacios, J., and Serrano, R. (1978) Proton permeability induced by polyene antibiotics. A plausible mechanism for their inhibition of maltose fermentation in yeast. *FEBS Lett.* **91**: 198-201.

Paget, G. E., and Walpole, A. L. (1960) The experimental toxicology of griseofulvin. *Arch. Dermat.* **81**: 750-757.

Paget, G. E., and Walpole, A. L. (1958) Some cytological effects of griseofulvin. *Nature* **182**: 1320-1321.

Pesti, M., Novak, E. K., Ferenczy, L., and Svoboda, A. (1981) Freeze fracture electron microscopical investigation of *Candida albicans* cells sensitive and resistant to nystatin. *Sabouraudia.* **19**: 17-26.

Plempel, M., Bartmann, K., Buchel, K. H., and Regel, E. (1969) Experimentelle Befunde uber ein neues oral wirksames Antimykotikum mit breitein Wirkungsspectrum. *Dt. med. Wschr.* **94**: 1356-1364.

Polak, A., and Scholer, H. J. (1980) Mode of action of 5-fluorocytosine. *Rev. Inst. Pasteur de Lyon.* **13**: 233-244.

Portillo, F., and Gancedo, C. (1985) Mitochondrial resistance to miconazole in *Saccharomyces cerevisiae. Mol. Gen. Genet.* **199**: 495-499.

Portillo, F., and Gancedo, C. (1984) Mode of action of miconazole on yeasts: Inhibition of mitochondrial ATPase. *Eur. J. Biochem.* **143**: 273-276.

Rast, D. M., and Bartnicki-Garcia, S. (1981) Effects of amphotericin B, nystatin, and other polyene antibiotics on chitin synthase. *Proc. Natl. Acad. Sci. USA* **78**: 1233-1236.

Ryder, N. S., Frank, I., and Dupont, M. C. (1986) Ergosterol biosynthesis inhibition by thiocarbamate antifungal agents, tolnaftate and tolciclate. *Antimicrob. Agents & Chemother.* **29**: 858-860.

Ryley, J. F., Wilson, R. G., and Barrett-Bee, K. J. (1984) Azole resistance in *Candida albicans. Sabouraudia. J. Med. Vet. Mycol.* **22**: 53-63.

Ryley, J. F., Wilson, R. G., Gravestock, M. B., and Poyser, J. P. (1981) Experimental approaches to antifungal chemotherapy. *Adv. Pharmacol. Chemother.* **18**: 47-176.

Sawistowska-Schroder, E. T., Kerridge, D., and Perry, H. (1984) Echinocandin inhibition of 1,3,-β-glucan synthase from *Candida albicans. FEBS Letts.* **173**: 134-136.

Scholer, H. J. (1980) Flucytosine. In *Antifungal chemotherapy*, Speller, ed., pp. 35-106. Chichester: John Wiley.

Shigematsu, M. L., Uno, J., and Akai, T. (1982) Effect of ketoconazole on isolated mitochondria from *Candida albicans. Antimicrob. Agents & Chemother.* **21**: 919-924.

Sloboda, R. D., Van Blaricon, G., Creasey, W. A., Rosenbaum, J. L., and Malewista, S. E. (1982) Griseofulvin: Association with tubulin and inhibition of microtubule assembly. *Biochem. Biophys. Res. Comm.* **105**: 882-888.

Smith, H. (1985). The therapeutic potential of inhibition or circumvention of the determinants of microbial pathogenicity. *Symp. Soc. Gen. Microbiol.* **38**: 367-393.

Sokol-Anderson, M., Brajtburg, J., and Medoff, J. (1986) Amphotericin B induced oxidative damage and killing of *Candida albicans. J. Infect. Dis.* **154**: 76-83.

Stiller, R. L., Bennett, J. E., Scholer, H. J., Wall, M., Polak, A., and Stevens, D. A. (1982) Susceptibility to 5-fluorocytosine and prevalence of serotype 402 *Candida albicans* isolates from the United States. *Antimicrob. Agents & Chemother.* **22**: 482–487.

Stutz, A. (1987) Allylamine derivatives—a new class of active substances in antifungal chemotherapy. *Angew. Chem. Int. Ed. Engl.* **26**: 120–128.

Sud, I. J., and Feingold, D. S. (1983) Effect of ketoconazole on the fungicidal action of amphotericin B in *Candida albicans. Antimicrob. Agents & Chemother.* **23**: 185–187.

Surarit, R., and Shepherd, M. G. (1987) The effects of azole and polyene antifungals on the plasma membrane enzymes of *Candida albicans. J. Med. Vet. Mycol.* **25**: 403–413.

Takeo, K., and Arai, T. (1987). Growing regions of the *Schizosaccharomyces* plasma membrane as selected sites of ultrastructural deformation by amphotericin B. *FEBS Microbiol. Lett.* **42**: 221–224.

Thomas, A. H. (1986) Suggested mechanisms for the antimycotic activity of the polyene antibiotics and the N-substituted imidazoles. *J. Antimicrob. Chemother.* **17**: 269–279.

Trinci, A. P. J., and Ryley, J. F. (eds.) (1984) Mode of action of antifungal agents. *Brit. Mycol. Soc. Symp.* 9.

Vanden Bossche, H., Willemsens, G., Marichal, P., Cools, W., and Lauwers, W. (1984) The molecular basis for the antifungal activities of N-substituted azole derivatives. Focus on R 51 211. *Brit. Mycol. Soc. Symp.* **9**: 320–341.

Vanden Bossche, H., Marichal, P., Gorrens, J., Bellens, D., Verhoeven, H., Coene, M.-C., Lauwers, W., and Janssen, P. (1987a) Interaction of azole derivatives with cytochrome P450 isozymes in yeast, fungi, plants, and mammalian cells. *Pestic. Sci.* **21**: 289–306.

Vanden Bossche, H., Willemsens, G., and Marichal, P. (1987b) Anti-*Candida* drugs—the biochemical basis of their activity. *CRC Crit. Rev. Microbiol.* **15**: 57–72.

Yu, R. J., and Blank, F. (1973) On the mechanism of action of griseofulvin in dermatophytes. *Sabouraudia.* **11**: 274–278.

Whelan, W. L., and Kerridge, D. (1984) Decreased activity of UMP: pyrophosphorylase associated with resistance to 5-fluorocytosine in *Candida albicans. Antimicrob. Agents & Chemother.* **26**: 570–574.

Whelan, W. L., Beneke, E. S., Rogers, A. L., and Soll, D. R. (1981) Segregation of 5-fluorocytosine resistant variants by *Candida albicans. Antimicrob. Agents & Chemother.* **19**: 1078–1081.

Williams, D. J., Marten, R. H., and Sarkany, I. (1958) Oral treatment of ringworm with griseofulvin. *Lancet* **ii**: 1212–1213.

CHAPTER 14

CHITIN METABOLISM: A TARGET FOR ANTIFUNGAL AND ANTIPARASITIC DRUGS

GRAHAM W. GOODAY

Department of Genetics and Microbiology, Marischal College, University of Aberdeen, Aberdeen, Scotland

Abstract—Chitin is an invariant essential component of the walls of all fungal pathogens of humans and other mammals. It also occurs as a structural component of the cyst walls of some pathogenic amoebae, the egg shells of parasitic nematodes, and many other invertebrates. It does not occur in vertebrates or vascular plants. It is synthesized by the enzyme chitin synthase, using uridine diphospho-*N*-acetylglucosamine as substrate. Chitinase activities are involved in morphogenesis of the chitin structures. Chitin metabolism is inhibited by specific antibiotics: polyoxins and nikkomycins as inhibitors of chitin synthase and allosamidins as inhibitors of chitinases. Polyoxins and nikkomycins are fungicidal, acaricidal, and nematocidal and prevent formation of chitinous cysts and eggs. Allosamidins are insecticidal.

1. CHITIN AND ITS OCCURRENCE

Chitin is the (1 → 4)-β-linked homopolymer of *N*-acetyl-D-glucosamine. The individual polymer chains can be of thought as helices, as each sugar unit is inverted with respect to its neighbors. This leads to their stabilization as rigid ribbons, by O3—H...O5 and O6—H...O7 hydrogen bonds. The most common form of chitin is α-chitin. Its unit cell is of two *N,N'*-diacetylchitobiose units of two chains in an antiparallel arrangement. Thus adjacent polymer chains run in opposite directions, held together by O6—H...O6 hydrogen bonds, and the chains are held in sheets by O7...H—N hydrogen bonds (Minke & Blackwell, 1978). This gives a statistical mixture of CH_2OH orientations, equivalent to half oxygens on each residue, each forming inter- and intramolecular hydrogen bonds. This results in two types of amide groups; all are involved in the interchain C=O...H—N bonds, while half of the groups also serve as acceptors for O6—H...O=C intramolecular bonds. This extensive intermolecular hydrogen bonding leads to a very stable structure, the individual polymer chains eventually giving rise to microfibrils if allowed to crystallize (Gooday, 1983a). A less common form of chitin is β-chitin, in which the unit cell is of one *N,N'*-diacetylchitobiose unit, giving a polymer stabilized as a rigid ribbon as for α-chitin, by O3—H...O5 intramolecular bonds (Gardner & Blackwell, 1975). Chains are then held together in sheets by C=O...H—N hydrogen bonding of the amide groups and by the CH_2OH side chains forming intersheet hydrogen bonds to the carbonyl oxygens on the next chains (O6—H...O7). This gives a structure of parallel poly-*N*-acetyl glucosamine chains with no intersheet hydrogen bonds. The parallel arrangement of polymer chains in β-chitin allows for more flexibility than does the antiparallel arrangement of α-chitin, but the resultant polymer still has immense strength (Lindsay & Gooday, 1985).

With only one exception, the β-chitin of diatoms, chitin is always found cross-linked to other structural components. In fungal walls it is found covalently bonded to glucans, either directly, as in *Candida albicans* (Surarit et al., 1988), or via peptide bridges (Sietsma et al., 1986). In insects and other invertebrates, the chitin is always associated with specific proteins, with both covalent and noncovalent bonding, to produce the observed ordered structures (Giraud-Gaille & Bouligand, 1986; Kramer & Koga, 1986; Blackwell & Weih, 1984). There are often also varying degrees of mineralization, in particular calcification, and sclerotization, involving interactions with phenolic and lipid molecules (Poulicek et al., 1986; Peter et al., 1986). In both fungi and invertebrates there are varying degrees of deacetylation, giving a continuum of structure between chitin (fully acetylated) and chitosan (fully deacetylated) (Datema et al., 1977; Davis & Bartnicki-Garcia, 1984; Aruchami et al., 1986; Gowri et al., 1986).

Chitin is the characteristic wall component of most fungi, and certainly in all the fungal pathogens of humans and other mammals. In the dimorphic human pathogenic fungi, there are distinct differences in chitin content between the yeast and mycelial forms: In *Candida albicans* there is severalfold more chitin in the mycelial walls (Chattaway et al., 1968), while for *Histoplasma capsulatum*, *Blastomyces dermatitidis*, and *Paracoccoides brasiliensis*, the reverse is the case (Domer et al., 1967; Kanetsuma & Carbonell, 1971; Kanetsuma et al., 1969).

In the fungal walls the chitin characteristically occurs as microfibrils in the innermost layer (Gooday & Trinci, 1980). The microfibrils of particular walls have characteristic structures and arrangements. Thus in dimorphic fungi such as *Candida albicans*, in the yeast and mycelial walls they occur as short stubby fibrils arranged randomly (Gow & Gooday, 1983; Gooday & Gow, 1983); in vegetative hyphal walls of the filamentous fungus *Neurospora crassa*, they are long and arranged randomly, except at apices of narrow elongating germ hyphae, where they tend to be arranged axially (Burnett, 1979), and in *Coprinus cinereus* they are long and randomly oriented in vegetative hyphal walls, but long and wound in shallow helices around the cells of the stipe of the mushroom (Gooday, 1975, 1979a). In the septa of both yeast and mycelial *Candida albicans* and of *Neurospora crassa*, the microfibrils are long and arranged predominantly tangentially (Gow et al., 1980; Gooday & Gow, 1983; Hunsley & Gooday, 1974). Chitins purified from these different sources, however, have indistinguishable chemical properties (Gow et al., 1987).

The chitin in the fungal wall also varies in its crystallinity, that is, degree of internal hydrogen bonding, its degree of covalent bonding to other wall components, such as glucans, and, especially in the zygomycetes, in its degree of deacetylation. Thus Vermeulen and Wessels (1984) describe the newly synthesized chitin in hyphal apices of *Schizophyllum commune* as being very susceptible to degradation by chitinase and solubilization by dilute mineral acid. They ascribe this to its nascent state, before extensive hydrogen bonding and covalent bonding have occurred.

Chitin occurs sporadically among protozoa. Typically it is a component of cyst walls. Thus it is a major component of the cyst walls of the sarcodinian intestinal parasite of snakes, *Entamoeba invadens* (Arroyo-Begovich & Carabez-Trego, 1982; Arroyo-Begovich et al., 1980) and of the mastigophoran human pathogen *Giardia lamblia*, a significant cause of diarrhoea (Ward et al., 1985). For both *Entamoeba* species and *Giardia lamblia*, cyst formation is of a great importance as the cysts are the major means of transmission from host to host. The cysts have high resistance to adverse conditions, especially to desiccation and to sterilizing agents such as chlorine. The chitin content of their walls surely makes an intrinsic contribution to the mechanisms of resistance. Chitin may also be a component of the wall of *Pneumocystis carinii*, an organism of uncertain affinity causing human pneumonia.

Chitin occurs in the egg shells of many nematodes, such as the large roundworm of humans, *Ascaris lumbricoides* (Jeuniaux, 1963), and chitin synthase has been reported in the eggs of *Ascaris suum* (Dubinsky et al., 1986). It also occurs in the ephemeral egg shells of the parasitic filarial nematodes, *Onchocerca gibsoni*, which infect cattle, and *Onchocerca volvulus*, the cause of river blindness in humans (Brydon et al., 1987; King et al., 1987). In other filarial nematodes, *Brugia malayi* and *Litomosoides carinii*, chitin is a component of the sheaths of the young microfilariae, which are derived by a stretching of the oocyte membranes (Fuhrman & Piessens, 1985; Peters et al., 1987).

Chitin has a wide distribution as a tough extracellular material among other invertebrates (Jeuniaux, 1963). For example, it is the characteristic component of the cuticles and peritrophic membranes of all of the arthropods, of the peritrophic membranes and chaetae of annelids, and of the shells of molluscs.

Chitin does not occur in vertebrates or vascular plants. Thus, analogously to the peptidoglycan metabolism of bacteria, chitin metabolism of fungi, protozoa, and invertebrates provides a target for chemotherapeutic agents. For fungal pathogens, as will be shown later, chitin synthesis is a lethal target; that is, its inhibition is fungicidal, not just fungistatic. For parasites transmitted by chitin-clad cysts or eggs, inhibition of chitin synthesis, while not of much direct benefit to the patient, would prevent transmission of the disease. For filarial nematodes, inhibition of chitin synthesis, while not killing the adult worms, should prevent the production of the microfilariae, and so in the case of *Onchocerca volvulus* should prevent the onset of blindness as well as transmission of the disease.

2. CHITIN METABOLISM

Chitin is synthesized by the one enzyme, chitin synthase (EC. 2.4.1.16), which has been characterized from many fungi and invertebrates (reviewed by Wessels & Sietsma, 1981; Gooday, 1983a; Kramer & Koga, 1986; Chen, 1987; Cohen, 1987; Cabib, 1987). The substrate is the nucleotide sugar, uridine diphospho-*N*-acetylglucosamine, UDP-GlcNAc. The stoichiometry is as follows:

$$2\text{UDP-GlcNAc} + (\text{GlcNAc})_n \rightarrow (\text{GlcNAc})_{n+2} + 2\text{UDP}$$

A divalent cation is required for activity. This is probably magnesium *in vivo*, but manganese or cobalt can sometime substitute *in vitro*. No primer has been identified. There is no evidence for the involvement of a lipid intermediate such as for peptidoglycan and glycoprotein syntheses. In 1972 we chose the basidiomycete *Coprinus cinereus* for study, and this proved to be an excellent source of the enzyme, giving high endogenous activities that could be solubilized readily with the saponin digitonin and subsequently purified (Gooday, 1973, 1977a, b, 1979a, 1983a; Gooday & Rousset-Hall, 1975; Gooday & Trinci, 1980; Montgomery et al., 1984; Montgomery & Gooday, 1985). The enzyme preparations from *Coprinus cinereus* have proved admirably suitable for the study of inhibitors of chitin synthesis (Gooday, 1975, 1977a, b, 1989a; Gooday et al., 1976; Rousset-Hall & Gooday, 1975; Adams & Gooday, 1980, 1983).

In most other cases enzyme preparations from different fungi are chiefly zymogenic, being activated, often manyfold, by treatment with proteases. For example, Hardy and Gooday (1983) describe activation by trypsin of microsomal and solubilized preparations of chitin synthase from *Candida albicans*. Enzyme specific activity was higher in mycelium than yeast, but in both cases treatment with trypsin resulted in manyfold activation. This phenomenon was first described by Cabib and Farkas (1971) with an enzyme preparation from *Saccharomyces cerevisiae* and investigated in detail since then (reviewed by Cabib, 1987). The major enzyme activity from this yeast, Chs1, has now been shown to have no direct role in chitin synthesis in normal vegetative growth, but rather may be a "repair enzyme" (Bulawa et al., 1986; Cabib, 1989). Instead, a minor activity, Chs2, is apparently the enzyme active *in vivo* (Sburlati & Cabib, 1986; Orlean, 1987). The two enzymes, however, have similar properties.

For a range of fungi, there is considerable evidence that the active enzyme and some of the zymogenic enzyme are sited as intrinsic proteins in the plasma membrane (reviews by Wessels & Sietsma, 1981; Gooday, 1983a, b; Cabib, 1987). Thus the active enzyme can be seen as accepting substrate and responding to effectors at the inner face of the membrane and feeding out polymer chains to the wall outside. The corollary is that most potential inhibitors will need to be transported into the cell before affecting the enzyme. This certainly seems true for the polyoxins and nikkomycins, as discussed later.

In many fungi, a significant portion of the zymogenic enzyme occurs as discrete intracellular particles, the chitosomes, discovered by Ruiz-Herrera and coworkers (1975) and Bracker and coworkers (1976), and investigated in detail since then (Hänseler et al., 1983; Ruiz-Herrera et al., 1984). The origin and fate of chitosomes are still unclear, but their most plausible role is as the mode of transport of zymogenic chitin synthase from its formation, perhaps in endoplasmic reticulum, to its activatible site in the plasma membrane. In hyphae it would then be activated for apical growth, for branching, and for septum formation (Gooday, 1983b).

The soluble product of chitin synthase, uridine diphosphate (UDP), is a competitive inhibitor of the enzyme from *Coprinus cinereus* (Rousset-Hall & Gooday, 1975; Gooday, 1977a). Associated with the chitin synthase in *Coprinus cinereus* is the enzyme uridine diphosphatase, hydrolyzing the UDP formed to UMP and inorganic phosphate. The UMP is much less inhibitory to chitin synthase than is UDP, and so the uridine diphosphatase may play a regulatory role in controlling chitin synthesis (Gooday, 1979a).

Chitin synthesizing systems are characteristically accompanied by chitin-degrading systems. Chitin is degraded to its monomer by the joint action of two enzymes: chitinase (EC. 3.2.1.14) hydrolyzes polymers and oligomers of *N*-acetyl-D-glucosamine to give *N,N'*-diacetylchitobiose as the major product, and *N*-acetyl-β-glucosaminidase (EC. 3.2.1.30, chitobiase) hydrolyzes this to give *N*-acetylglucosamine (Gooday, 1989b). In some cases the roles of chitinase activities are clearly the gross lysis of structural chitin, such as in the ink-cap fungi, *Coprinus* species, and puffballs, *Lycoperdon* species, and during ecdysis in arthropods. In fungi, however, there are also growth-associated chitinases, with activities expressed during spore germination and exponential hyphal growth in *Mucor* species and in *Candida albicans* (Gooday et al., 1986; D. M. Rast, R. Furter, and G. W. Gooday, unpublished results; Barrett-Bee & Hamilton, 1984). Humphreys & Gooday (1984a, b, c) describe a membrane-bound partially zymogenic chitinase in growing hyphae of *Mucor mucedo.* It has been suggested that these are specific morphogenetic chitinase activities (Gooday et al., 1986; Gooday 1989a). Bartnicki-Garcia (1973) presents a unitary model of cell wall growth in which lytic enzymes play a vital role in maintaining a balance between wall synthesis and wall lysis during hyphal apical growth, so that the apex is in a plastic state to allow insertion of new chitin into the wall. Gooday (1989a), suggests three more positive roles for chitinases in wall growth. The first is the regulation of the formation of the crystalline α-chitin in its fully hydrogen-bonded antiparallel form. Vermeulen and Wessels (1984,1986) have shown that synthesis and crystallization of chitin chains are two separate processes separated in space and time in hyphal apices. The second role is the modeling of the microfibrils to give their final form characteristic of the particular fungal cell type. Gow and Gooday (1983) emphasize the range or form of chitin found in different fungal walls. The third role could be cross-linking of chitin to other wall components through glycosidic linkages, as chitinases like other polysaccharases can have transglycosylase activities (Usai et al., 1987).

Gooday et al. (1988) describe chitinase activity in female filarial nematodes, *Onchocerca gibsoni*, which they suggest is involved in egg shell formation and/or hatching. Chitinase has been implicated in excystment of protozoa and hatching of the eggs of the nematode *Ascaris suum* (Ward & Fairburn, 1972).

Thus the process of chitin deposition during morphogenesis is seen as involving chitinase activities as well as chitin synthase. Chitinase should then also be a target for antifungal and antiparasitic drugs, with the possible advantage that such compounds, unlike inhibitors of chitin synthase, might not require uptake into cells to be active.

3. POLYOXINS AND NIKKOMYCINS

The polyoxins and nikkomycins are two classes of closely related nucleoside-di- and -tripeptide antibiotics which are very specific competitive inhibitors of chitin synthase, mimicking its substrate UDP-GlcNAc (Fig. 14-1). The polyoxins were characterized in the 1960s as a family of metabolites from the soil microbe, *Streptomyces cacaoi* var. *asoensis* (Isono et al., 1965, 1969). The nikkomycins were characterized in the 1970s as a family of metabolites from *Streptomyces tendae* (Dähn et al., 1976; Hagenmaier et al., 1979, 1981; König et al., 1980; Friedler et al., 1982). The nikkomycins have also been described as the neopolyoxins, by Kobinata et al. (1980) and Uramoto et al. (1980, 1982), from a new strain of *Streptomyces caocoi* var. *asoensis.*

Both polyoxins and nikkomycins were isolated as antifungal antibiotics and inhibit a wide range of different fungi (Gooday, 1979b, 1989a). Both groups are powerful competitive inhibitors of chitin synthase (Endo & Misato, 1969; Endo et al., 1970; Müller et al., 1981; Furter & Rast, 1985). Using a cell-free preparation of chitin synthase from *Neurospora crassa*, Gow and Selitrennikof (1984) showed that polyoxin B, nikkomycin Z, and UDP competed with each other and the substrate UDP-GlcNAc for binding to chitin syn-

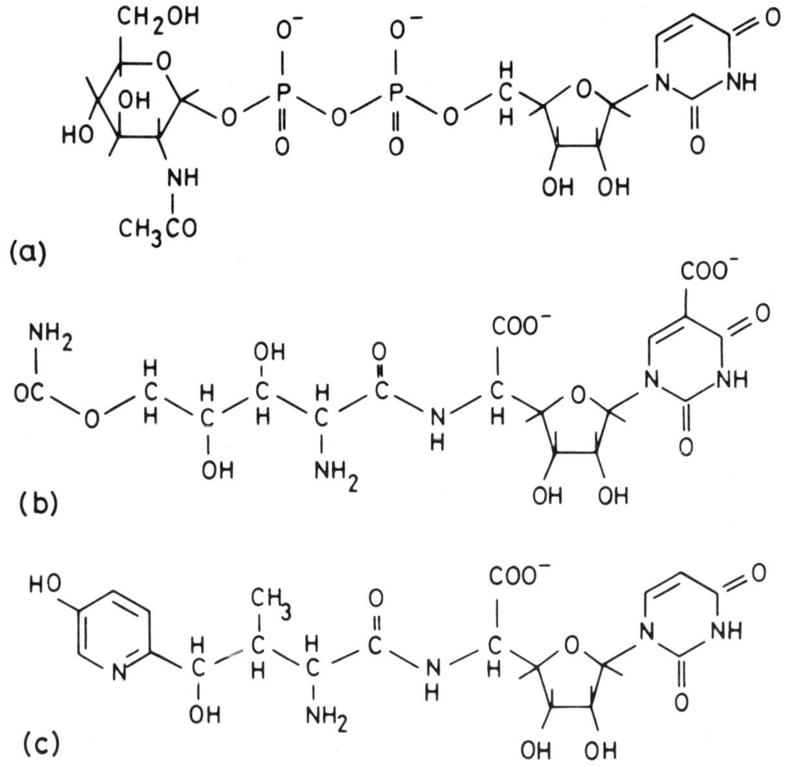

(a)

(b)

(c)

FIG. 14-1. (A) UDP-*N*-acetylglucosamine, (B) polyoxin D, (C) nikkomycin Z.

thase. All cell-free chitin synthase systems from fungi, and many of those from invertebrates, that have been tested to date have been shown to be susceptible to these antibiotics, with Ki values typically in the order of a few micromolar, that is, several hundredfold less than values for K_m (Gooday 1979b; Kramer & Koga, 1986; Cohen, 1987).

As chitin synthase is an integral protein in the plasma membrane, accepting substrate from the cytosol, the polyoxins and nikkomycins require transport into the fungal cell for their inhibitory activity. Evidence for this comes from observations that the enzyme chitin synthase from a wide range of fungi is approximately equally susceptible to inhibition, but that the intact fungi show a very wide range of susceptibility (Gooday 1989a). When polyoxins were used in the field in Japan as fungicides against black spot of pear *Alternaria kikuchiana*, resistant strains emerged (Nishimura et al., 1973). Hori et al. (1974) showed that the chitin synthase from resistant strains was still susceptible to polyoxin B. Hori and coworkers (1977) showed that the uptake of tritiated polyoxin A by a susceptible strain was antagonized by peptides such as glycyl-glycine, in a competitive manner. Resistant strains of fungus showed diminished uptake. The uptake of polyoxins and nikkomycins has been studied in detail for the human pathogen *Candida albicans*. Payne and Shallow (1985) and McCarthy and colleagues (1985) showed that strains and mutants resistant to polyoxin showed cross-resistance to nikkomycin and also to the toxic peptide bacilysin (tetaine). These authors and Yaden and colleagues (1984) showed that mutants resistant to nikkomycin had changed patterns of peptide uptake. McCarthy and colleagues (1985) showed that the uptake of two peptides that antagonize nikkomycin action, alanyl-alanine and leucyl-glycine, was impaired in resistant mutants. Yadan and colleagues (1984) and Gonneau and colleagues (1986) showed that uptake of tritiated nikkomycin Z was antagonized by dimethionine and trimethionine, while uptake of ^{14}C-dimethionine was antagonized by nikkomycin Z. A nikkomycin-resistant mutant showed impaired uptake of both nikkomycin and dimethionine.

Both polyoxins and nikkomycins are active against a wide taxonomic spectrum of or-

Table 14-1. *Representative Effects of Polyoxins and Nikkomycins on Different Organisms*

Organism	Effects	References
Fungi		
Chytridiomycete: *Allomyces macrogynus*	Swelling and bursting of rhizoids and hyphae	Youatt et al. (1988)
Zygomycete; *Mucor rouxii*	Swelling and bursting of hyphae	Bartnicki-Garcia & Lippman (1972) Müller et al. (1981); Furter & Rast (1985)
Ascomycete: *Neurospora crassa*	Swelling and bursting of hyphae	Endo et al. (1970); G. W. Gooday (unpublished)
Hemiascomycete: *Saccharomyces cerevisiae*	Exploded/refringent cell pairs	Bowers et al. (1974)
Deuteromycete: *Candida albicans*	Bulbous chains of cells, death	Adams & Gooday (1983); Becker et al. (1983)
Basidiomycete: *Coprinus cinereus*	Swelling and bursting of hyphae; no stipe elongation, autolysis	Gooday (1972); Gooday et al. (1976)
Protista		
Sarcodina; *Entamoeba invadens*	Cyst formation inhibited	Avron et al. (1982)
Diatom: *Thalassiosira fluviatilis*	Spine formation inhibited	Gooday et al. (1985); Morin et al. (1986)
Animalia		
Nematode: *Meloidogyne javanica*	Egg formation inhibited	Spiegel & Chet (1985)
Mite: *Tetranychis articae*	Moulting and egg laying inhibited	Mothes & Seitz (1982)
Insect: *Melanoplus sanguinipes*	Death during moulting	Vardanis (1978)

ganisms (Table 14-1). Worth noting from this table is their activity against the fungus *Candida albicans* and the protozoan *Entamoeba invadens*. Also worth noting is the action of nikkomycin against the chitin spine formation in centric diatoms, as this is β-chitin and not α-chitin as the other examples quoted here. The β-chitin in these diatoms is in the form of pure polysaccharide spines extending from the peripheries of the cells, allowing them to float in the water column. Polyoxin and nikkomycin prevent this spine formation, and so the cells sink to the bottom of the culture vessel. In the case of *Saccharomyces cerevisiae*, both chitin synthase enzymes so far identified, the Chs2, involved in active growth, and the Chs1, possibly a repair enzyme, are about equally susceptible to inhibition by polyoxin D (Sburlati & Cabib, 1986; Orlean, 1987). Treatment of growing cells of this yeast with polyoxin D results in two responses, "exploded pairs" with bursting at the site of budding and partially lysed "refringent pairs" (Bowers et al., 1974). Polyoxin D also inhibits septation and separation of buds of yeast cells of *Candida albicans* leading to cell death, but four different strains tested showed very different sensitivities (Becker et al., 1983). Both yeast cells and mycelia of this dimorphic fungus are susceptible (Becker et al., 1983; Hilenski et al., 1986). The polyoxins, and much more powerfully, nikkomycins X and Z are active against yeast cells and mycelium of the dimorphic fungus *Mucor rouxii* (Bartnicki-Garcia & Lippman, 1972; Müller et al., 1981; Furter & Rast, 1985). The antibiotics caused abnormal swellings and bursting of both growth forms. Sporangiospores were more sensitive to nikkomycins than yeast or mycelium. They showed enhanced swelling, and cell death at the presumptive time of germ tube emergence (Furter & Rast, 1985).

It is clear that in culture, in the right experimental conditions, inhibition of chitin synthesis by these antibiotics is a fungicidal activity. Thus growing vegetative hyphae of the *Neurospora crassa* and *Coprinus cinereus* respond to both polyoxin D and to nikkomycin X/Z by ballooning at the apices, multiple apical branching, "beading" of the hyphae, and finally bursting (G. W. Gooday, unpublished results). Youatt and colleagues (1988) have investigated the effects of polyoxin and nikkomycin on the zoospores of the chytrid fungus *Allomyces macrogynus.* Ungerminated zoospores, which lack chitin, swam for up to two days in the presence of both antibiotics, emphasizing the specificity of their action for chitin synthesis, but germination and outgrowth of spores was inhibited, and the spores and hyphae soon disintegrated.

Neither polyoxins nor nikkomycins have any reported significant toxicity to vertebrates or higher plants (Isono et al., 1967; Fiedler et al., 1982; Adams & Gooday, 1983). They have no reported activity against any other enzyme system involving UDP-GlcNAc, such as glycoprotein biosynthesis. This great specificity for chitin synthase reinforces the appeal of chitin synthesis as a target. Efforts have been made to improve the antifungal potential of polyoxins and nikkomycins by producing semisynthetic or totally synthetic analogs. In particular a major aim has been to increase activity against human pathogenic fungi, especially *Candida albicans.* To date, however, none of these analogs has been as active as the natural products (Gooday, 1989a). The polyoxins have been formulated as agricultural sprays and used widely in Japan for many years against plant pathogens (Misato & Kakiki, 1977; Misato et al., 1977). Nikkomycins also are active in the field against plant pathogens (Fiedler et al., 1982). Becker and colleagues (1988) report the results of experiments testing the effects of polyoxin and nikkomycin on survival of mice experimentally infected with *Candida albicans* to give systemic candidiosis. In their regime, polyoxin D gave no protection, while treatment with nikkomycin increased the survival times of the mice. In their experiments no mouse died of candidal infection while receiving nikkomycin, but stopping the drug treatment resulted in reestablishment of the infection and death of mice.

The action of polyoxins and nikkomycins against protozoa and invertebrates shown in Table 14-1 demonstrates the potential of chitin synthase as a target in the control of a wide range of pathogens, parasites, and pests.

4. ALLOSAMIDINS

Recently, the first antibiotics specifically active against chitinases were described. These are the allosamidins, produced by *Streptomyces* sp. no. 1713 (Sakuda et al., 1986, 1987a, b; Fig. 14-2). Independently Somers and colleagues (1987) isolated the same metabolite, designated as A82516, from *Streptomyces* strain A82516. Both laboratories were using a screen to detect compounds with potential insecticidal activity, in the first case using chitinase from silkworm pupae, *Bombyx mori*, and in the second case using chitinase from *Streptomyces griseus.* Both allosamidins and A82516 are insecticidal to larvae. The allosamidins are pseudotrisaccharides consisting of a disaccharide of *N*-acetylallosamine linked to a novel amino cyclitol derivative, named as allosamizoline. Methylallosamidin, methylated at the 6-hydroxyl group of the nonreducing end of the disaccharide, is a co-metabolite.

A notable feature of allosamidin is its very different activities against chitinases from different sources. Thus Koga and colleagues (1987) report good activity against insect chi-

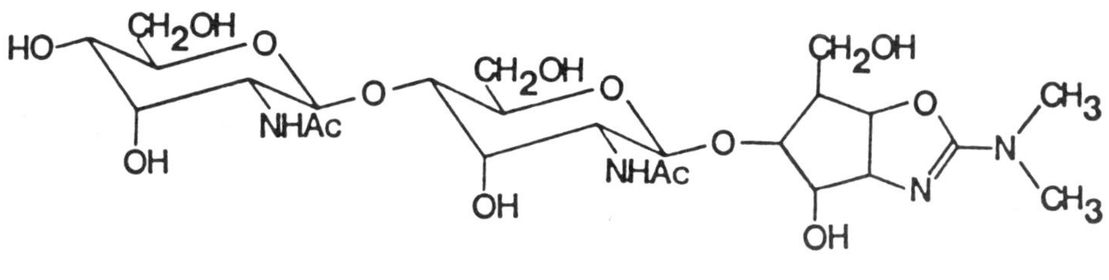

FIG. 14-2. Allosamidin.

tinase from *Bombyx mori*, poor activity against bacterial chitinases from *Streptomyces griseus* and *Serratia marcescens*, and no detectable activity against the plant chitinase from yam, lysozymes from white or human urine, or insect B-*N*-acetylglucosaminidase from *Bombyx mori.* We have shown that allosamidin is active against secreted chitinases from the fungi *Neurospora crassa* and *Aspergillus nidulans* and very powerfully active against the chitinase of the nematode *Onchocerca gibsoni* (Gooday 1989a; Gooday et al., 1988). It is also active against two different chitinase enzymes from the fish turbot *Scophthalmus maximus.* The enzyme in the blood plasma (probably a defense enzyme) was much more sensitive than that from the stomach (a food processing enzyme) (F. D. C. Manson and G. W. Gooday, unpublished results).

5. CONCLUSIONS

From the action of polyoxins and nikkomycins on fungi, protozoa, and invertebrates, and the action of allosamidin and A82516 on insects, it is clear that chitin metabolism is a worthwhile lethal target in these organisms. We should now be able to develop more specific screening procedures to throw up novel compounds from microbes with this target. These in turn should spur development of novel synthetic compounds as chemotherapeutic agents against fungi, protozoa, and parasites.

REFERENCES

Adams, D. J., and Gooday, G. W. (1983) Chitin synthesis as a target—current progress. Abh. Akad. Wiss. DDR., VIth Int. Symp. Systemische Fungizide und Antifungale Verbindungen, pp. 39–45.

Adams, D. J., and Gooday, G. W. (1980) A rapid chitin synthase preparation for the assay of potential fungicides and insecticides. *Biotechnology Lett.* **2**: 75–78.

Arroyo-Begovich, A., and Carabez-Trego, A. (1982) Location of chitin in the cyst wall of *Entamoeba invadens* with colloidal gold tracers. *J. Parasitol.* **68**: 253–258.

Arroyo-Begovich, A., Carabez-Trego, A., and Ruiz-Herrera, J. (1980) Identification of the structural component in the cyst wall of *Entamoeba invadens. J. Parasitol.* **66**: 735–741.

Aruchami, M., Sundara-Rajulu, G., and Gowri, N. (1986). Distribution of deacetylase in arthropoda. In *Chitin in nature and technology*, R. Muzzarelli, C. Jeuniaux, and G. W. Gooday, eds., pp. 263–265. New York: Plenum Press.

Avron, B., Deutsch, R. M., and Mirelman, D. (1982). Chitin synthesis inhibitors prevent cyst formation by Entamoeba trophozoites. *Biochem. Biophys. Res. Comm.* **108**: 815–821.

Barrett-Bee, K., and Hamilton, M. (1984) The detection and analysis of chitinase activity from the yeast form of *Candida albicans. J. Gen. Microbiol.* **130**: 1857–1861.

Bartnicki-Garcia, S. (1973) Fundamental aspects of hyphal morphogenesis. In *Microbial differentiation* J. M. Ashworth and J. E. Smith, eds., pp. 245–268. Cambridge: Cambridge University Press: New York: Academic Press.

Bartnicki-Garcia, S., and Lippman, E. (1972) Inhibition of *Mucor rouxii* by polyoxin D: Effects on chitin synthetase and morphological development. *J. Gen. Microbiol.* **71**: 301–309.

Becker, J. M., Marcus, S., Tullock, J., Miller, D., Krainer, E., Khare, R. K., and Naider, F. (1988) Use of chitin-synthesis inhibitor nikkomycin to treat disseminated candidiosis in mice. *J. Infect. Dis.* **157**: 212–214.

Becker, J. M., Covert, N. L., Shenbagamurthi, P., Steinfeld, A. S., and Naider, F. (1983) Polyoxin D inhibits growth of zoopathogenic fungi. *Antimicrob. Agents Chemotherapy* **23**: 926–929.

Blackwell, J., and Weih, M. A. (1984) The structure of chitin-protein complexes. In *Chitin, chitosan, and related enzymes*, J. P. Zikakis, ed., pp. 257–272. New York: Academic Press.

Bowers, B., Levin, G., and Cabib, E. (1974) Effect of polyoxin D on chitin synthesis and septum formation in *Saccharomyces cerevisiae. J. Bacteriol.* **119**: 564–575.

Bracker, C. E., Ruiz-Herrera, J., and Bartnicki-Garcia, S. (1976) Structure and transformation of chitin synthetase particles (chitosomes) during microfibril synthesis *in vitro. Proc. Nat. Acad. Sci. USA* **73**: 4570–4574.

Brydon, L. J., Gooday, G. W., Chappell, L. H., and King, T. P. (1987) Chitin in egg shells of *Onchocerca gibsoni* and *Onchocerca volvulus. Mol. Biochem. Parasitol.* **25**: 267–272.

Bulawa, C. E., Slater, M., Cabib, E., Au-Young, J., Sburlati, A., Adair, W. C., and Robbins, P. W. (1986) The *S. cerevisiae* structural gene for chitin synthase is not required for chitin synthesis *in vivo. Cell* **46**: 213–225.

Burnett, J. H. (1979) Aspects of the structure and growth of hyphal walls. In *Fungal walls and hyphal growth*, J. H. Burnett and A. P. J. Trinci, eds., pp. 1–25. Cambridge: Cambridge University Press.

Cabib, E. (in press) Chitin synthesis in yeast. In *The Biochemistry of cell walls and membranes in fungi*, M. Goosey, P. Kahn, and A. P. J. Trinci, eds.

Cabib, E. (1987) The synthesis and degradation of chitin. *Adv. Enzymol.* **59**: 59–101.

Cabib, E., and Farkas, V. (1971) The control of morphogenesis: An enzymatic mechanism for the initiation of septum formation in yeast. *Proc. Nat. Acad. Sci. USA* **68**: 2052–2056.

Chattaway, F. N., Holmes, M. R., and Barlow, A. J. E. (1968) Cell wall composition of the mycelial and blastospore forms of *Candida albicans. J. Gen. Microbiol.* **51**: 367–376.

Chen, A. C. (1987) Chitin metabolism. *Arch. Insect Biochem. Physiol.* **6**: 267–277.
Cohen, E. (1987) Chitin biochemistry: Synthesis and inhibition. *Ann. Rev. Entomol.* **32**: 71–93.
Dähn, U., Hagenmaier, H., Höhne, H., König, W. A., Wolf, G., and Zähner, H. (1976) Stoffwechselprodukte von Mikroorganismen. 154 Mitteilung. Nikkomycin, ein neuer Hemmstoff de Chitin synthese bei Pilzen. *Arch. Microbiol.* **107**: 143–160.
Datema, R., Ende, M. van den, and Wessels, J. G. H. (1977) The hyphal wall of *Mucor mucedo* 2. Hexosamine-containing polymers. *Eur. J. Biochem.* **80**: 621–626.
Davis, L. L., and Bartnicki-Garcia, S. (1984) The co-ordination of chitosan and chitin synthesis in *Mucor rouxii. J. Gen. Microbiol.* **130**: 2095–2102.
Domer, J. E., Hamilton, J. G., and Karkin, J. C. (1967) Comparative study of the cell walls of the yeastlike and mycelial phases of *Histoplasma capsulatum. J. Bacteriol.* **94**: 466–474.
Dubinsky, P., Rybos, M., and Turcekova, L. (1986) Properties and localization of chitin synthase in *Ascaris suum* eggs. *Parasitology* **92**: 219–225.
Endo, A., and Misato, T. (1969) Polyoxin D, a competitive inhibitor of UDP-*N*-acetylglucosamine: Chitin *N*-acetylglucosaminyltransferase in *Neurospora crassa. Biochem. Biophys. Res. Comm.* **37**: 718–722.
Endo, A., Kakiki, K., and Misato, T. (1970) Mechanism of action of the antifungal agent polyoxin D. *J. Bacteriol.* 104: 189–196.
Fiedler, H. P., Kurth, R., Langhärig, J., Delzer, J., and Zähner, H. (1982) Nikkomycins: Microbial inhibitors of chitin synthetase. *J. Chem. Tech. Biotechnol.* **32**: 271–280.
Fuhrman, J. A., and Piessens, W. F. (1985) Chitin synthesis and sheath morphogenesis in *Brugia malayi* microfilariae. *Mol. Biochem. Parasitol.* **17**: 93–104.
Furter, R., and Rast, D. M. (1985) A comparison of the chitin synthase-inhibitory and antifungal efficacy of nucleoside-peptide antibiotics: Structure-activity relationships. *FEMS Microbiol. Lett.* **28**: 205–211.
Gardner, K. H., and Blackwell, J. (1975) Refinement of the structure of β-chitin. *Biopolymers* **14**: 1581–1595.
Giraud-Gaille, M. M., and Bouligand, Y. (1986) Chitin-protein molecular organization in arthropod. In *Chitin in nature and technology*, R. Muzzarelli, C. Jeuniaux, and G. W. Gooday, eds., pp. 29–35. New York: Plenum Press.
Gonneau, M., Yadan, J. C., Sarthou, P., and Le Goffic, F. (1986) Nikkomycin X as inhibitor of *Candida albicans* growth. In *Chitin in nature and technology*, R. Muzzarelli, C. Jeuniaux, and G. W. Gooday, eds., pp. 203–205. New York and London: Plenum Press.
Gooday, G. W. (1989a) Inhibition of chitin metabolism. In *The biochemistry of cell walls and membranes in fungi*, in press. M. Goosey, P. Kuhn, and A. P. J. Trinci, eds., Berlin: Springer-Verlag.
Gooday, G. W. (1989b) Enzymic determination of chitin. In *Methods of enzymic analysis.* D. J. Manners and R. J. Sturgeon, eds., pp. Vol. X of *Methods in carbohydrate chemistry*, in press. R. L. Whistler and J. N. BeMiller, eds., London: Academic Press.
Gooday, G. W. (1983a) The microbial synthesis of cellulose, chitin, and chitosan. *Prog. Indust. Microbiol.* **18**: 85–127.
Gooday, G. W. (1983b) The hyphal tip. In *Fungal differentiation: A contemporary synthesis*, J. E. Smith, ed., pp. 315–356. New York: Marcel Dekker.
Gooday, G. W. (1979a) Chitin synthesis and differentiation in *Coprinus cinereus.* In *Fungal walls and hyphal growth*, J. H. Burnett and A. P. J. Trinci, eds., pp. 203–223. Cambridge: Cambridge University Press.
Gooday, G. W. (1979b) The action of polyoxin on fungi. Abh. Akad. Wiss. DDR. Vth. Int. Symp. Systemfungizide, pp. 159–168.
Gooday, G. W. (1977a) The first Fleming lecture. Biosynthesis of the fungal wall: Mechanisms and implications. *J. Gen. Microbiol.* **99**: 1–11.
Gooday, G. W. (1977b) The enzmyology of hyphal growth. In *The filamentous fungi*, J. E. Smith and D. R. Berry, eds., pp. 51–77. Fungal Development. London: Arnold.
Gooday, G. W. (1975) The control of differentiation in fruit bodies of *Coprinus cinereus. Rept. Tottori Mycol. Inst.* (Japan) **12**: 151–160.
Gooday, G. W. (1973) Activity of chitin synthetase during the development of fruit bodies of the toadstool *Coprinus cinereus. Biochem. Soc. Trans.* **1**: 1105–1107.
Gooday, G. W. (1972) Effect of polyoxin D on morphogenesis in *Coprinus cinereus. Biochem. J.* **129**: 17–18p.
Gooday, G. W., Brydon, L. J., and Chappell, L. H. (1988) Chitinase in female *Onchocerca gibsoni* and its inhibition by allosamidin. *Mol. Biochem. Parasitol.*, **29**: 223–225.
Gooday, G. W., Humphreys, A. M., and McIntosh, W. H. (1986) Roles of chitinase in fungal growth. In *Chitin in nature and technology*, R. Muzzarelli, C. Jeuniaux, and G. W. Gooday, eds., pp. 83–91. New York: Plenum Press.
Gooday, G. W., Woodman, J., Casson, E. A., and Browne, C. A. (1985) Effect of nikkomycin on chitin spine formation in the diatom *Thalassiosira fluviatilis* and observations of its peptide uptake. *FEMS Microbiol. Lett.* **28**: 335–340.
Gooday, G. W., and Gow, N. A. R. (1983) A model of the hyphal septum of *Candida albicans. Experimental Mycology* **7**: 370–373.
Gooday, G. W., and Trinci, A. P. J. (1980) Wall structure and biosynthesis in fungi. In *The eukaryotic microbial cell*, G. W. Gooday, D. Lloyd, and A. P. J. Trinci, eds., pp. 207–251. 30th Symposium of Society for General Microbiology, Cambridge University Press.
Gooday, G. W., Rousset-Hall, A. de, and Hunsley, D. (1976) The effect of polyoxin D on chitin synthesis in *Coprinus cinereus. Trans. Br. Mycol. Soc.* **67**: 193–200.
Gooday, G. W., and Rousset-Hall, A. de (1975) Properties of chitin synthetase from *Coprinus cinereus. J. Gen. Microbiol.* **89**: 137–145.
Gow, N. A. R., Gooday, G. W., Russell, J. D., and Wilson, M. J. (1987) Infrared and X-ray diffraction data on chitins of variable structure. *Carbohydrate Research* **165**: 105–110.
Gow, L. A., and Selitrennikof, C. P. (1984) Chitin synthetase of *Neurospora crassa*: inhibition by nikkomycin, polyoxin, and UDP. *Curr. Microbiol.* **11**: 211–216.

Gow, N. A. R., and Gooday, G. W. (1983) Ultrastructure of chitin in hyphae of *Candida albicans* and other dimorphic and mycelial fungi. *Protoplasma* **115**: 52–58.

Gow, N. A. R., Gooday, G. W., Newsam, R. J., and Gull, K. (1980) Ultrastructure of the septum in *Candida albicans. Curr. Microbiol.* **4**: 357–359.

Gowri, N., Aruchami, M., and Sundara-Rajulu, G. (1986) Natural deacetylation of the cuticle in *Sacculina rotundata.* In *Chitin in Nature and Technology*, R. Muzzarelli, C. Jeuniaux, and G. W. Gooday, eds., pp. 266–268. New York: Plenum Press.

Hagenmaier, H., Keckeisen, A., Dehler, W., Fiedler, H., Zähner, H., and König, W. A. (1981) Stoffwechselprodukte von Mikroorganismen, 199. Konstitution saufklärung der Nikkomycine I, J, M, und N. *Liebigs Ann. Chem.* 1981: 1018–1024.

Hagenmaier, H., Keckeisen, A., Zähner, H., and König, W. A. (1979) Stoffwechselprodukte von Mikroorganismen, 182. Aufklärung der Struktur des Nukleosidantibiotikums Nikkomycin X. *Liebigs Ann. Chem.* 1979: 1494–1502.

Hänseler, E., Nyhlen, L. E., and Rast, D. M. (1983) Isolation and properties of chitin synthetase from *Agaricus bisporus* mycelium. *Exp. Mycol.* **7**: 17–30.

Hardy, J. C., and Gooday, G. W. (1983) Stability and zymogenic nature of chitin synthase from *Candida albicans. Curr. Microbiol.* **9**: 51–54.

Hilenski, L. K. L., Naider, F., and Becker, J. M. (1986) Polyoxin D inhibits colloidal gold-wheat germ agglutinin labeling of chitin in dimorphic forms of *Candida albicans. J. Gen. Microbiol.* **132**: 1441–1457.

Hori, M., Kakiki, K., and Misato, T. (1977) Antagonistic effect of dipeptides on the uptake of polyoxin A by *Alternaria kikuchiana. J. Pestic. Sci.* **2**: 139–150.

Hori, M., Eguchi, J., Kakiki, K., and Misato, T. (1974) Studies on the mode of action of polyoxins. VI. Effect of polyoxin B on chitin synthesis in polyoxin-sensitive and -resistant strains of *Alternaria kikuchiana. J. Antibiotics* **27**: 261–266.

Humphreys, A. M., and Gooday, G. W. (1984a) Properties of chitinase activities from *Mucor mucedo*: Evidence for a membrane-bound zymogenic form. *J. Gen. Microbiol.* **130**: 1359–1366.

Humphreys, A. M., and Gooday, G. W. (1984b) Phospholipid requirement of microsomal chitinase from *Mucor mucedo. Current Microbiol.* **11**: 187–190.

Humphreys, A. M., and Gooday, G. W. (1984c) Chitinase activities from *Mucor mucedo.* In *Microbial cell wall synthesis and autolysis*, C. Nombela, ed., pp. 269–273. Amsterdam: Elsevier.

Hunsley, G., and Gooday, G. W. (1974) Structure and development of septa in *Neurospora crassa. Protoplasma* **82**: 126–146.

Isono, K., Asahi, K., and Suzuki, A. (1969) Studies on polyoxins, antifungal antibiotics. XIII. The structure of polyoxins. *J. Am. Chem. Soc.* **91**: 7490–7505.

Isono, K., Nagutsu, J., Kobinata, K., Sasaki, K., and Suzuki, S. (1967) Studies of polyoxins, antifungal antibiotics. V. Isolation and characterization of polyoxins C, D, E, F, G, H, and I. *Agric. Biol. Chem.* **31**: 190–199.

Isono, K., Nagatsu, J., Kawashiwa, Y., and Suzuki, S. (1965) Studies on polyoxins, antifungal antibiotics. I. Isolation and characterization of polyoxins A and B. *Agr. Biol. Chem.* **29**: 848–854.

Jeuniaux, C. (1963). *Chitine et chitinolyse.* Paris: Masson.

Kanetsuma, F., and Carbonell, L. M. (1971) Cell wall composition of the yeastlike and mycelial forms of *Blastomyces dermatitidis. J. Bact.* **106**: 946–948.

Kanetsuma, F., Carbonell, L. M., Morena, R. E., and Rodriquez, J. (1969) Cell wall composition of the yeast and mycelial forms of *Paracoccoides brasiliensis. J. Bact.* **97**: 1036–1041.

King, T. P., Brydon, L., Gooday, G. W., and Chappell, L. H. (1987) Silver enhancement of lectin-gold and enzyme-gold cytochemical labeling of eggs of the nematode *Onchocerca gibsoni. Histochem. J.* **19**: 281–287.

Kobinata, K., Oramoto, M., Nishii, M., Kusakabe, H., Nakamura, G., and Isono, K. (1980) Neopolyoxin A, neopolyoxin B, and neopolyoxin C, new chitin synthetase inhibitors. *Agric. Biol. Chem.* **44**: 1709–1722.

Koga, D., Isogai, A., Sakuda, S., Matsumoto, S., Suzuki, A., Kimmura, A., and Ide, A. (1987) Specific inhibition of *Bombyx mori* chitinase by allosamidin. *Agric. Biol. Chem.* **51**: 471–467.

König, W. A., Hass, W., Dehler, W., Fiedler, H. P., and Zähner, H. (1980) Stoffwechselprodukte von Mikroorganismen, 189. Strutkturaufklárung und Partialsynthese des Nukleosidantibiotikums Nikkomycin B. *Liebigs Ann. Chem.* 1980: 622–628.

Kramer, K. J., and Koga, D. (1986) Insect chitin. Physical state, synthesis, degradation, and metabolic regulation. *Insect. Biochem.* **16**: 851–877.

Lindsay, G. J. H., and Gooday, G. W. (1985) Action of chitinase on spines of the diatom *Thalassiosira fluviatilis. Carbohydrate Polymers* **5**: 131–140.

McCarthy, P., Troke, P. F., and Gull, K. (1985) Mechanism of action of nikkomycin and the peptide transport system of *Candida albicans. J. Gen. Microbiol.* **131**: 775–780.

Minke, R., and Blackwell, J. (1978) The structure of α-chitin. *J. Mol. Biol.* **120**: 167–181.

Misato, T., and Kakiki, K. (1977) Inhibition of fungal cell wall synthesis and cell membrane function. In *Antifungal compounds*, M. R. Siegal and H. Sisler, eds., Vol. 2., pp. 277–300. New York, Basel: Marcel Dekker.

Misato, T., Ko, K., and Yamaguchi, U. (1977) Use of antibiotics in agriculture. *Adv. Appl. Microbiol.* **21**: 53–88.

Montgomery, G. W. G., and Gooday, G. W. (1985) Phospholipid-enzyme interactions of chitin synthase of *Coprinus cinereus. FEMS Microbiol. Lett.* **27**: 29–33.

Montgomery, G. W. G., Adams, D. J., and Gooday, G. W. (1984) Studies in the purification of chitin synthase form *Coprinus cinereus. J. Gen. Microbiol.* **13**: 291–297.

Morin, L. G., Smucker, R. A., and Herth, W. (1986) Effects of two chitin synthesis inhibitors on *Thalassiosira fluviatilis* and *Cyclotèlla cryptica. FEMS Microbiol. Lett.* **37**: 263–268.

Mothes, U., and Sietz, K. (1982) Action of the microbial metabolite and chitin synthesis inhibitor nikkomycin on the mite *Tetranychus urticae. Pestic. Sci.* **13**: 426–441.

Müller, H., Furter, R., Zähner, H., and Rast, D. M. (1981) Metabolic products of microorganisms 203. Inhibition of chitosomal chitin synthetase and growth of *Mucor rouxii* by nikkomycin Z, nikkomycin X, and polyoxin A: A comparison. *Arch. Micobiol.* **130**: 195–197.

Nishimura, M., Kohmoto, K., and Udagawa, H. (1973) Field emergence of fungicide-tolerant strains of *Alternaria kikuchiana. Rept. Tottori Mycol. Inst.* **10**: 677–686.

Orlean, P. (1987) Two chitin synthases in *Saccharomyces cerevisiae. J. Biol. Chem.* **262**: 5732–5739.

Payne, J. W., and Shallow, D. A. (1985) Studies on drug targeting in the pathogenic fungus *Candida albicans*: Peptide transport mutants resistant to polyoxins, nikkomycins, and bacilysin. *FEMS Microbiol. Lett.* **28**: 55–60.

Peter, M. G., Kegel, G., and Keller, R. (1986) Structural studies on sclerotized insect cuticle. In *Chitin in nature and technology*, R. Muzzarelli, C. Jeuniaux, and G. W. Gooday, eds., pp. 21–28. New York: Plenum Press.

Peters, W., Schraermeyer, U., and Zahner, H. (1987) Formation and degradation of chitin during development of microfilariae. *Trop. Med. Parasit.* **38**: 70.

Poulicek, M., Voss-Foucart, M. F., and Jeuniaux, C. (1986) Chitinoproteic complexes and mineralization in mollusk skeletal structures. In *Chitin in nature and technology*, R. Muzzarelli, C. Jeuniaux, and G. W. Gooday, eds., pp. 7–12. New York: Plenum Press.

Rousset-Hall, A. de, and Gooday, G. W. (1975) A kinetic study of a solubilized chitin synthetase preparation from *Coprinus cinereus. J. Gen. Microbiol.* **89**: 146–154.

Ruiz-Herrera, J., Sing, V. O., Van der Woude, W. J., and Bartnicki-Garcia, S. (1975) Microfibril assembly by granules of chitin synthetase. *Proc. Nat. Acad. Sci. USA* **72**: 2706–2710.

Ruiz-Herrera, J., Bracker, C. E., and Bartnicki-Garcia, S. (1984) Sedimentation properties of chitosomes from *Mucor rouxii. Protoplasma* **122**: 178–190.

Sakuda, S., Isogai, A., Matsumoto, S., and Suzuki, A. (1987a) Search for microbial insect growth regulators. II. Allosamidin, a novel insect chitinase inhibitor. *J. Antibiot.* **40**: 296–300.

Sakuda, S., Isogai, A., Makita, T., Matsumoto, S., Koseki, K., Kodama, H., and Suzuki, A. (1987b) Structures of Allosamidins, novel insect chitinase inhibitors, produced by actinomycetes. *Agric. Biol. Chem.* **51**: 3251–3259.

Sakuda, S., Isogai, A., Matsumoto, S., and Susuki, A. (1986) The structure of allosamidin, a novel insect chitinase inhibitor, produced by *Streptomyces* sp. *Tetrahedron Lett.* **27**: 2475–2478.

Sburlati, A., and Cabib, E. (1986) Chitin synthetase 2, a presumptive participant in septum formation in *Saccharomyces cerevisiae. J. Biol. Chem.* **261**: 15147–15152.

Sietsma, J. H., Vermeulen, C. A., and Wessels, J. G. H. (1986) The role of chitin in hyphal morphogenesis. In *Chitin in nature and technology*, R. Muzzarelli, C. Jeuniaux, and G. W. Gooday, eds., pp. 63–69. New York: Plenum Press.

Somers, P. J. B., Yao, R. C., Doolin, L. E., McGowan, M. J., Fukuda, D. S., and Mynderse, J. S. (1987) Method for the detection and quantitation of chitinase inhibitors in fermentation broths: Isolation and insect life cycle effect of A82516. *J. Antibiot.* **40**: 1751–1756.

Spiegel, Y., and Chet, I. (1985) Chitin synthestase inhibitors and their potential to control the root-knot nematode *Meloidogyne javanica. Nematologica* **31**: 480–482.

Surarit, R., Gopal, P. K., and Shepherd, M. G. (1988) Evidence for a glycosidic linkage between chitin and glucan in the cell wall of *Candida albicans. J. Gen. Microbiol.* **134**: 1723–1730.

Uramoto, M., Kobinata, K., Isono, K., Higashijima, T., Miyazawa, T., Jenkins, E. E., and McCloskey, J. A. (1982) Chemistry of the neopolyoxins, pyrimidine, and imidazoline nucleoside peptide antibiotics. *Tetrahedron* **38**: 1559–1608.

Uramoto, M., Kobinata, K., Isono, K., Higashijima, T., Miyazawa, T., Jenkins, E. E., and McCloskey, J. A. (1980) Structures of neoployoxins A, B, and C. *Tetrahedron Lett.* **21**: 3395–3398.

Usai, T., Hayashi, Y., Nanjo, F., Sakai, K., and Ishido, Y. (1987) Transglycosylation reaction of a chitinase purified from *Nocardia orientalis. Biochm. Biophys. Acta* **923**: 302–309.

Vardanis, A. (1978) Polyoxin fungicides: Demonstration of insecticidal activity due to inhibition of chitin synthesis. *Experientia* **34**: 228–229.

Vermeulen, C. A., and Wessels, J. G. H. (1986) Chitin biosynthesis by a fungal membrane preparation. Evidence for a transient non-crystalline state of chitin. *Eur. J. Biochem.* **158**: 411–415.

Vermeulen, C. A., and Wessels, J. G. H. (1984) Ultrastructural differences between wall apices of growing and non-growing hyphae of *Schizophyllum commune. Protoplasma* **120**: 123–130.

Ward, K. A., and Fairburn, D. (1972) Chitinase in developing eggs of *Ascaris suum* (Nematoda). *J. Parasitol.* **58**: 546–549.

Ward, H. O., Alroy, J., Lev, B. I., Keusch, G. T., and Pereira, M. E. A. (1985) Identification of chitin as a structural component of *Giardia* cysts. *Infect. Immun.* **49**: 629–634.

Wessels, J. G. H., and Sietsma, J. H. (1981) Fungal cell walls: A survey. In *Plant carboyhydrates.* II. *Extracellular carbohydrates.* W. Tanner and F. A. Loewus, eds., pp. 352–394 (Encyclopedia of Plant Physiology, New Series, Vol. 13B). Berlin, Heidelberg, New York: Springer.

Yadan, J., Gonneau, M., Sarthou, P., and Le Goffic, F. (1984) Sensitivity to nikkomycin in *Candida albicans*: Role of peptide permeases. *J. Bacteriol.* **160**: 884–888.

Youatt, J., Gow, N. A. R., and Gooday, G. W. (1988) Bioelectric and biosynthetic aspects of cell polarity in *Allomyces macrogynus. Protoplasma* **146**, 118–126.

CHAPTER 15

A STUDY OF PEPTIDE TRANSPORT IN *CANDIDA ALBICANS*

William D. Kingsbury
Department of Medicinal Chemistry, Smith Kline & French Laboratories, Swedeland, Pennsylvania, United States

Abstract — As an approach to the development of antifungal agents, a novel peptide carrier system was designed, based on the chemical instability of α-substituted glycine analogs. The initial studies were undertaken with 5-fluorouracil (5-FU)-containing peptides. These peptides were shown to deliver 5-FU into fungal cells specifically and only via peptide permeases. This effort provided the framework for the development of a series of unique detector peptides that permitted the nature of fungal peptide permeases to be investigated. It is anticipated that the results of these studies will be important in the future optimization and design of antimicrobial agents that operate through a peptide transport mechanism.

1. INTRODUCTION

Microorganisms have been shown to possess specialized transport systems for the uptake of peptides (Payne & Gilvarg, 1978). In *Candida albicans* the factors that determine the recognition of peptides by microbial peptide transport systems have been the subject of numerous investigations (Becker & Naider, 1980; Payne & Gilvarg, 1978; Payne, 1980). A significant observation that has emerged from these studies, primarily in bacteria, is that peptide transport systems generally possess little demonstrable side chain specificity. This is likely an accommodation to the diversity of side chain combinations that occur in peptides assembled from the naturally occurring amino acids. Early indications that this process could be exploited therapeutically was demonstrated in *E. coli* where normally impermeant amino acid analogs, not recognized by the more selective amino acid transport systems, were shown to enter these cells by a peptide carrier mechanism when incorporated into the backbone of a peptide. Following transport, cytoplasmic peptidases hydrolyze the peptide to release the constituent amino acids (Payne, 1980). Many natural and synthetic examples involving peptides that contain growth inhibitory amino acids have been reported (Ringrose, 1980) and considerable interest has been expressed in utilizing this approach as a means of developing novel chemotherapeutic agents (Ames et al., 1973; Fickel & Galvarg, 1973). The synthesis and development of the wide-spectrum antimicrobial agent alaphosphin (Allen et al., 1978) (L-alanyl-L-1-aminoethylphosphonic acid) is a powerful example of the peptide transport concept.

2. TRANSPORT CONCEPT

In an attempt to broaden the overall scope of the peptide transport approach so that inhibitory agents other than amino acid analogs could be brought into microbial cells, a more versatile peptide delivery system in which the toxophoric agent is attached to the α-carbon of a glycine residue within a peptide chain was developed. Intracellular cleavage of the peptide by cytoplasmic peptidases results in the formation of an unstable intermediate that decomposes with release of the attached toxophoric group.

The new transport concept (shown in Table 15-1) is based on the inherent chemical instability of α-substituted glycines, *1*, where the linked α-substituent is a good leaving group (XR = $-$Cl, $-$Br, $-$OAc, $-$SR, $-NR_2$). Compounds of this type have been found to decompose rapidly with the expulsion of the α-substituent (i.e., *1* $\rightarrow$ *2*). However, stabilization can be achieved through acylation of the glycyl nitrogen; for example, the N-acyl-α-acetoxyglycine *3* is a stable molecule (Horikawa et al., 1976). Theoretically, attachment of an appropriate acyl group that would stabilize such molecules, be compatible with pep-

TABLE 15-1.

$$\underset{\substack{1\\ \alpha\text{-substituted glycine}\\ \text{(unstable)}}}{H_2N{-}\overset{\overset{\displaystyle XR}{|}}{C}H{-}CO_2H} \longrightarrow \underset{2}{RXH + HN = CHCO_2H}$$

$$\underset{\substack{3\\ \text{acylated }\alpha\text{-substituted glycine}\\ \text{(stable)}}}{CH_3CONH\overset{\overset{\displaystyle XR}{|}}{C}HCO_2H}$$

tide transport, and be released readily within the cell could provide the basis for a novel form of drug delivery in which the α-substituent would be the drug delivered into microbial cells freed of the need for its own transport. However, N-terminal acyl derivatives of type 3 or peptides generated from extensions at the carboxy terminus of *3* would be poorly accepted by most microbial peptide permeases since a free terminal amino group is required for optimal transport (Payne & Gilvarg, 1978). Furthermore, peptidase activity would be unlikely to deacylate such peptides thus preventing the formation of the unstable α-substituted glycine intermediate. On the other hand, if the stabilizing acyl group is derived from the carbonyl group of an amino acid, the resulting dipeptide should serve as a substrate for the microbial permeases as well as for the intracellular peptidases, as indicated in Table 15-2 (Kingsbury et al., 1984b). Thus, transport of the dipeptide would be followed by hydrolysis producing the unstable α-substituted glycine unit that degrades releasing the α-substituent within the cell. To assess the feasibility of this approach, 5-fluorouracil, the biologically active metabolite of the clinically useful drug 5-fluorocytosine (Waldorf & Polale, 1983), was selected as a pharmacologically interesting toxophoric group to study, since a biological response would be guaranteed if 5-FU was brought into the cells of the test organism (Kingsbury et al., 1984a).

It is possible to distinguish between the activity of free 5-FU and the 5-FU peptide by examining the ability of noninhibitory peptides to antagonize the uptake, and thus the biological activity of the peptide-inhibitor conjugate. Under these conditions, no antagonism of 5-FU activity should occur since its entry is independent of peptide transport. Initial biological evaluation was performed using the diastereoisomeric mixture *8* (Table 15-3) under two separate sets of assay conditions. In one, *C. albicans* was grown in a defined medium that is free of peptides while in the other growth was followed in a complex medium known to contain peptides. The results of these tests imply that *8* enters the cells of the test organisms by peptide-mediated transport; 5-FU is active when tested in both media, but *8* is active only in the absence of other peptides. The inhibitory effects of the 5-FU peptide

TABLE 15-2.

$$H_2N\overset{\overset{\displaystyle R}{|}}{C}HCONH\overset{\overset{\displaystyle XR}{|}}{C}HCO_2H \xrightarrow[\text{2. Intracellular peptidase}]{\text{1. Cellular entry}} H_2N\overset{\overset{\displaystyle R}{|}}{C}HCO_2H + H_2N\overset{\overset{\displaystyle XR}{|}}{C}HCO_2H$$

$$\downarrow$$

$$H_2\overset{+}{N} = CH\dot{C}O_2H + {}^{-}XR$$

TABLE 15-3.

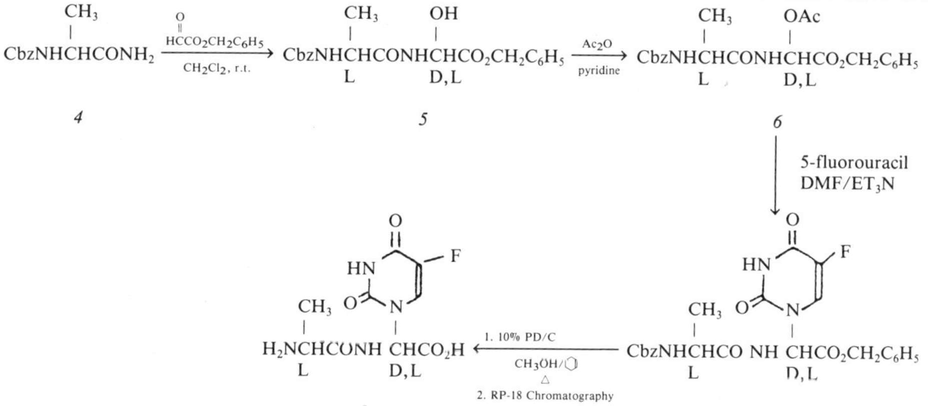

CbzNHCH(CH_3)CONH$_2$ (4) $\xrightarrow[CH_2Cl_2,\ r.t.]{HC(O)CO_2CH_2C_6H_5}$ CbzNHCH(CH_3)CONHCH(OH)$CO_2CH_2C_6H_5$ (L, D,L) (5) $\xrightarrow[pyridine]{Ac_2O}$ CbzNHCH(CH_3)CONHCH(OAc)$CO_2CH_2C_6H_5$ (L, D,L) (6)

6 $\xrightarrow{\text{5-fluorouracil, DMF/ET}_3\text{N}}$ CbzNHCH(CH_3)CO NH CH(5-fluorouracil-1-yl)$CO_2CH_2C_6H_5$ (L, D,L) (7)

7 $\xrightarrow{\text{1. 10\% PD/C, CH}_3\text{OH/cyclohexene, }\Delta\text{; 2. RP-18 Chromatography}}$ $H_2NCH(CH_3)CONH$ CH(5-fluorouracil-1-yl)CO_2H (L, D,L) (8)

8
8a, (L,L)
8b, (L,D)

conjugate *8* measured as a function of concentration together with the ability of dialanine to antagonize its activity are in accord with the initial observations and support peptide transport mediated entry of peptide *8* into microbial cells.

Since the synthesis of the 5-FU peptides produced a separable mixture of diastereoisomers, *8a* and *8b*, each diastereomer could be tested for biological activity. In view of the convincing evidence that illustrates that the peptide permeases are stereospecific, allowing only the transport of L,L-dipeptides (Wofinbarger & Marzluf, 1975; Nisbet & Payne, 1979), the L,L-dipeptide should be inhibitory while the L,D-dipeptide should be inactive. The biological results demonstrate that only one of the diastereomers was inhibitory, a finding that is in agreement with peptide permease-mediated entry and also allows stereochemical assignments to be made for each isomer.

While exploring the use of this carrier system we prepared L-alanyl-L-2-thiophenyl-glycine (*9*, Ala-α-TPG) and L-alanyl-L-2-thiophenyl-glycine-L-alanine (*10*, Ala-α-TPG-Ala), as shown in Table 15-4 (Kingsbury et al., 1984a; Kingsbury & Boehm, 1986). Studies with this peptide revealed that the rate of cleavage, and thus thiophenol (TP) release, by cell extracts of *E. coli*, could be followed spectrophotometrically using Ellman's reagent (Kingsbury et al., 1984a).

The rational development of antifungal peptide drugs may be accelerated by a clearer elucidation of the number of specificity of the peptide permeases in the target organism. To achieve this, specific and reproducible techniques for this study of fungal peptide permeases must be developed. Early studies of peptide transport were dependent upon the use of a limited number of radiolabeled peptides (Becker & Naider, 1977; Wofinbarger & Marzluf, 1975). However, Nisbet and Payne (1979) developed a fluoroescamine method for studying peptide uptake and more recently this technique has been developed into a con-

TABLE 15-4.

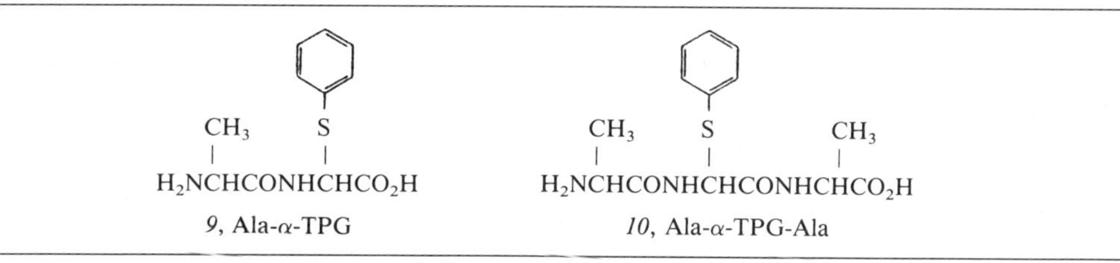

tinuous monitoring system (Payne and Nisbet, 1981). Although these techniques allow the uptake of any peptide possessing a free amino terminus to be studied, the rapid screening of a wide variety of peptides for their affinity to their permeases is not possible.

The use of peptides containing α-TPG in the study of fungal peptide transport is therefore a valuable addition to existing techniques. However, it is only valid when peptide uptake, and not hydrolysis or thiophenol efflux, is the rate-limiting step in the generation of extracellular thiophenol. Our hypothesis was that the detector peptides should be transported by the cell's peptide permeases and cleaved by intracellular peptidases. The released α-substituted glycine residue is unstable and breaks down to release thiophenol, glyoxylate, and ammonia. Since thiophenol is lipophilic, it passes freely through the cytoplasmic membrane. An equilibrium situation is prevented by the presence of extracellular Ellman's reagent which removes all molecules containing thiol residues from the extracellular environment, thus both producing a color reaction and preventing sequestration of the released thiophenol. This thiol reagent does, however, have the potential of disrupting membrane-dependent processes or of inhibiting enzymes in which a cysteinyl-sulfhydryl group is of importance. Ellman's reagent was found to have no influence upon the rate of thiophenol release at the concentration employed. However, when used in great excess (1 mM), a significant reduction in the rate of color generation was observed. This process is not fully understood, but it is analogous to the effect of another thiol reagent, N-ethylmaleimide, which has been shown to inhibit trimethionine uptake in *C. albicans* (Logan et al., 1979).

The proposed methodology requires that there be no extracellular peptidase activity and that the rate of intracellular hydrolysis be sufficient to prevent the accumulation of the stable peptide within the cytoplasm. The absence of extracellular hydrolytic activity toward small peptides has previously been reported for *Candida albicans* (Logan et al., 1979; Lichliter et al., 1976) and should be reestablished for any strain used in studies of this nature. It has been shown that the release of thiophenol from the detector peptides by intact cells is highly sensitive to the presence of sodium azide, an ATPase inhibitor which is known to affect peptide transport (Davies, 1980). No mechanism of peptidase activity, independent of membrane translocation, has been shown to be sensitive to this inhibitor, and it can therefore be assumed that extracellular hydrolysis is not of importance in thiophenol generation by this procedure.

The use of permeabilized cells permits the study of intracellular enzymes in a less disrupted environment than is present in a broken cell preparation and allows solutes to pass freely into the cell. A recent report (Ram et al., 1983) optimized the conditions for permeabilizing *C. albicans*, and this technique was adopted. When permeabilized, the cells showed a greatly increased rate of thiophenol release from the detector peptides, a result which implies that a membrane function, presumably a permease, is mediating transmembrane permeation and hence limiting the substrate available for intracellular degradation.

The sodium azide sensitivity observed for intact cells during thiophenol generation confirmed membrane transport as being essential to the process and refutes the involvement of extracellular or periplasmic peptidases. Bestatin, an aminopeptidase inhibitor, completely inhibited detector hydrolysis in permeabilized cells, indicating that these cells are, to a large extent, dependent upon aminopeptidase rather than carboxypeptidase activity.

The rate of thiophenol release from cells is equivalent to the rate of peptide uptake as determined by the fluoroescamine technique. This indicates that thiophenol release is not the rate-limiting step and that the rate of color generation is a true measurement of peptide uptake. These novel peptides can therefore be used in the study of peptide transport in the lower eukaryotes, provided that the necessary controls are performed to negate extracellular hydrolysis or intracellular sequestration.

The demonstration of competition between naturally occurring peptides and the detectors would indicate that transport is taking place *via* the peptide permeases and confirmatory evidence for this was obtained using *C. albicans* 12NIK5. This mutant is unable to transport dipeptides while oligopeptide transport remains unaffected (McCarthy, 1983). This evidence, in conjunction with other factors such as the low degree of competition between oligopeptides and the dipeptide detector, Ala-α-TPG, has led us to conclude that there are multiple peptide permeases present in *C. albicans*. Since the dipeptide detector is not degraded by intact *C. albicans* 124NIK5, it can be stated with some certainty that such peptides are utilizing the eukaryotic peptide permeases. When permeabilized, NIK5 is able to degrade the dipeptide, indicating that the mutation of the peptide permease has no effect upon the subsequent peptidase activity. This suggests that peptide transport and hydrolysis are separate events in *C. albicans*.

These novel peptides can be used as a simple, rapid assay method for studying peptide transport in lower eukaryotes. They provide data which were previously available only through the use of complex techniques. Alteration of the amino acid residues present in the detector peptides will provide further data concerning the substrate specificity and multiplicity of peptide permeases and may allow the development of effective antifungal drugs through the exploitation of this warhead delivery system.

REFERENCES

Allen, J. G., Atherton, F. R., Hall, M. J., Hassall, C. H., Holmes, S. W., Lambert, R. W., Nisbet, L. J., and Ringrose, P. S. (1978) Phosphonopeptides, a new class of synthetic antibacterial agents. *Nature* **272**: 56.

Ames, B. N., Ames, G., F.-L., Young, J. D., Tsuchiya, D., and Lecocq, J. (1973) Illicit transport, the oligopeptide permease. *Proc. Natl. Acad. Sci. USA* **70**: 456.

Becker, J. M., and Naider, F. (1977) Peptide transport in yeast: Uptake of radioactive trimethionine in *Saccharomyces cerevisiae*. *Arch. Biochem. Biophys.* **178**: 245–255.

Becker, J. M., and Naider, F. (1980) Transport and utilization of peptides by yeast. in *Microorganisms and nitrogen sources*, J. W. Payne, ed., pp. 257–279 and references therein. New York: John Wiley.

Davies, M. B. (1980) Peptide uptake in *Candida albicans*. *J. Gen. Microbiol.* **121**: 181–186.

Fickel, T. E., and Gilvarg, C. (1973) Transport of impermeant substances in *Escherichia coli* by way of oligopeptide permease. *Nature New Biol.* **241**: 161.

Horikawa, H., Iwasaki, T., Matsumoto, K., and Miyoshi, M. (1976) A new synthesis of 2-alkoxy- and 2-acetoxy-2-amino acids by anodic oxidation. *Tetrahedron Lett.* no. 3, 191–194.

Kingsbury, W. D., and Boehm, J. C. (1986) Synthesis of α-thiophenylglycine peptides. *Int. J. Peptide Protein Res.* **27**: 659.

Kingsbury, W. D., Boehm, J. C., Nehta, R. J., Grappel, S. F., and Gilvarg, C. (1984a) A novel peptide delivery system involving peptidase activated prodrugs as antimicrobial agents. Synthesis and biological activity of peptidyl derivatives of 5-fluorouracil. *J. Med. Chem.* **27**: 1447.

Kingsbury, W. D., Boehm, J. C., Perry, D., and Gilvarg, C. J. (1984b) Portage of various compounds into bacteria by attachment to glycine residues in peptides. *Proc. Natl. Acad. Sci. USA* **81**: 4573.

Lichliter, W. D., Naider, F., and Becker, J. M. (1976) Basis for the design of anticandidal agents from studies of peptide utilization in *Candida albicans*. *Antimicrob. Ag. Chem.* **10**: 483–490.

Logan, D. A., Becker, J. M., and Naider, F. (1979) Peptide transport in *Candida albicans*. *J. Gen. Microbiol.* **114**: 179.

McCarthy, P. J. (1983) Ph.D. dissertation, University of Kent at Canterbury.

Nisbet, T. M., and Payne, J. W. (1979) Peptide uptake in *Saccharomyces cerevisiae*. Characteristics of a transport system shared by dipeptides and tripeptides. *J. Gen. Microbiol.* **115**: 127–133.

Payne, J. W. (1980) Transport and utilization of peptides by bacteria. In *Microorganisms and nitrogen sources*, J. W., Payne, ed., pp. 211–256 and references therein. New York: John Wiley.

Payne, J. W., and Nisbet, T. M. (1981) Continuous monitoring of substrate uptake by microorganisms. *J. App. Biochem.* **3**: 447–458.

Payne, J. W., and Gilvarg, C. (1978) Transport of peptides in bacteria. In *Bacterial Transport*, B. P. Rosen, ed., pp. 325–383 and references therein. New York: Marcel Dekker.

Ram, S. P., Sullivan, P. A., and Shepherd, M. G. (1983) The *in situ* assay of *Candida albicans* enzymes during yeast growth and germ tube formation. *J. Gen. Microbiol.* **129**: 2367–2378.

Ringrose, P. S. (1980) Peptides as antimicrobial agents. In *Microorganisms and nitrogen sources*, J. W. Payne, ed., pp. 641–692 and references therein. New York: John Wiley.

Waldorf, A. R., and Polale, A. (1983) Mechanisms of action of 5-fluorocytosine *Antimicrob. Agents Chemother.* **23**: 79–85.

Wofinbarger, L., and Marzluf, G. A. (1975) Specificity and regulation of peptide transport in *Neurospora crassa*. *Arch. Biochem. Biophys.* **171**: 637–644.

CHAPTER 16

THE RATIONAL DESIGN OF FUNGAL LANOSTEROL C14 DEMETHYLASE INHIBITORS

M. S. Marriott

Glaxo Group Research Ltd., Greenford Road, Greenford, United Kingdom

Abstract – The rational design of medically important inhibitors of fungal lanosterol C14 demethylase is discussed in terms of structure-activity relationships relevant to intrinsic potency and *in vitro* and *in vivo* activity. While much is known in these three areas, emerging data on interactions with mammalian steroid and xenobiotic metabolizing cytochromes P_{450} suggest our ability to design selective agents is still at an early stage.

1. INTRODUCTION

Azole-containing (imidazole, triazole) antifungal drugs have been known for some time (Borgers, 1985) and have been the subject of intense research for both medical and agricultural use (Vanden Bossche, 1985; Baldwin, 1986). While early examples were reported to have a variety of actions (Iwata et al., 1973; Yamaguchi & Iwata, 1979), more recent compounds appear to owe their antifungal activity exclusively to inhibition of lanosterol C14 demethylation (Marriott & Richardson, 1988). Thus, initial work on the design of novel azoles was rather unstructured, and it is only relatively recently that a more rational approach has been possible. Design features in a medically important azole antifungal vary enormously from the desirable properties of one intended for agricultural use. This chapter will concentrate on the rational design of azole C14 demethylase inhibitors of medical importance.

2. MODE OF ACTION

Vanden Bossche and colleagues (1978) were the first to show that removal of the methyl group at C14 of the lanosterol nucleus was sensitive to the action of miconazole. Subsequently, several authors have confirmed that imidazole- and triazole-containing antifungals are potent inhibitors of C14 demethylase (Henry & Sisler, 1979; Pye & Marriott, 1982). The process by which the methyl group is removed involves three rounds of oxidation (Fig. 16-1) leading to the release of formic acid (Gibbons et al., 1979), and it is generally assumed that all stages are accomplished by the same enzyme (Aoyama et al. 1984; Aoyama et al., 1987). Aoyama and colleagues (1984) have purified lanosterol C14 demethylase from *Saccharomyces cerevisiae* and have demonstrated conversion of lanosterol to C14 desmethyl lanosterol in a reconstituted system.

C14 demethylase is a cytochrome P_{450}-dependent mono-oxygenase and binding of azoles induces a type II spectral shift in this cytochrome, indicating ligand binding to the heme moiety (Yoshida & Aoyama, 1986; Yoshida & Aoyama, 1987). Thus, the lone pair of electrons on the azole nitrogen act as the sixth ligand, displacing oxygen and inhibiting enzyme activity (Baldwin, 1986), Fig. 16-2. Not surprisingly, therefore, it is important that this nitrogen is unhindered, and indeed substitution on either side results in a loss of activity. Computer-derived models of azole interaction with heme are useful for understanding their mode of action. Of more value is recent work on the cloning of C14 demethylase from various sources (Kalb et al., 1986; Chen et al., 1987). Figure 16-3 compares the derived amino acid sequence of the heme-binding region of yeast cytochrome P_{450DM} and bovine steroid 17α hydroxylase (Zuber et al., 1986). Clearly, similarities and dissimilarities exist and, to date, it is the fortuitous exploitation of these differences that has led to the discovery of selective C14 demethylase inhibitors. In the future, it is possi-

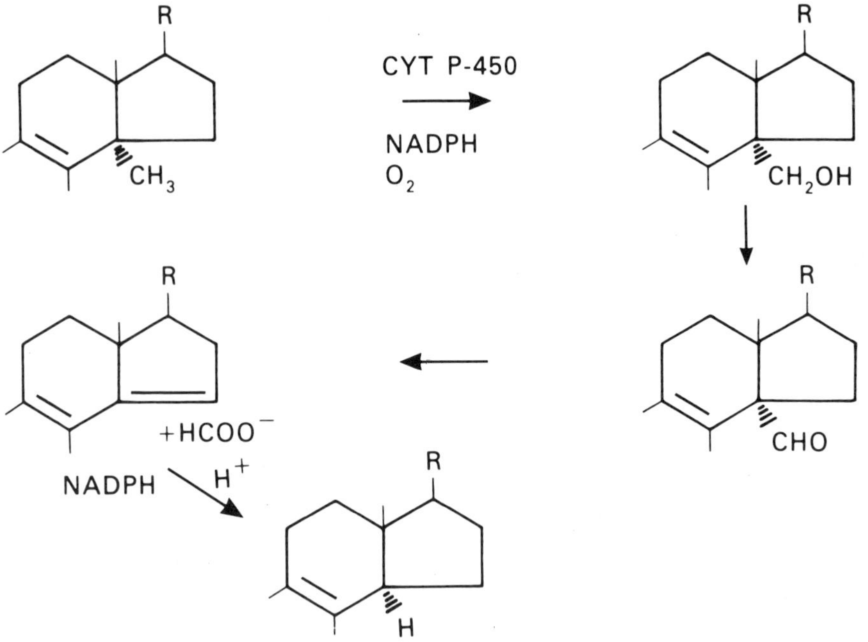

Fig. 16-1. Proposed mechanism for the removal of the methyl group at position 14 of lanosterol.

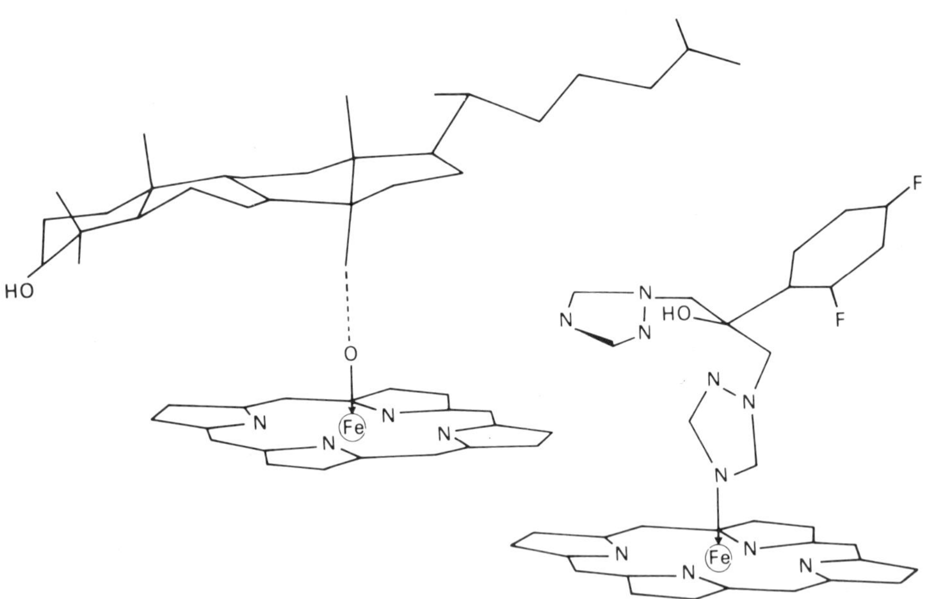

Fig. 16-2. Simulated computer model of lanosterol and fluconazole interacting with the heme moiety of cytochrome P_{450DM}.

Bovine	F	G	A	G	P	R	S	C	V	G	E	M	L	A	R	Q	E	L	F	L	F
S. cerevisiae	F	G	G	G	R	H	R	C	I	G	E	H	F	A	Y	C	Q	L	G	V	L
C. tropicalis	F	G	G	G	R	H	R	C	I	G	E	Q	F	A	Y	V	Q	L	G	T	I

Fig. 16-3. Amino acid sequences of the heme-binding regions of bovine 17α hydroxylase, *S. cerevisiae* C14 demethylase, and *C. tropicalis* C14 demethylase. Amino acids are represented by the single-letter code.

ble that more detailed knowledge of the molecular architecture of cytochromes P_{450}, especially fungal cytochrome P_{450DM}, will lead to a more rational approach.

3. INTRINSIC ACTIVITY

The computer model of Marchington (see Fig. 16-2 and Baldwin, 1986) suggests that, when bound to cytochrome P_{450}, an azole antifungal is occupying some or all of the substrate binding pocket. While this suggests that lipophilic compounds will be more active, potent inhibitory activity is found in agents differing by more than five log P units. There does, however, appear to be a minimum lipophilic motif present in most medically important azole antifungals (Fig. 16-4) consisting of an N-linked imidazole or triazole and a (usually halogen) substituted phenyl group. Modifications to this occur in clotrimazole and agriculturally useful azoles.

The usual phenyl substitution pattern is 2,4 dichloro, although other halogens or halogen equivalents are acceptable (Marriott & Richardson, 1988). Thus, these authors have studied the effect of substitution pattern on activity in a series of 2-substituted-1,3-bis-triazolylpropan-2-ol derivatives. Halogen substitution (F, Cl, Br, I, CF_3) at positions 2−, 4−, or 2,4− of the phenyl ring resulted in good activity, but 3−, 2,3−, 3,4−, and 3,5-substituted derivatives were inactive (Table 16-1). However, meta-substitution was not always associated with a loss of activity, since 2,5− and 2,4,5-trihalo-substituted phenyl derivatives were active. This suggests some subtle conformational effect preventing efficient access to the substrate binding site, although this was not examined rigorously. The same authors also studied other substituted phenyl derivatives, including replacement of the halophenyl by alkyl, aralkyl, or heterocyclyl groups. With the exception of 5-chloropyrid-2-ol (Table 16-2) this resulted in almost a complete loss of activity.

4. *IN VITRO* VERSUS *IN VIVO* ACTIVITY

Activity against the target enzyme is no guarantee of activity against intact fungi. Pye and Marriott (1982) demonstrated that a relatively simple modification (addition of a hydroxyl group) could have a profound effect on *in vitro* activity, presumably by preventing access to the enzyme (Table 16-3). Bawden and colleagues (1983) studied the effect of

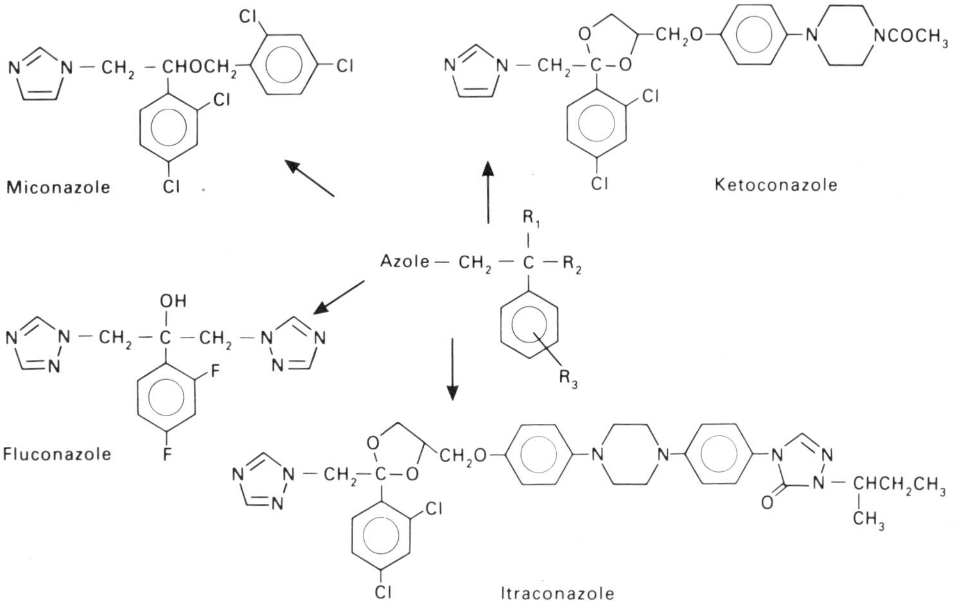

FIG. 16-4. Basic structural motif present in most medically important azole antifungals.

TABLE 16-1. *Effect of Halogen Substitution on the Antifungal Properties of Bis-Triazole Alcohols*

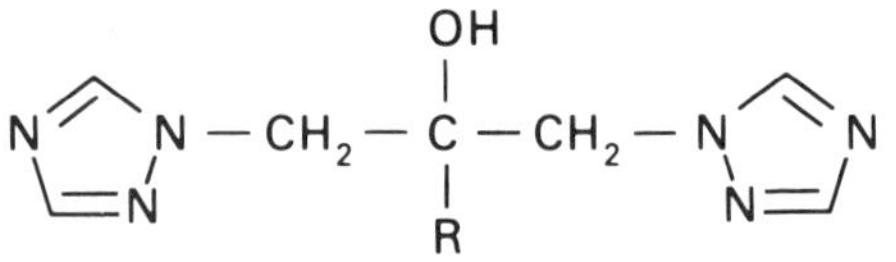

OH
N—CH$_2$—C—CH$_2$—N
R

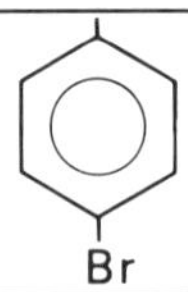

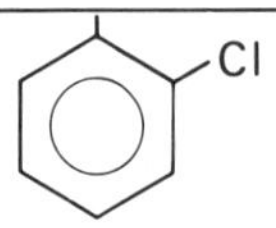

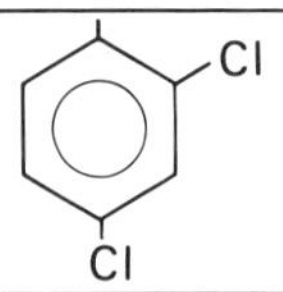

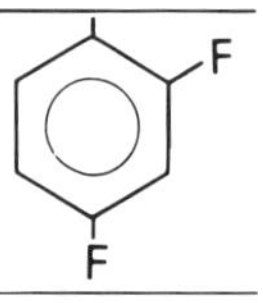

R		Br	Cl	Cl, Cl	F, F
ED_{50}†	5.7	0.1	0.2	0.1	0.1
R	Cl	F, F	F, F	Cl, Cl	F, F, Br
ED_{50}†	>10	>10	>10	2.0	0.1

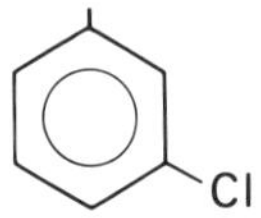

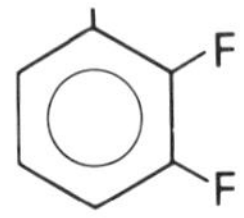

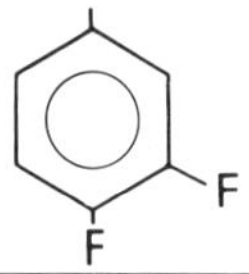

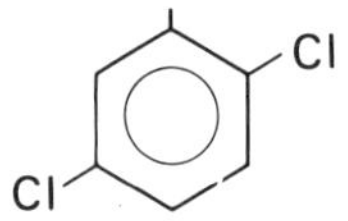

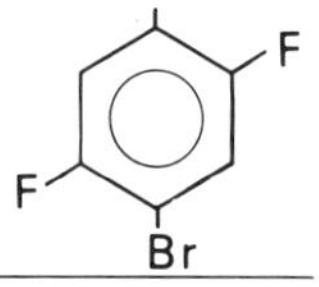

Data are from Marriott and Richardson (1988). ED_{50} refers to oral activity (mg/kg) in a murine model of systemic candidosis (Richardson et al., 1985) and accurately reflects the *in vitro* antifungal activity of the compounds.

TABLE 16-2. *Effect of Replacing Halophenyl Substituent with Other Lipophilic Groups on the Antifungal Properties of Bis-Triazole Tertiary Alcohols*

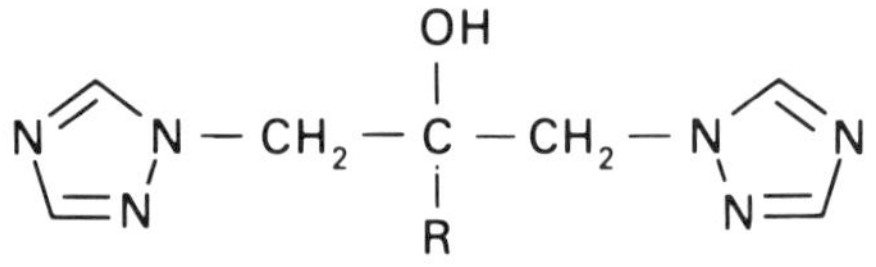

OH
N—CH$_2$—C—CH$_2$—N
R

R	CF_3	Me, Cl	CH_2, Cl	S, Br	N, Cl
ED_{50}†	0.1	>10	>10	1.9	0.1

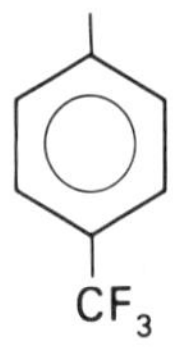

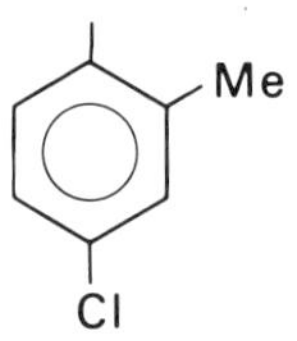

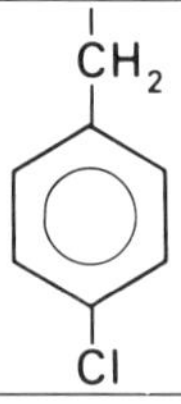

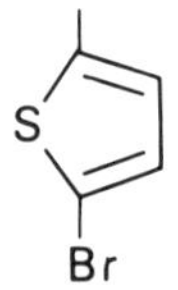

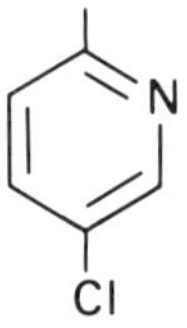

For explanation of data, see Table 16-1.

log P_0 on the activity of a series of alkyl-substituted imidazolyl tertiary alcohols. They found an optimum log P_0 for activity against *Candida albicans*, *Candida* spp., dermatophytes, and *Aspergillus* (Fig. 16-5). Under the assay conditions used, the azoles were fungistatic; that is, they were probably exerting an antifungal effect through inhibition of C14 demethylase rather than direct membrane damage (fungicidal). The results are, therefore, a combination of intrinsic activity and ability to reach the target site.

TABLE 16-3. *Effect of Hydroxyl Substitution on the Activity of an Imidazolyl Tertiary Alcohol*

	UK-38,667	UK-38,754
Candida C14 Demethylase (IC_{50}, μM)	0.05	0.05
Whole cell C14 demethylase (IC_{50}, μM)	0.1	20
MIC ($\mu g/ml$)	12.5	>100

Data from Pye and Marriott (1982).

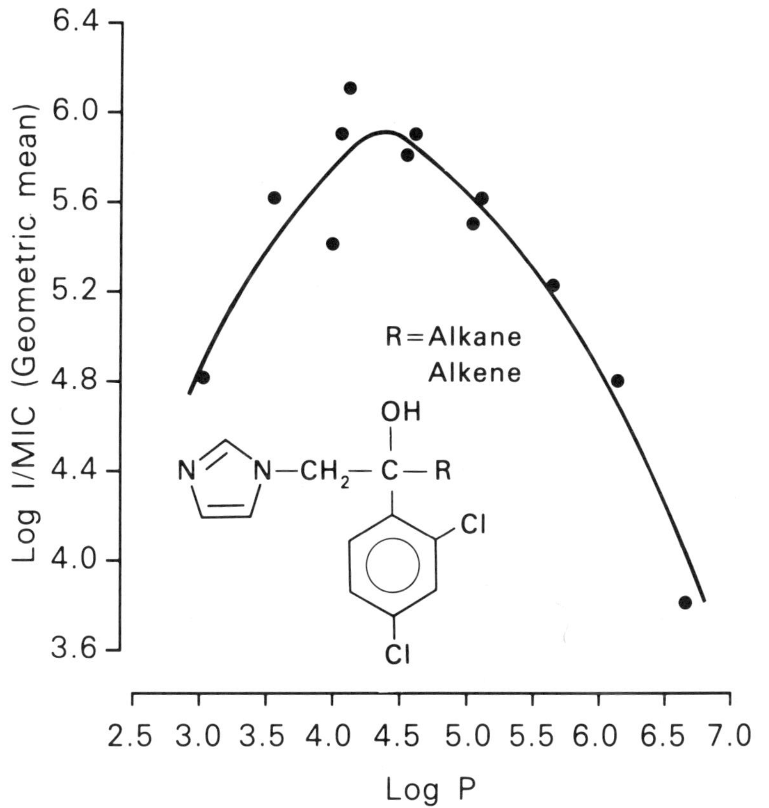

FIG. 16-5. Influence of log P_0 on the activity of a series of alkyl-substituted imidazolyl tertiary alcohols against *Aspergillus fumigatus*. Antifungal activity is expressed as the reciprocol of geometric mean MIC ($\mu g/ml$).

In the same way that potent enzyme inhibition does not necessarily lead to antifungal activity, inhibition of whole cells does not always translate into activity *in vivo*. Early imidazoles were inactive orally and only weakly active parenterally. This was due to rapid metabolism by the liver, leading to a large first-pass effect after oral dosing and a short serum half-life (Table 16-4). Ketoconazole was the first azole to have good oral bioavailability but still has a relatively short half-life in laboratory animals (Table 16-4) and in humans (Van Tyle, 1984). Figure 16-6 highlights some of the principal metabolic sites of a typical azole antifungal, and the remaining examples in Table 16-4 illustrate how these have been overcome.

The points to emerge from these examples are that triazole is less susceptible to oxidative metabolism than is imidazole, substitution (especially para) of the phenyl ring prevents hydroxylation of this group, and a free hydrogen on the "central" carbon should be avoided. It is also important that the remainder of the molecule should be compatible with activity without being a metabolic liability. In the case of the itraconazole side chain, which presents several additional metabolic sites, attack is slow and the compound has a prolonged serum half-life, although protein binding is undoubtedly an important contributory factor. Fluconazole, on the other hand, has a second triazole, which performs the same function; that is, it is compatible with activity and metabolically stable. Substitution of the

Table 16-4. *Some Pharmacokinetic Properties of Imidazole- and Triazole-Containing Antifungals*

	Mouse Bioavailability	Kinetics Half-life
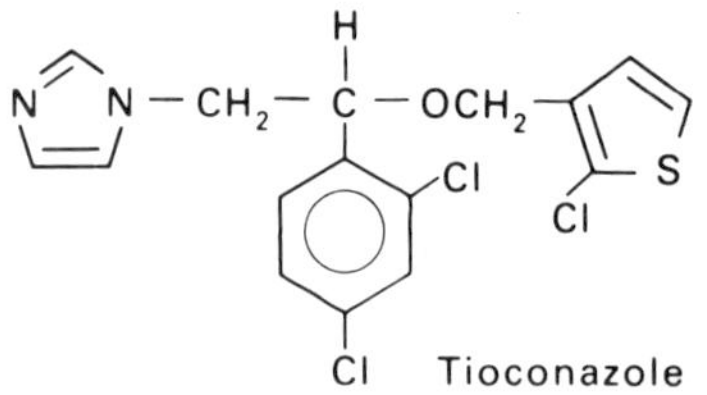 Tioconazole	~ 50%	<1 hr
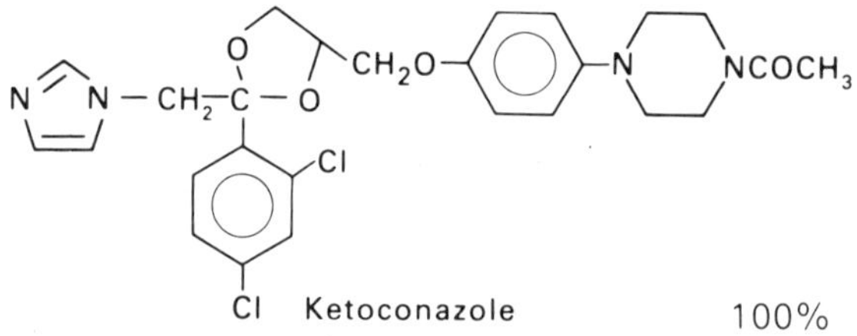 Ketoconazole	100%	1.5 hr
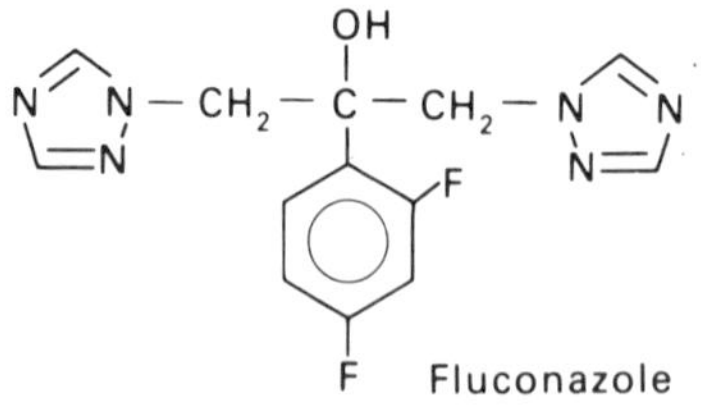 Fluconazole	100%	4.5 hr
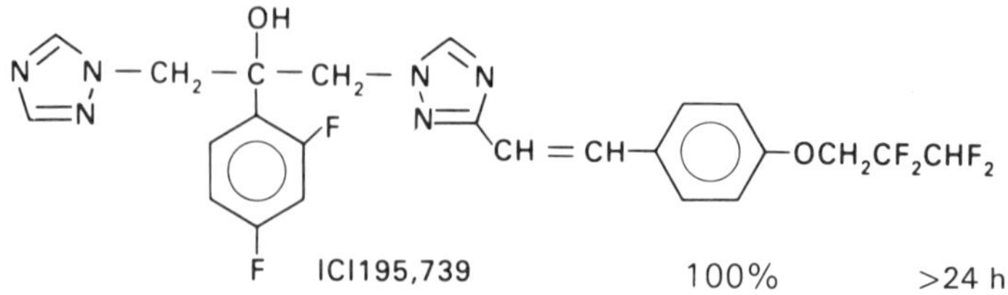 ICI195,739	100%	>24 hr

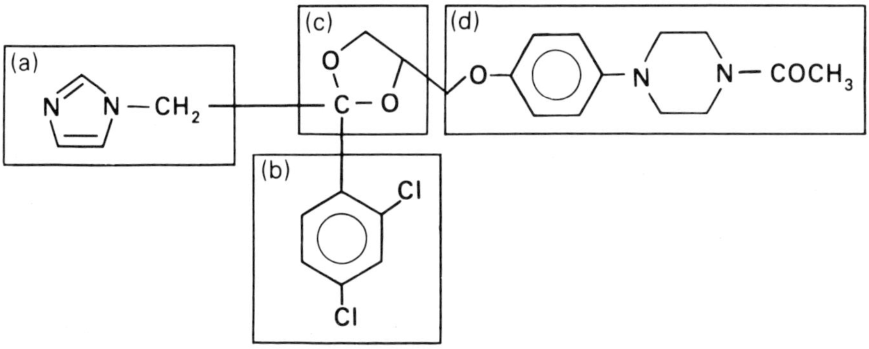

(a) Triazole less prone to oxidative N-de-alkylation than imidazole
(b) Halo substituents on phenyl ring reduce aromatic hydroxylation
(c) Dioxolane or tertiary alcohol more stable than -CH
(d) "Right hand" substituent should not be a metabolic liability

FIG. 16-6. Potential metabolic sites on typical azole antifungal, ketoconazole.

second triazole as in ICI 195, 739, further reduces metabolism leading to an extremely extended half-life.

Fluconazole (log P, 0.5) and ketoconazole (log P, 3.7) or itraconazole (log P, 5.5) represent more or less opposite ends of a spectrum of antifungal and physicochemical parameters. Fluconazole is only weakly lipophilic, is not bound to plasma proteins to any significant extent, and is cleared predominantly as unchanged drug in the urine. Thus, dosing with fluconazole leads to sustained, high concentrations of unbound drug which more than compensate for the difference in observed *in vitro* activity between it and ketoconazole or itraconazole (Fig. 16-7).

Ketoconazole and itraconazole, although more potent *in vitro*, are highly protein-bound and provide sustained, but low, concentrations of free drug. Hence, provided all relevant parameters are taken into account, it is possible to correlate *in vitro* and *in vivo* activity.

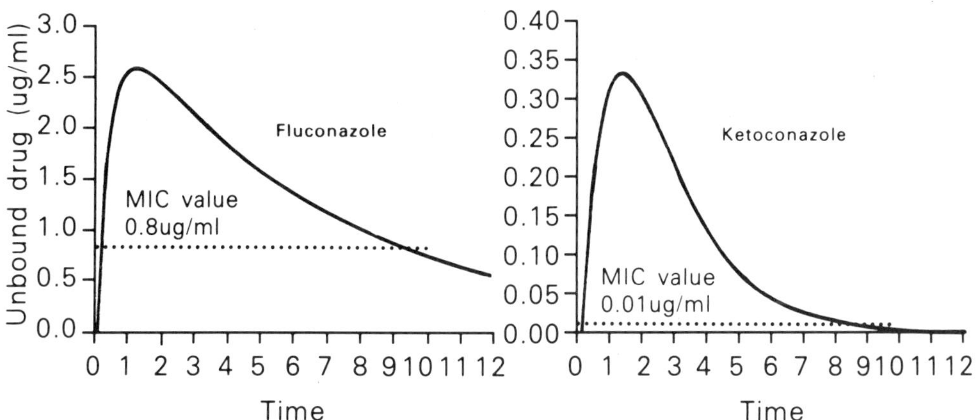

FIG. 16-7. Murine pharmacokinetics of ketoconazole and fluconazole at equiactive doses. Data refer to unbound drug in plasma and show that at doses giving equivalent antifungal protection in a murine model of vaginal candidosis, concentrations of unbound drug remain above the respective MIC's for equal periods of time.

However, the lesson to be learned for the medicinal chemist is that there are at least two ways to achieve *in vivo* activity.

5. SELECTIVITY AND SIDE EFFECTS

Cytochrome P_{450} is a common component of mono-oxygenases involved in steroid interconversions and drug metabolism. Not surprisingly, therefore, azole antifungals have been found to inhibit several of these enzymes, producing side effects such as gynecomastia due to lowering of testosterone levels on prolonged dosing (DeFelice et al., 1981; Pont et al., 1982). Inhibition of testosterone biosynthesis by ketoconazole, probably due to aromatase inhibition (Fig. 16-8), has been used to therapeutic advantage in the treatment of prostatic cancer (Amery et al., 1986). However, selectivity is obviously a key issue in the design of novel azole antifungals. Table 16-5 illustrates the inhibitory activity of different azoles against yeast and mammalian C14 demethylase and aromatase. The data indicate, first, that inhibitory potency against either enzyme is a function of the structure of the azole and, second, that the same enzyme from different species can show variable sensitivity. While this is not surprising for species such as yeast and rat with wide taxonomic separation, Table 16-6 shows that similar differences in sensitivities exist for aromatase, 17α hydroxylase and 11β hydroxylate from rat, cow, sheep, and humans. Table 16-6 also indicates that different enzymes from the same species can show differential sensitivities

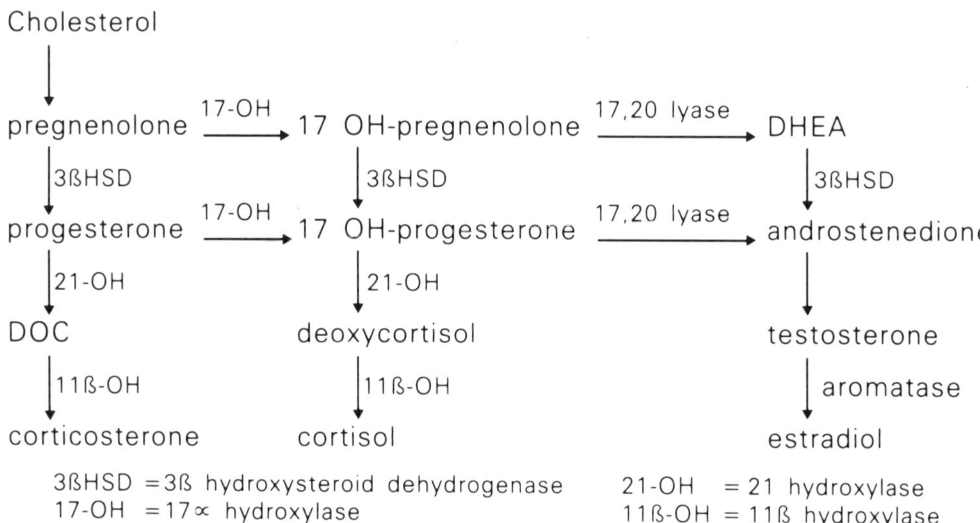

FIG. 16-8. Steroid interconversions and the enzymes involved. Data in Tables 16.5, 16.6, and 16.7 refer to inhibition of these enzymes by azole antifungals.

TABLE 16-5. *Inhibition of Yeast and Mammalian Lanosterol C14 Demethylase and Mammalian Aromatase by Azole Antifungals*

Enzyme	Candida C14 Demethylase (a) (IC_{50}, μM)	Rat C14 Demethylase (b) (IC_{50}, μM)	Sheep Placental Aromatase (c) (IC_{50}, μM)
Miconazole	0.20	–	0.5
Econazole	0.09	–	0.03
Ketoconazole	0.05	3.5	5.0
Fluconazole	0.05 (b)	>1000	–

From (a) Pye and Marriott (1982), (b) Marriott et al. (1986), (c) France et al. (1987).

TABLE 16-6. *Inhibition of Mammalian Aromatases, 17α Hydroxylases, and 11β Hydroxylases by Ketoconazole*

Enzyme species	Aromatase (IC_{50}, μM)	17α Hydroxylase (K_i, μM)	11β hydroxylase (IC_{50}, μM)
Sheep	5.0 (a)	–	–
Rat	1.0 (b)	160 (c)	4.0 (e)
Cow	–	–	1.3 (f)
Human	100 (b)	0.04 (d)	0.01 (d)

(a) France et al. (1987), (b) Disney et al. (1987), (c) Ayub and Levell (1987), (d) Couch et al. (1987), (e) Shaw et al. (1988), (f) Nagai et al. (1986).

to a specific azole, and this point is further emphasized in Table 16-7, which gives the inhibitory activity of ketoconazole against human adrenal steroid metabolizing enzymes.

The data presented in Tables 16-5, 16-6, and 16-7 have been assembled from several publications by different authors and may be criticized on that account. Nevertheless, the differences in selectivity are so striking that the conclusions are no doubt valid. This has profound implications for the rational design of selective C14 demethylase inhibitors, suggesting that absolute selectivity can only be determined by comparison with human enzymes. Table 16-8 shows that the same observations can be made for enzymes involved in metabolism of xenobiotics, and recent work by Purba and Back (1986) and La Delfa and colleagues (1988) emphasizes that the ability to inhibit a murine enzyme does not lead to side effects in humans if the equivalent human enzyme is insensitive.

6. OTHER IMPORTANT PROPERTIES

Table 16-9 lists some other important properties to be considered when designing the ideal azole drug. Some of these are simply of practical value, such as aqueous solubility, since this allows formulation for intravenous administration, an important asset for treat-

TABLE 16-7. *Inhibition of Human Adrenal Steroid Metabolizing Enzymes by Ketoconazole*

Enzyme	K_i (μM)
3-β-hydroxysteroid dehydrogenase	12
17-α-hydroxylase	0.04
17,20-lyase	0.08
21-hydroxylase	38
11-β-hydroxylase	0.01

Data from Couch et al. (1987).

TABLE 16-8. *Inhibition of Rat Liver Cytochrome P_{450} Drug Metabolizing Enzymes by Certain Azole Antifungals*

Enzyme azole	7 ethoxycourmarin 0-deethylase (IC_{50}, μM)	Aminopyrine N-demethylase (IC_{50}, μM)
Ketoconazole	6 (a)	27 (c)
Econazole	<1 (b)	7 (b)
Fluconazole	31 (a)	–

From (a) Houston et al. (1988), (b) Murry and Zaluzny (1988), (c) Meredith et al. (1985).

Table 16-9. *Other Important Design Features of an Ideal Antifungal Drug*

1. Aqueous solubility
2. Low serum protein binding
3. Good tissue distribution, including penetration to CSF
4. Nonhepatotoxic
5. Fungicidal action

ing the seriously ill patient. Others such as hepatotoxicity require further attention. Probably all azoles have some effects on the liver (Tachibana et al., 1988), although these are usually only mild changes of an adaptive nature. Occasional frank hepatotoxicity has been seen with ketoconazole, but this appears to be an idiosyncratic reaction (Henning et al., 1983; Van Tyle, 1984). Buchi and colleagues (1986) have recently suggested a model for detecting hepatotoxic potential in azoles, but as yet no detailed SAR is available.

Fungicidal activity presents a particularly exciting challenge. Itraconazole is fungicidal against certain strains of *Aspergillus* (Van Cutsem et al., 1984), and this appears to be related to structural features of the compound and is not associated with membrane damage (M.S. Marriott, K. Richardson, and P.F. Troke, unpublished observations). This raises several important questions. First, is there a second target within the *Aspergillus* cell sensitive to itraconazole? If so, what is the nature of this target? and does it exist in all fungi? Should this be the case, can an azole be designed with selective, broad-spectrum fungicidal activity? Clearly, this is a major challenge for the design of the next generation of azole antifungals.

7. CONCLUSIONS

Fungal infections, particularly those in immuno-compromised patients, continue to increase, a situation accentuated by the advent of the acquired immune deficiency syndrome. Amphotericin B remains the drug of choice for the treatment of many systemic fungal infections, although nephrotoxicity places severe restrictions on its use. Significant progress has been made from early, topically active azoles such as clotrimazole, to the new, long-acting, systemic agents such as itraconazole and fluconazole. Nevertheless, neither drug can be said to match amphotericin B in terms of potency, although both are considerably less toxic. There remains, therefore, scope for an improved, systemically active antifungal drug.

Recent advances in the molecular biology of yeast cytochrome P_{450DM} will greatly influence our understanding of the interaction of azoles with this important fungal enzyme. However, data on their interaction with mammalian cytochromes P_{450} indicate subtle, but significant, differences in structure and sensitivity, making rational design of selective agents more problematic. It would appear that only the use of human enzymes may be of value in assessing selectivity in future. Finally, the possibility that an additional target exists which can lead to specific fungicidal action, unrelated to the membrane damaging effects of earlier azoles, is intriguing and worthy of further investigation.

REFERENCES

Amery, W. K., De Coster, R., and Caers, I. (1986). Ketoconazole: From an antimycotic to a drug for prostate cancer. *Drug Dev. Res.* **8**: 299–307.

Aoyama, Y., Yoshida, Y., Sonoda, Y., and Sato, Y. (1987). Metabolism of 32-hydroxy-24,25-dihydrolanosterol by purified cytochrome P-450_{14DM} from yeast. *J. Biol. Chem.* **262**: 1239–1243.

Aoyama, Y., Yoshida, Y., and Sato, R. (1984). Yeast cytochrome P_{450} catalyzing lanosterol C14-demethylation. *J. Biol. Chem.* **259**: 1661–1666.

Ayub, M., and Levell, M. J. (1987). Inhibition of testicular 17α-hydroxylase and 17-20-lyase but not 3β-hydroxysteroid dehydrogenase-isomerase or 17β-hydroxysteroid oxidoreductase by ketoconazole and other imidazole drugs. *J. Steroid Biochem.* **28**: 521–531.

Baldwin, B. C. (1986). Role of biochemical studies in the discovery of agricultural fungicides. In *In vitro and in vivo evaluation of antifungal agents*, K. Iwata and H. Vanden Bossche, eds., pp 185–195. Amsterdam: Elsevier.

Bawden, D., Gymer, G. E., Marriott, M. S., and Tute, M. S. (1983). Quantitative structure-activity relationships in a group of imidazole antimycotic agents. *Eur. J. Med. Chem.* **18**: 91–96.

Borgers, M. (1985). Antifungal azole derivatives. In *The scientific basis of antimicrobial chemotherapy*, D. Greenwood and F. O'Grady, eds., pp. 133–154. Cambridge: Cambridge University Press.

Buchi, K. N., Gray, P. D., and Tolman, K. G. (1986). Ketoconazole hepatotoxicity: An *in vitro* model. *Biochem. Pharmacol.* **35**: 2845–2847.

Chen, C., Turi, T. G., Sanglard, D., and Loper, J. C. (1987). Isolation of the *Candida tropicalis* gene for P_{450} lanosterol demethylase and its expression in *Saccharomyces cerevisiae*. *Biochem. Biophys. Res. Commun.* **146**: 1311–1317.

Couch, R. M., Muller, J., Perry, Y. S., and Winter, J. S. D. (1987). Kinetic analysis of inhibition of human adrenal steroidogenesis by ketoconazole. *J. Clin. Endocrinol. Metab.* **65**: 551–554.

DeFelice, R., Johnson, D. G., and Galgiani, J. N. (1981). Gynecomastia with ketoconazole. *Antimicrob. Agents Chemother.* **19**: 1073–1074.

Disney, G., Tarbit, M. H., and Burnet, F. (1987). Rat ovarian and human placental aromatases display different sensitivities to inhibition by ketoconazole. *Biochem. Soc. Trans.* **16**: 29.

France, J. T., Mason, J. I., Magness, R. R., Murry, B. A., and Rosenfeld, C. R. (1987). Ovine placental aromatase: studies of activity levels, kinetic characteristics, and effects of aromatase inhibitors. *J. Steroid. Biochem.* **28**: 155–160.

Gibbons, G. F., Pullinger, C. R., and Mitropoulos, K. A. (1979). Studies on the mechanisms of lanosterol 14α-demethylation. *Biochem. J.* **183**: 309–315.

Henning, H., Kasper, B., and Lüders, C. J. (1983). Ketoconazol-induzierte Hepatitis, eine Kasuistik. *Z. Gastroenterologie* **21**: 709–715.

Henry, M. J., and Sisler, H. D. (1979). Effects of miconazole and dodecylimidazole on sterol biosynthesis in *Ustilago maydis*. *Antimicrob. Agents Chemother.* **15**: 603–607.

Houston, J. B., Humphrey, M. J., Matthew, D. E., and Tarbit, M. H. (1988). Comparison of two azole antifungal drugs, ketoconazole and fluconazole, as modifiers of rat hepatic monoxygenase activity. *Biochem. Pharmacol.* **37**: 401–408.

Iwata, K., Yomaguchi, M., and Hiratani, A. M. (1973). Mode of action of clotrimazole. *Sabouraudia* **11**: 158–166.

Kalb, V. F., Loper, J. C., Dey, C. R., Woods, C. W., and Sutter, T. R. (1986). Isolation of a cytochrome P_{450} structural gene from *Saccharomyces cerevisiae*. *Gene* **45**: 237–245.

La Delfa, I., Zhu, Q. M., Mo, Z., and Blascke, T. F. (1988). Potent and reversible *in vivo* inhibition of antipyrine metabolism in mice by fluconazole, a new bis-triazole antifungal. *Clin. Res.* **36**: 118A.

Marriott, M. S., and Richardson, K. (1988). The discovery and mode of action of fluconazole. In *Recent trends in the discovery, development and evaluation of antifungal agents*, R. A. Fromtling, ed., pp. 81–92. Barcelona: J. R. Prous.

Marriott, M. S., Pye, G. W., Richardson, K., and Troke, P. F. (1986). The activity of fluconazole (UK-49,858), a novel bis-triazole antifungal and ketoconazole against fungal and mammalian sterol C14 demethylases. In *In vitro and in vivo evaluation of antifungal agents*, K. Iwata and H. Vanden Bossche, eds., pp. 143–146. Amsterdam: Elsevier.

Meredith, C. G., Maldano, A. L., and Speeg, K. V. (1985). The effect of ketoconazole on hepatic oxidative drug metabolism in the rat *in vivo* and *in vitro*. *Drug Met. Disp.* **13**: 156–162.

Murry, M., and Zaluzny, L. (1988). Comparative effects of antithrombotic and antimycotic N-substituted imidazoles on rat hepatic microsomal steroid and xenobiotic hydroxylases *in vitro*. *Biochem. Pharmacol.* **37**: 415–420.

Nagai, K., Miyamori, I., Ikeda, M., Koshida, H., Takeda, R., Suhara, K., and Katagiri, M. (1986). Effect of ketoconazole (an imidazole antimycotic agent) and other inhibitors of steroidogenesis on cytochrome P_{450}-catalyzed reactions. *J. Steroid Biochem.* **24**: 321–323.

Pont, A., Williams, P. L., Azhar, S., Reitz, R. E., Bochra, C., Smith, E. R., and Stevens, D. A. (1982). Ketoconazole blocks testosterone synthesis. *Arch. Intern. Med.* **142**: 2137–2140.

Pye, G. W., and Marriott, M. S. (1982). Inhibition of sterol C14 demethylation by imidazole-containing antifungals. *Sabouraudia* **20**: 325–329.

Purba, H. S., and Back, D. J. (1986). Effect of fluconazole (UK-49,858) on antipyrine metabolism. *Brit. J. Clin. Pharmac.* **21**: 603P.

Richardson, K., Brammer, K. W., Marriott, M. S., and Troke, P. F. (1985). Activity of UK-49858, a bistriazole derivative, against experimental infections with *Candida albicans* and *Trichophyton mentagraphytes*. *Antimicrob. Agents Chemother.* **27**: 832–835.

Shaw, J. T. B., Tarbit, M. H., and Troke, P. F. (1988). Cytochrome P-450–mediated sterol synthesis and metabolism: Differences in sensitivity to fluconazole and other azoles. In *Recent trends in the discovery, development, and evaluation of antifungal agents*, R. A. Fromtling, ed., pp. 125–139. Barcelona: J. R. Prous.

Tachibana, M., Noguchi, Y., and Monro, A. M. (1988). Toxicology of fluconazole in experimental animals. In *Recent trends in the discovery, development, and evaluation of antifungal agents*, R. A. Fromtling, ed., pp. 93–102. Barcelona: J. R. Prous.

Van Cutsem, J., Van Geven, F., Van de Ven, M. A., Borgers, M., and Janssen, P. A. J. (1984). Itraconazole, a new triazole that is orally active in aspergillosis. *Antimicrob. Agents Chemother.* **26**: 527–534.

Vanden Bossche, H. (1985). Biochemical targets for antifungal azole derivatives: Hypothesis on the mode of action. In *Current topics in medical mycology*, M. R. McGinnis, ed., Vol. 1, pp. 313–351. New York: Springer-Verlag.

Vanden Bossche, H., Willemsens, G., Cools, W., Lauwers, W. F. J. and Le Jeune, L. (1978). Biochemical effects of miconazole on fungi, II. Inhibition of ergosterol biosynthesis in *Candida albicans*. *Chemi-Biol. Interact.* **21**: 59–78.

Van Tyle, J. H. (1984). Ketoconazole: Mechanisms of action, spectrum of activity, pharmacokinetics, drug interactions, adverse reactions, and therapeutic use. *Pharmacology* **4**: 343–373.

Yamaguchi, H., and Iwata, K. (1979). Effect of fatty acyl group and sterol composition on sensitivity of lecithin liposomes to imidazole antimycotics. *Antimicrob. Agents Chemother.* **15**: 706–711.

Yoshida, Y., and Aoyama, Y. (1987). Interaction of azole antifungal agents with cytochrome P-450_{14DM} purified from *Saccharomyces cerevisiae* microsomes. *Biochem. Pharmacol.* **36**: 229–235.

Yoshida, Y., and Aoyama, Y. (1986). Interaction of azole fungicides with yeast cytochrome P-450 which catalyzes lanosterol 14α-demethylation. In *in vitro and in vivo evaluation of antifungal agents*, K. Iwata, and H. Vanden Bossche, eds. pp. 123–134. Amsterdam: Elsevier.

Zuber, M. X., John, M. E., Okamura, T., Simpson, E. R., and Waterman, M. R. (1986). Bovine adrenocortical cytochrome $P450_{17\alpha}$. Regulation of gene expression by ACTH and elucidation of primary sequence. *J. Biol. Chem.* **261**: 2475–2482.

CHAPTER 17

ALLYLAMINE DERIVATIVES – INHIBITORS OF FUNGAL SQUALENE EPOXIDASE

ANTON STÜTZ
Sandoz Forschungsinstitut, Vienna, Austria

Abstract – The allylamine antimycotics are potent and selective inhibitors of squalene epoxidase in a range of fungi pathogenic in humans. The first representative of this new class of antimycotics, naftifine, was discovered by accident. The exploration of structure–activity relationships on the basis of naftifine and new synthetic strategies led to the discovery of terbinafine, the first pharmaceutical agent to contain an (E)-1,3-enyne structural element. Terbinafine exhibits considerable higher activity than does the original lead structure naftifine both *in vitro* and *in vivo*: it is also up to one order of magnitude more effective than standard preparations in various chemotherapeutical animal tests after topical and oral administration.

The most potent squalene epoxidase inhibitor identified so far is a terbinafine derivative, in which the naphthalene part has been exchanged by 3-chloro-7-benzo(b)thiophene. This compound also shows significantly increased activity against *Candida albicans* and other pathogenic fungi. Recently homopropargylamino and benzylamino compounds related to the allylamine derivatives have also been found to be potent squalene epoxidase inhibitors.

Squalene epoxidase from mammalian liver is orders of magnitude less sensitive to the allylamine derivatives. This selectivity appears to be mostly due to intrinsic differences between the respective epoxidase systems.

1. INTRODUCTION

The discovery of the first representative of this new class of antifungal agents, naftifine, was basically accidental. In 1974 this compound was obtained as the result of an unexpected chemical reaction during a synthesis program for CNS-active compounds at Sandoz-Wander, Berne (Berney & Schuh, 1978). Since it was a novel compound (Fig. 17-1), it was also tested as part of a general screening program at the Sandoz Research Institute in Vienna, where it was found to be highly active *in vitro* and *in vivo* against a number of pathogenic fungi (Georgopoulos et al., 1981; Petranyi et al., 1981). Subsequent investigations on the profile of its activity revealed a novel mode of action (Paltauf et al., 1982;

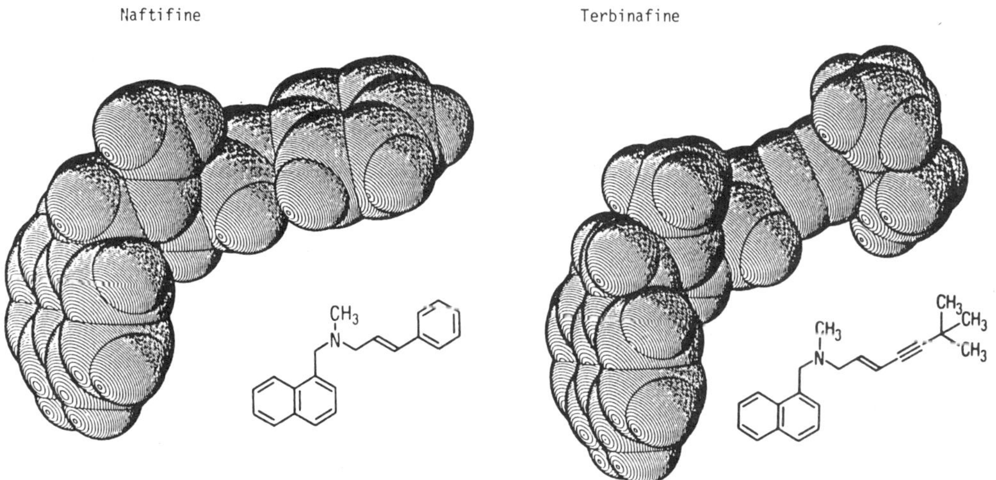

FIG. 17-1. Naftifine and terbinafine, representatives of antifungal allylamine derivatives. Computer graphic representation of the three-dimensional structures derived from X-ray analysis of the hydrochlorides.

Ryder et al., 1984) and promising results with respect to the antifungal spectrum, the type of activity, and pharmacokinetic properties. In extended preclinical and clinical trials, naftifine proved to be an efficacious antimycotic for topical application in dermatomycoses (Clayton et al., 1985). It was first marketed in 1985 as a topical agent for mycoses of the skin (EXODERIL®).

The discovery of the antifungal activity of naftifine was at the same time the starting point for intensive studies on structure–activity relationships (Stütz & Petranyi, 1984; Petranyi et al., 1984; Stütz et al., 1986) resulting in the development of terbinafine (Fig. 17-1), a derivative with considerably enhanced antimycotic properties.

In this chapter some aspects of the work leading to the discovery of terbinafine are described, followed by characteristic properties of this compound and recent structure–activity findings. More detailed descriptions of the SAR studies and synthetic procedures developed have been given elsewhere (Stütz, 1987, 1988).

2. FROM NAFTIFINE TO TERBINAFINE

Early variations of the naftifine molecule showed that the antifungal activity was specifically linked to certain structural elements which could not be related to any known classes of antifungals (Stütz et al., 1986). Because of the tertiary allylamine function common to all these active compounds, they were termed "allylamine derivatives."

A comparison of active versus inactive compounds (Grassberger et al., 1986) shown in Fig. 17-2 makes clear the necessity of further structural requirements for antifungal activity, that is, the 1-substituted naphthalene ring, and that the aromatic ring systems must not be interchanged. In addition conformational aspects also seem to be of importance, since incorporation of the flexible structure of naftifine into different ring systems leads to only two biologically active semirigid analogues (Stütz, 1987).

In a systematic study (Stütz, 1987) the 3-phenylallyl (cinnamyl) group in naftifine was replaced by alkyl chains with an increasing number of conjugated double bonds, and these compounds were tested against various human-pathogenic microorganisms. Biological activity reached a clearly defined maximum with two conjugated double bonds. Fig. 17-3 reveals that the antifungal activity of the (E,E)-2,4-alkadienyl derivative is comparable to that of the lead structure naftifine both *in vitro* and *in vivo*. Substitution of the double bond (Stütz & Petranyi, 1984) between C4 and C5 by a triple bond improved the activities *in vitro* and *in vivo*, especially after oral administration. In the latter case 75 mg/kg of both naftifine or the 2,4-alkadienyl derivative, for example, were ineffective in the guinea pig-trichophytosis model by mycological criteria, whereas the same dose of the (E)-2-alken-4-ynyl-derivative completely cured the animals. The trans configuration is essential for this effect: The corresponding cis isomer is less active by several orders of magnitude. Similarly analogs with an inverted enyne group or with two conjugated triple bonds show low activity only (Fig. 17-3).

In further modifications the alkyl substituent adjacent to the triple bond in (E)-2-alkenynyl-derivatives was varied (Fig. 17-4). Increased branching finally improved the oral efficacy by one order of magnitude in the form of the tert-butyl compound (terbinafine) (Stütz & Petranyi, 1984). The tert-butyl group is, moreover, a prerequisite for activity *in vitro* against *Aspergillus fumigatus* and *Candida albicans*.

Within these studies the conjugated trans-enyne group has proved to be an important structural modification for improving the antimycotic activity of allylamines, particularly after oral administration, and represents a novel structural element in pharmaceutical agents.

3. TERBINAFINE

3.1. Mode of Action and Selectivity

Terbinafine and the allylamines interfere in the biosynthesis of ergosterol (Fig. 17-5) and specifically inhibit the oxidation of squalene to squalene-2,3-epoxide (K_i for squalene epoxidase from *Candida albicans*: 3×10^{-8}M) (Ryder, 1985, 1987). The result is a de-

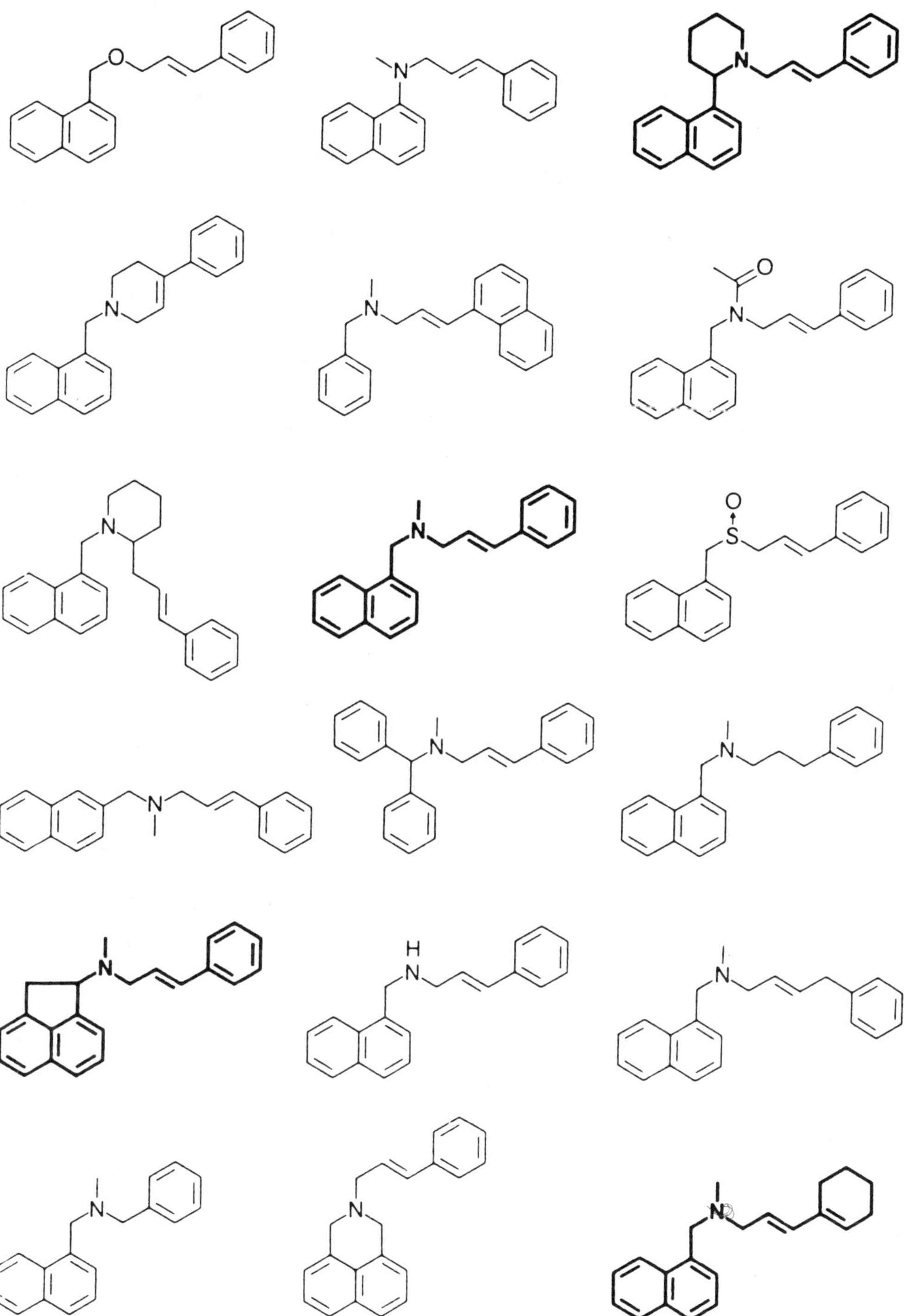

FIG. 17-2. Basic structural modifications of naftifine. The structures in heavy print are of comparable effectiveness *in vitro* and *in vivo*. The others are inactive. Reprinted with permission of Triangle.

crease of ergosterol in the fungal cell while squalene accumulates. Comparative studies with rat liver squalene epoxidase have shown that terbinafine is highly selective for the fungal system (Ryder & Dupont, 1985). Squalene epoxidase is a key enzyme in sterol biosynthesis and the first enzyme in this reaction pathway that requires molecular oxygen. Specific inhibition of this enzyme was demonstrated for the first time with the allylamine derivatives.

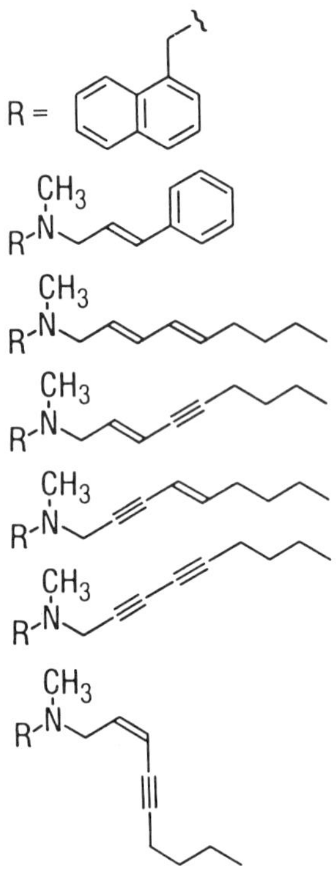

	MIC (mg/l)					IN VIVO ACTIVITY (% myc. cure)				
	Trich. ment.	Epid. fl.	Micr. can.	Spor. sch.	Cand. par.	TOPICAL* 0.125%	0.5%*	ORAL** 37.5	75	150
R =										
$R{-}N(CH_3)$	0.05	0.2	0.1	1.6	1.6	35	65	—	—	48
$R{-}N(CH_3)$	0.05	0.2	0.1	3.1	1.6	40	69	—	—	43
$R{-}N(CH_3)$	0.01	0.01	0.01	1.6	0.4	83	100	83	100	100
$R{-}N(CH_3)$	0.2	1.6	0.2	> 100	> 100					
$R{-}N(CH_3)$	0.2	3.1	0.8	100	100					
$R{-}N(CH_3)$	0.2	100	0.2	50	100					

*PEG solution **mg/kg/day

guinea pig dermatophytosis model

FIG. 17-3. *In vitro* and *in vivo* (guinea pig trichophytosis model) activities of allylamine derivatives (Stütz & Petranyi; 1984). MIC: lowest concentration of the substance that completely inhibits fungal growth. *Trich. Ment.: Trichophyton mentagrophytes; Epid. fl.: Epidermophyton floccosum; Micr. Can.: Microsporum canis; Spor. Sch.: Sporothrix schenckii; Cand. par.: Candida parapsilosis.*

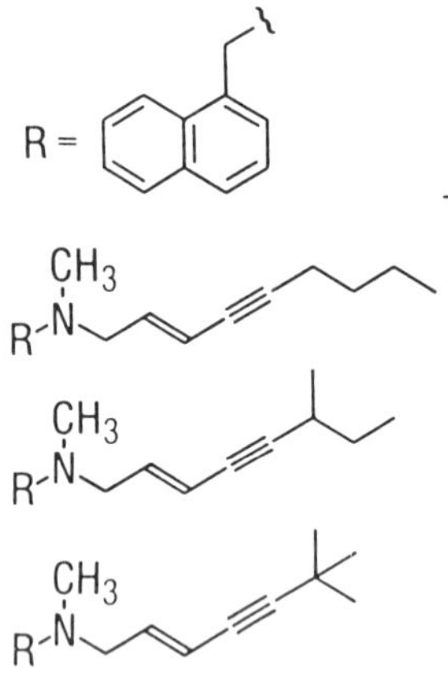

	MIC (mg/l)*							ORAL ACTIVITY (%myc. cure)	
	Trich. ment.	Epid. fl.	Micr. can.	Spor. sch.	Asp. fum.	Cand. alb.	Cand. par.	5*	10*
R =									
$R{-}N(CH_3)$	0.01	0.01	0.01	1.6	100	100	0.4	0	15
$R{-}N(CH_3)$	0.01	0.006	0.006	0.8	100	100	0.4	23	75
$R{-}N(CH_3)$	0 006	0.006	0.006	0.4	0.8	25	0.4	98	100

*tube dilution in Sabouraud broth *mg/kg/day

FIG. 17-4. *In vitro* and *in vivo* activities (guinea pig–trichophytosis model) of (E)-2-alken-4-ynyl derivatives (Stütz & Petranyi, 1984). For abbreviations, see Fig. 17-3: *Asp. fum.: Aspergillus fumigatus; Cand. alb.: Candida albicans.* Daily dose (mg/kg).

In contrast to azole antimycotics, terbinafine and other allylamines are essentially not inhibitors of cytochrome P-450, as was proved in model systems representative for drug metabolism as well as for steroidal hormone synthesis (Schuster, 1985). It may therefore be expected that oral administration of allylamine derivatives will not result in incompatibilities and altered steroidal hormone levels of the type observed with azole derivatives. The results of the current clinical studies with terbinafine are consistent with this assumption (Jones, 1987; Villard & Jones, 1989).

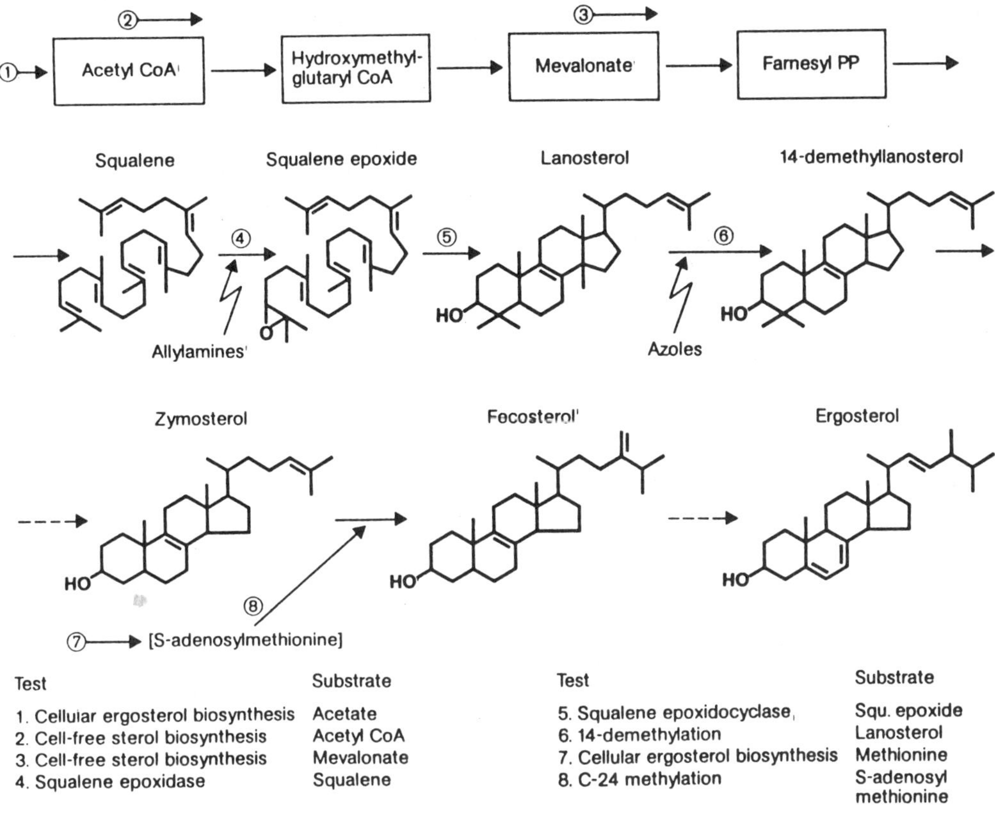

FIG. 17-5. Simplified representation of the biosynthesis of ergosterol (Grassberger et al., 1986). Reprinted with permission of Triangle.

3.2. ACTIVITY *IN VITRO* AND *IN VIVO*

In vitro terbinafine exerts a broad spectrum of activity against a wide range of pathogenic fungi (Table 17-1) (Petranyi et al., 1984, 1987a). Activity is exceptionally high against dermatophytes and good against filamentous and dimorphic fungi, in general. The response of yeasts to this compound is variable between different species and strains. The filamentous form of *C. albicans* is more susceptible than the yeast form (MIC ranges in 19 strains: 0.1 to 0.8 mg/l for terbinafine) (Schaude et al., 1987).

The spectrum of activity was confirmed in independent studies *in vitro* (Goudard et al., 1986; Shadomy et al., 1985) and showed terbinafine to be highly active against further important pathogens such as *Histoplasma capsulatum* and *Cryptococcus neoformans* (geometric mean MIC's 0.061 mg/l and 0.731 mg/l, respectively). In addition, the allylamines are active against a wide range of less common fungal pathogens (Clayton, 1987). Terbinafine action is *primarily fungicidal* against dermatophytes, aspergilli, biphasic fungi, and *Candida parapsilosis* and fungistatic against *Candida albicans* (Petranyi et al., 1987a; Shadomy et al., 1985).

The oral effectiveness of terbinafine is dramatically increased in comparison with naftifine as shown by their ED_{50} values in the oral guinea pig trichophytosis model (Petranyi et al., 1984, 1987b).

	ED_{50} (mg/kg/d)
Naftifine	292.0
Terbinafine	2.8

In comparative tests (Petranyi et al., 1984) terbinafine was superior to the standards griseofulvin and ketoconazole by a factor of 10.

Table 17-1. *Terbinafine: Spectrum of the Antifungal Activity and Minimum Inhibitory Concentrations (MIC, mg/l)*

Species tested	No.	MIC (mg/l) range
Trichophyton mentagrophytes	7	0.003–0.01
Trichophyton rubum	4	0.003–0.006
Trichophyton schoenleinii	1	0.006
Trichophyton tonsurans	1	0.003
Trichophyton verrucosum	1	0.003
Epidermophyton floccosum	3	0.003–0.006
Microsporum canis	3	0.006–0.01
Microsporum gypseum	1	0.006
Microsporum persicolor	1	0.003
Microsporum racemosum	1	0.006
Aspergillus fumigatus	3	0.1–1.56
Aspergillus niger	1	0.05
Sporothrix schenckii	4	0.1–0.4
Candida albicans	4	25–100
Candida guilliermondii	3	6.25–100
Candida krusei	4	100–>100
Candida parapsilosis	4	0.8–1.6
Candida tropicalis	5	100–>100
Candida pseudotropicalis	2	50
Torulopsis glabrata	3	>100
Pityrosporum ovale	5	0.2–0.8
Pityrosporum orbiculare	1	0.8

From Petranyi et al. (1987a).

A new infection model (Petranyi, 1985) with a predominantly epidermal dermatophytosis on the dorsal surface of the external auditory meatus of the guinea pig also demonstrates the superior oral efficacy of terbinafine in comparison with griseofulvin. While griseofulvin (10×60 mg/kg) produces only a transient drop in the elevated skin temperature, terbinafine (10×20 mg/kg) leads to its normalization throughout the period of observation (Grassberger et al., 1986). This effect may be the result of the fungicidal activity of terbinafine.

Terbinafine was shown to be more effective than the standards after topical application. Complete mycological cure of guinea pig trichophytosis and microsporosis was observed after treatment with 0.06 and 0.5% solutions of terbinafine, respectively, for seven days. Under the same experimental conditions, not even 2% solutions of the standards econazole or tolnaftate effected a complete mycological cure. A guinea pig skin infection caused by *Candida albicans* was cured after topical application of a 1% terbinafine solution for five days (Petranyi et al., 1984, 1987b).

Terbinafine was put through extensive toxicity tests in laboratory animals. The substance proved to be readily absorbed from the gastrointestinal tract and to be well tolerated. No teratogenic or embryotoxic effects were observed (Petranyi et al., 1983; Ganzinger et al., 1983).

3.3. Clinical Results

Clinical trials including about 2000 patients have already established high efficacy of terbinafine in cutaneous dermatophyte and yeast infections both on topical and oral application (Jones, 1987; Villard & Jones, 1989).

In a recent double-blind study (Savin, 1989) 26 patients with mocassin-type *Tinea pedis* were treated with terbinafine or griseofulvin. The average duration of disease, mainly caused by *Trichophyton rubrum*, had been 9 years. During 6 weeks of treatment a marked difference in mycologically negative results was observed; at the end of therapy 75% negative cultures and microscopic study of lesion scrapings were recorded in the terbinafine group, 29% in the griseofulvin group. At follow-up 2 weeks after treatment 88% of the terbinafine-treated patients were negative versus 43% in the griseofulvin group. The superiority of terbinafine was also apparent in terms of visible symptoms. In particular the chronic inflammation disappeared in all but one patient up to 10 months after therapy. At this time only about 30% of those treated with griseofulvin were cured in comparison to 96% of patients treated with terbinafine. In addition, this short course of treatment led to improvement in over 80% of patients with nail disease associated with the chronic *Tinea pedis* (Savin, 1989). In another study of 11 patients with onychomycosis treated for 6 months, all patients were cured (Zaias et al., 1989).

4. RECENT SAR FINDINGS

Since the discovery of terbinafine our research within allylamine antimycotics was focused mainly on two aspects:

1. Attempts to improve further activity against *Candida albicans*.
2. Attempts to identify new structural types of this class of compounds.

Recent results (Stütz, 1988; Stütz et al., 1988; Stütz & Nussbaumer, 1989) indicate that progress in both aspects may be possible:

1. Substitution of the naphthalene part in terbinafine by a 3-chloro-benzo[b]thiophene ring bearing the side chain in position 7 significantly increases activity against *Candida albicans* (geometric mean MIC's 0.61 mg/l versus terbinafine 28.8 mg/l; 29 clinical isolates) and other species *in vitro* (compound A in Fig. 17-6) (Petranyi et al., 1988). This effect seems to be specifically linked to the substitution pattern in the heteroaromatic ring system. Compound A is the most potent squalene epoxidase inhibitor so far identified (Ryder, 1988).
2. The oral efficacy of compound B (Fig. 17-6), the oxa analog of terbinafine, is comparable to griseofulvin in the guinea pig trichophytosis model.
3. Both the homopropargylamine derivative C and the benzylamino compound D (Fig. 17-6) are highly effective *in vitro* and *in vivo*.

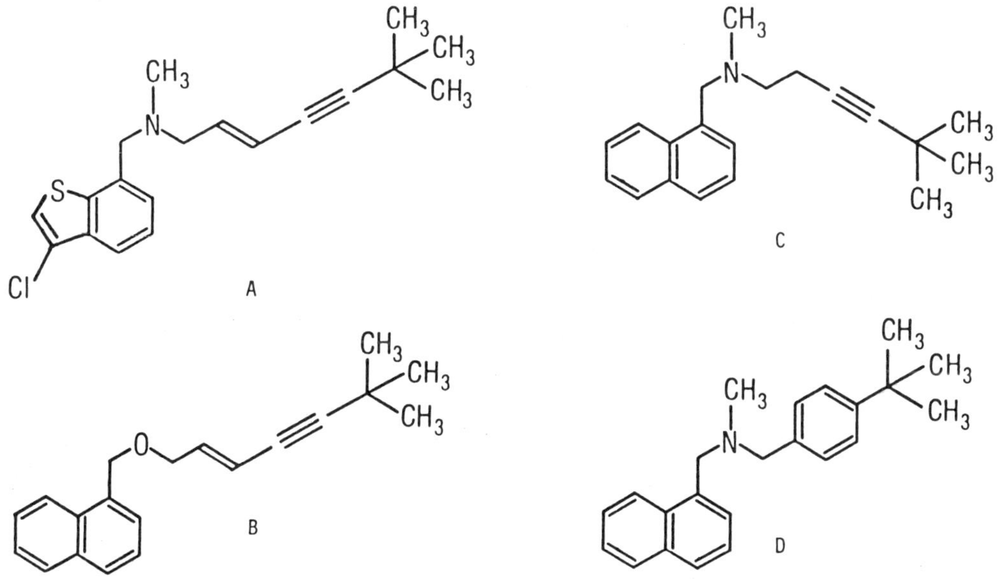

A

B

C

D

FIG. 17-6. Allylamine-related compounds of recent interest.

Since all these compounds act by the same mode of action as former allylamine derivatives do, the structural requirements and limitations of this class of antimycotics need to be redefined in a more general way and may open new perspectives for the future design of antifungal compounds.

REFERENCES

Berney, D., and Schuh, K. (1978) Heterocyclic spiro-naphthalenones. Part I: Synthesis and reactions of some spiro [(1H-naphthalenone)-1,3′-piperidines]. *Helv. Chim. Acta* **61**: 1262–1273.

Clayton, Y. M. (1987) In *Recent trends in the development and evaluation of antifungal agents*, R. A. Fromtling, ed., pp. 433–439. Barcelona: J. R. Prous.

Clayton, Y. M., Meinhof, W., and Seeliger, H. (eds.) (1985) *Topische Therapie der Dermatomykosen, Mykosen* **28**: Suppl. 1. Berlin: Grosse Verlag.

Ganzinger, U., Stephen, A., Hitzenberger, G., Baumgartner, R., Madoerin, M., Mekler, P. H., Richardson, B. P., Brüggemann S., Suter, W., Racine, R., Donatsch, P., Schatz F., and Haberl, H. (1983) SF 86-327: Evaluation of toxicity in laboratory animals, tolerance and pharmacokinetics after oral application to man. In *Proc. Int. Congr. Chemother. 13th*, K. H. Spitzy and K. Karrer, eds., **116**: pp. 52–58. Vienna: Verlag H. Egermann.

Georgopoulos, A., Petranyi, G., Mieth, H., and Drews, J. (1981) *In vitro* activity of naftifine, a new antifungal agent. *Antimicrob. Agents Chemother.* **19**: 386–389.

Goudard, M., Buffard Y., Ferrari, H., and Regli, P. (1986) Spectre d'action in vitro d'un nouvel antifongique dérivé de la naftifine: La terbinafine (SF 86-327). *Path. Biol.* **34**: 680–683.

Grassberger, M. A., Mieth, H., Petranyi, G., Ryder, N. S., and Stütz, A. (1986) Aspects of antimycotic research exemplified by the allylamines. *Triangle, Sandoz J. Med. Sci.* **25**(2/3): 71–84.

Jones, T. C. (1987) Allylamines—A new class of antifungal drugs with high efficacy in cutaneous dermatophyte and yeast infections. In *New development in antifungal therapy*, Proc. 15th Intern. Congr. Chemother., pp. 71–73, Vol. 1. Landsberg/Leck: Ecomed.

Paltauf, F., Daum, G., Zuder, G., Högenauer, G., Schulz, G., and Seidl, G. (1982) Squalene and ergosterol biosynthesis in fungi treated with naftifine, a new antimycotic agent. *Biochim. Biophys. Acta* **712**: 268–273.

Petranyi, G. (1985) Präklinische Evaluation von Exoderil (Naftifin). I. Experimentelle Untersuchungsergebnisse zum antifungalen Wirkungsprofil. *Mykosen* **28** (Suppl. 1): 37–43.

Petranyi, G., Meingassner, J. G., and Schaude, M. (1988) Experimental chemotherapeutic activity of SDZ 87-469, a new allylamine antimycotic. In *Abstracts, X Congress of the International Society for Human and Animal Mycology*, Barcelona, June 27–July 1, 1988, p. 88.

Petranyi, G., Meingassner, J. G., and Mieth, H. (1987a) Antifungal activity of the allylamine derivative terbinafine *in vitro*. *Antimicrob. Agents Chemother.* **31**: 1365–1368.

Petranyi, G., Meingassner, J., and Mieth, H. (1987b) Activity of terbinafine in experimental fungal infections in laboratory animals. *Antimicrob. Agents Chemother.* **31**: 1558–1561.

Petranyi, G., Ryder, N. S., and Stütz, A. (1984) Allylamine derivatives, a new class of synthetic antifungal agents inhibiting fungal squalene epoxydase. *Science* **224**: 1239–1241.

Petranyi, G., Stütz, A., and Ganzinger, U. (1983) SF 86-327: A new antifungal allylamine derivative: preclinical and preliminary clinical data. In *Proc. 13th Int. Congr. Chemother.*, K. H. Spitzy and K. Karrer, eds., **20**, pp. 21–30. Vienna: Verlag H. Egermann.

Petranyi, G., Georgopoulos, A., and Mieth, H. (1981) *In vivo* antimycotic activity of naftifine. *Antimicrob. Agents Chemother.* **19**: 390–392.

Ryder, N. S. (1988) Squalene epoxidase—enzymology and inhibition. In *Proc. Harden Meeting on Biochemistry of Cell Walls and Membranes of Fungi*, Oxford, April 24–27, 1988, in press.

Ryder, N. S. (1987) Squalene epoxidase as the target of antifungal allylamines. *Pestic. Sci.* **21**: 281–288.

Ryder, N. S. (1985) Specific inhibition of fungal sterol biosynthesis by SF 86-327, a new allylamine antimycotic agent. *Antimicrob. Agents Chemother.* **27**: 252–256.

Ryder, N. S., and Dupont, M.-C. (1985) Inhibition of squalene epoxidase by allylamine antimycotic compounds. *Biochem. J.* **230**: 765–770.

Ryder, N. S., Seidl, G., and Troke, P. F. (1984) Effect of the antimycotic drug naftifine on growth of and sterol biosynthesis in *Candida albicans*. *Antimicrob. Agents Chemother.* **25**: 483–487.

Savin, R. (1989) Successful treatment of chronic *Tinea pedis* (moccasin type) with terbinafine (Lamisil). *Clin. Exp. Dermatol.* **14**: 116–119.

Schaude, M., Ackerbauer, H., and Mieth, H. (1987) Inhibitory effect of antifungal agents on germ tube formation in Candida albicans. *Mykosen* **30**: 281–287.

Schuster, I. (1985) The interaction of representative members from two classes of antimycotics—the azoles and the allylamines—with cytochromes P-450 in steroidogenic tissues and liver. *Xenobiotica* **15**: 529–546.

Shadomy, S., Espinel-Ingroff, A., and Gebhart, R. J. (1985) *In vitro* studies with SF 86-327, a new orally active allylamine derivative. *Sabouraudia* **23**: 125–132.

Stütz, A. (1988) Synthesis and structure-activity correlations within allylamine antimycotics. *Ann. N. Y. Acad. Sci.* **544**: 46–62.

Stütz, A. (1987) Allylamine derivatives—a new class of active substances in antifungal chemotherapy. *Angew. Chem. Int. Ed. Engl.* **26**: 320–328.

Stütz, A., Nussbaumer, P., and Petranyi, G. (1988) SDZ 87-469: Synthesis and structure-activity relationships of a novel allylamine antimycotic. In *Abstracts, X Congress of the International Society for Human and Animal Mycology*, Barcelona, June 27–July 1, 1988, p. 89.

Stütz, A., and Nussbaumer, P. (1989) SDZ87-469. Drugs of the future, in press.

Stütz, A., Georgopoulos, A., Granitzer, W., Petranyi, G., and Berney, D. (1986) Synthesis and structure-activity relationships of naftifine-related allylamine antimycotics. *J. Med. Chem.* **29**: 112–125.

Stütz, A., and Petranyi, G. (1984) Synthesis and antifungal activity of (E)-N-(6,6-dimethyl-2-hepten-4-ynyl)-N-methyl-1-naphthalene-methanamine (SF 86-327) and related allylamine derivatives with enhanced oral activity. *J. Med. Chem.* **27**: 1539–1543.

Villard, V., and Jones, T. (1989) Clinical efficacy and tolerability of terbinafine (Lamisil) – a new topical and systemic fungicidal drug for treatment of dermatomycoses. *Clin. Eyp. Dermatol.* **14**: 124–127.

Zaias, N., Serrano, L., and Ganzinger, U. (1987) Effectiveness and safety of SF 86-327 (terbinafine) in treatment of T. rubrum onychomycosis. *17th World Congr. of Dermatol.*, Berlin, May 24–29, 1987 (Abs.), p. 550.

INDEX